CORNEAL TOMOGRAPHY IN CLINICAL PRACTICE (PENTACAM SYSTEM)
Basics and Clinical Interpretation

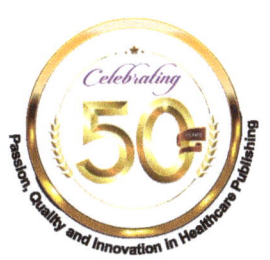

Disclaimer

The information provided via this book is intended for general information purposes.

The information provided via this book is published to assist you, but it is not to be relied upon as authoritative.

The author accepts no liability whatsoever for any direct or consequential loss arising from any use of the information contained in this book.

For any corrections, suggestions and recommendations, readers can email the author at
mazen.sinjab@yahoo.com

CORNEAL TOMOGRAPHY IN CLINICAL PRACTICE (PENTACAM SYSTEM)

Basics and Clinical Interpretation

THIRD EDITION

Mazen M Sinjab
MD MSc ABOphth PhD FRCOphth (London) CertLRS (London)
Founder and Owner
Al Zahra Medical Group
Damascus, Syria
mazen.sinjab@yahoo.com
www.mazensinjab.com

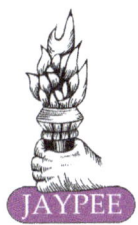

JAYPEE BROTHERS MEDICAL PUBLISHERS
The Health Sciences Publisher
New Delhi | London | Panama

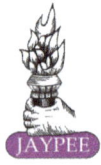
Jaypee Brothers Medical Publishers (P) Ltd

Headquarters
Jaypee Brothers Medical Publishers (P) Ltd
4838/24, Ansari Road, Daryaganj
New Delhi 110 002, India
Phone: +91-11-43574357
Fax: +91-11-43574314
Email: jaypee@jaypeebrothers.com

Overseas Offices
J.P. Medical Ltd
83 Victoria Street, London
SW1H 0HW (UK)
Phone: +44 20 3170 8910
Fax: +44 (0)20 3008 6180
Email: info@jpmedpub.com

Jaypee-Highlights Medical Publishers Inc
City of Knowledge, Bld. 235, 2nd Floor
Clayton, Panama City, Panama
Phone: +1 507-301-0496
Fax: +1 507-301-0499
Email: cservice@jphmedical.com

Jaypee Brothers Medical Publishers (P) Ltd
Bhotahity, Kathmandu, Nepal
Phone: +977-9741283608
Email: kathmandu@jaypeebrothers.com

Website: www.jaypeebrothers.com
Website: www.jaypeedigital.com

© 2019, Jaypee Brothers Medical Publishers

The views and opinions expressed in this book are solely those of the original contributor(s)/author(s) and do not necessarily represent those of editor(s) of the book.

All rights reserved. No part of this publication may be reproduced, stored or transmitted in any form or by any means, electronic, mechanical, photocopying, recording or otherwise, without the prior permission in writing of the publishers.

All brand names and product names used in this book are trade names, service marks, trademarks or registered trademarks of their respective owners. The publisher is not associated with any product or vendor mentioned in this book.

Medical knowledge and practice change constantly. This book is designed to provide accurate, authoritative information about the subject matter in question. However, readers are advised to check the most current information available on procedures included and check information from the manufacturer of each product to be administered, to verify the recommended dose, formula, method and duration of administration, adverse effects and contraindications. It is the responsibility of the practitioner to take all appropriate safety precautions. Neither the publisher nor the author(s)/editor(s) assume any liability for any injury and/or damage to persons or property arising from or related to use of material in this book.

This book is sold on the understanding that the publisher is not engaged in providing professional medical services. If such advice or services are required, the services of a competent medical professional should be sought.

Every effort has been made where necessary to contact holders of copyright to obtain permission to reproduce copyright material. If any have been inadvertently overlooked, the publisher will be pleased to make the necessary arrangements at the first opportunity. The **CD/DVD-ROM** (if any) provided in the sealed envelope with this book is complimentary and free of cost. **Not meant for sale.**

Inquiries for bulk sales may be soliciated at: jaypee@jaypeebrothers.com

Corneal Tomography in Clinical Practice (Pentacam System): Basics and Clinical Interpretation

First Edition: 2009
Second Edition: 2012
Third Edition: **2019**

ISBN 978-93-86261-10-6

Printed at

Dedicated to

My dear Father "Mohammad"
(may God rest his soul)
who planted in my soul the love of excellence.
I will mention his name with my name all my life

To my Mother "Almasah"
(may God rest her soul)
who planted in my heart loving the poor and helping others

To my Wife "Ruba"
(may God save her)
whose unwavering support was critical for all my success.

A Message from the Other World

Man is born and has been granted "The Life"
To live is an only one chance that cannot be repeated.

We have been created without our choice,
and we are going to die without our choice as well,
but to make our life is our choice.

Success does not need to be created, it just needs to be made
Making success needs five tools, sincerity, honest, humility, persistence and patience
But, to deliver success to others, an additional tool is essential; it is loving others.

"Make your success and deliver it to others; life is very short."

Preface to the Third Edition

Seven years were necessary for a giant textbook to be born. Since the second edition in 2012, we have witnessed a lot of changes in many concepts of corneal topography. A number of concepts and parameters became void, and many new came to light. Even devices are currently more accurate than before and are provided with totally new softwares.

With the new term "Corneal Tomography," corneal topography withdrew to a small space in the wide theater of corneal imaging. "Topography" is now used to describe the data generated by placido-based devices from the anterior corneal surface, while "Tomography" is a term given to the data generated from the whole cornea by either slit-scanning technology or Scheimpflug-based technology.

Tomography is a revolution in corneal imaging. From limbus to limbus, both corneal surfaces are captured and analyzed in addition to the distance between them, namely the corneal thickness map. Moreover, the anterior segment is evaluated to the depth that the slit light can reach. All of that changed the way of thinking in diagnoses and decision making, and defining some diseases such as ectatic corneal diseases.

A good quality of the tomographic capture is the key for the right decision and accurate research. It is the responsibility of the technicians who capture the patients, and the responsibility of the optometrists who usually do a primary interpretation, before it finally comes to the hands of ophthalmologists, who carry the major responsibility on their shoulders. That encouraged me to establish "Screening Guidelines", and to build up the "Practical Subjective Scoring System".

This third edition is divided into 7 sections and 24 chapters, discussing, in detail with many clinical examples, Corneal Optics and Geometry, Measuring Corneal Geometry, Screening Guidelines, Overview for Corneal Maps and Profiles, Corneal Power Maps, Elevation Maps, Belin/Ambrósio Enhanced Ectasia Display, Corneal Thickness Maps and Profiles, Geometric Tomography and Corneal Topometry, Corneal Astigmatism, Objective Corneal Dioptric Power, Astigmatic Dissociation, Basics of Wavefront Analysis and Measurements, Zernike Analysis, Fourier Analysis, Factors of False Findings, Enantiomorphism, Practical Subjective Scoring System, Tomographic Characteristics of Ectatic Corneal Diseases, Grading Systems of Ectatic Corneal Diseases, Progression Criteria, Entities Misdiagnosed as Ectasia, Holladay Report, and Corneal Tomography and Corneal Aberrometry in Cataract Surgery.

Because I committed myself to a systematic approach in all my books, the practical methodology that I follow is an imprint. The systematic methodology starts with presenting the basic information without elaborating. After that, it goes through the contents in a way that satisfies the needs of practitioners, be them ophthalmologists, optometrists, or technicians.

Although the second edition was, at that time, a revolution in the amount of and the methodology of delivering the information, this third edition is completely different in many points. It is more informative and up-to-date. It contains much more clinical examples. It presents many new concepts that, up to my knowledge, have ever been discussed before neither in textbooks nor in conferences.

Mazen M Sinjab

Preface to the First Edition

Taking the right decision in laser refractive surgery depends to a great extent on good reading of corneal topography and its clinical interpretation. This is very important for having the aimed results and avoiding postoperative complications.

The data in this book were obtained and gathered from the user manual of the Pentacam, international conferences, refractive journals, personal contacts with many refractive professors and of course self-experience.

The strategy in compiling this little book is combining excellence in pictorial quality with a concise but ordered text.

I have aimed the book at all those who need some initial assistance in reading and clinical interpretation of corneal topography. As the ophthalmology editor, I take full responsibility for any error and look forward to being further educated.

Mazen M Sinjab

Contents

Section 1: Introduction

1. Corneal Optics and Geometry   3
   The Optical System of the Human Eye   3
   Corneal Geometry   4

2. Measuring Corneal Geometry   8
   Curvature-based Devices (Topographers)   8
   Elevation-based Devices (Tomographers)   10
   Topography versus Tomography   11
   Hybrid Devices (Topo-Tomographers)   12

3. Screening Guidelines   13
   The Four-composite Map   13
   General Settings   13
   Color Scale   17
   Maps Overlay   20
   Reference Body Shape   23
   Preparing the Eye for the Capture   23
   Checking the Quality of the Capture   23
   Specific Settings for Holladay Report   25

Section 2: Corneal Maps and Profiles

4. Overview   33
   Corneal Parameters   33

5. Corneal Power Maps   36
   Factors Affecting Corneal Power Measurement   36
   Maps Measuring Corneal Power   38
   Patterns of Corneal Curvature   43
   Clinical Differences between Sagittal and Tangential Curvature Maps   47

6. Elevation Maps   51
   Principle of the Elevation Maps   51
   The Reference Surface   51

7. Belin/Ambrosio Enhanced Ectasia — 60
The Belin/Ambrosio Ectasia Display 60
Pachymetric Data 66
Numeric Values 66
Applications of Belin/Ambrosio Enhanced Ectasia 66

8. Corneal Thickness Maps and Profiles — 67
Corneal Thickness Map (Pachymetry Map) 67
Corneal Thickness Spatial Profile and Percentage Thickness Increase 73
Pachymetric Progression Index 79
The Relative Pachymetry 79

9. Geometric Tomography and Corneal Topometry — 82
Corneal Toricity 82
Corneal Asphericity 82
Corneal Asymmetry 85

Section 3: Understanding Corneal Refraction

10. Corneal Astigmatism — 91
Definitions and Classifications of Astigmatism 91
Etiology of Irregular Astigmatism 93
Evaluation of Irregular Astigmatism 100

11. Objective Corneal Dioptric Power — 103
Calculating Objective Corneal Dioptric Power 103
Clinical Examples 104

12. Astigmatic Dissociation — 108
Etiology 108
Types of Dissociation 109
Clinical Examples 110
Summary of Guidelines 113

Section 4: Wavefront Analysis

13. Basics of Wavefront Analysis and Measurements — 117
Principles of Wavefront and Wavefront Analysis 117
Types of Aberrations 118
Measurement of Aberrations 118
Changes of Aberrations with Age 120
Clinical Application of Wavefront Technology 120

14. Zernike Analysis — 122
Constant Aberrations 122
Lower-order Aberrations 123
Higher-order Aberrations 129

15. Fourier Analysis — 137
Fourier Analysis of Corneal Wavefront 137

Section 5: A Systematic Interpretation of Corneal Tomography

16. Factors of False Findings — 143
Contact Lenses 143
Misalignment 144
Large Angle Kappa or Lambda 148
Tear Film Disturbance 148
Posterior Surface Astigmatism 149
Corneal Opacities and Pathologies 149
Previous Corneal Surgeries 149
Bad Exposure to the Camera 152
Pregnancy 152

17. Enantiomorphism — 153

18. Practical Subjective Scoring System — 160
Image Quality Control 160
Practical Subjective Scoring System (PS3) 161
Decision Tree Based on PS3 163

Section 6: Corneal Tomography in Ectatic Corneal Diseases

19. Tomographic Characteristics of Ectatic Corneal Diseases — 167
Tomographic Definition of Ectatic Corneal Diseases 167

20. Grading Systems of Ectatic Corneal Diseases — 177
Amsler-Krumeich Classification 177
Alio-Shabayek Modification 177
Modification of Ishii and Associates 177
Belin ABCD Keratoconus Staging 178

21. Progression Criteria — 181
Parameters of Progression 181

22. Entities Misdiagnosed as Ectasia — 191
Source of Entities Misdiagnosed as Ectasia 191
Patterns of Entities Misdiagnosed as Ectasia 191

Section 7: Miscellaneous

23. Holladay Report — 207
Holladay Report 207
Holladay Detailed Equivalent K-reading Report 209
Clinical Examples 211

24. Corneal Tomography and Corneal Aberrometry in Cataract Surgery 223
Preoperative Screening Process 223
Preoperative Planning Process 224
Postoperative Planning Process 225

Bibliography 227

Index 237

Abbreviations

AB/IS	:	Asymmetric bowtie inferior steep
AB/SRAX	:	Asymmetric bowtie with skewed radial axis index
AB/SS	:	Asymmetric bowtie superior steep
AC	:	Anterior chamber
ACA	:	Anterior chamber angle
ACD	:	Anterior chamber depth
ACV	:	Anterior chamber volume
AK	:	Astigmatic keratotomy
AS-OCT	:	Anterior segment optical coherence tomography
ATR	:	Against-the-rule
AZ	:	Ablation zone
BAD	:	Belin/Ambrósio enhanced ectasia display
BFS	:	Best fit sphere
BFTE	:	Best fit toric ellipsoid
BVD	:	Back vertex distance
CCT	:	Central corneal thickness
CDVA	:	Corrected distance visual acuity
CL	:	Contact lens
CP	:	Corneal periphery
CR	:	Cycloplegic refraction
CTK	:	Central toxic keratopathy
CTSP	:	Corneal thickness spatial profile
CXL	:	Corneal cross-linking
D	:	Diopter
DLK	:	Diffuse lamellar keratitis
e	:	Eccentricity
EBMD	:	Epithelial basement membrane dystrophy
ECD	:	Ectatic corneal disease
EKR	:	Equivalent K-reading power
EME	:	Entity misdiagnosed as ectasia
EOZ	:	Efficient optical zone
EP	:	Entrance pupil
Epi-LASIK	:	Epipolis laser in situ keratomileusis
Femto-LASIK	:	Femtosecond laser in situ keratomileusis
FFKC	:	Forme fruste keratoconus

HOA	:	Higher order aberration
I	:	Inferior
ICR	:	Intracorneal ring
IOL	:	Intraocular lens
IS	:	Inferior steep
K_1	:	Flat keratometry -reading
K_2	:	Steep keratometry -reading
KC	:	Keratoconus
KCS	:	Keratoconus suspect
KG	:	Keratoglobus
Km	:	Mean K-reading
Kmax	:	Maximum K-reading
Kref	:	Reference K-reading
LASEK	:	Laser subepithelial keratomileusis
LASIK	:	Laser in situ keratomileusis
LKP	:	Lamellar keratoplasty
LOA	:	Lower order aberration
LOS	:	Line of sight
LRI	:	Limbal relaxing incision
LVC	:	Laser vision correction
MA	:	Manifest astigmatism
MFIOL	:	Multifocal intraocular lens
MR	:	Manifest refraction
MRc	:	Manifest refraction corrected at corneal plane
MTF	:	Modulation transfer function
OA	:	Optical axis
OD	:	Right eye
ODP	:	Objective sphero-cylindric dioptric power
OS	:	Left eye
OSD	:	Ocular surface disease
OTF	:	Optical transfer function
PA	:	Pupillary axis
PHT	:	Pinhole test
PIOL	:	Phakic intraocular lens
PKP	:	Penetrating keratoplasty
PMD	:	Pellucid marginal degeneration
PMT	:	Post-mydriatic test
PPI	:	Pachymetric progression index
PRK	:	Photorefractive keratectomy
PS3	:	Practical subjective scoring system
PSF	:	Point spread function
PTA	:	Percent of tissue altered
PTF	:	Phase transfer function
PTI	:	Percentage thickness increase
PVA	:	Potential visual acuity
QS	:	Quality specification

RGP	:	Rigid gas permeable
RI	:	Refractive index
RK	:	Radial keratotomy
RMS	:	Root mean square
RS	:	Reference surface
S	:	Superior
SA	:	Spherical aberration
SB/SRAX	:	Symmetric bowtie with skewed radial axis index
SB	:	Symmetric bowtie
SBK	:	Sub-Bowman keratomileusis
SD	:	Standard deviation
SE	:	Spherical equivalent
Sim-K	:	Simulated keratometry
SMILE	:	Small incision lenticule extraction
SR	:	Strehl ratio
SS	:	Superior steep
TA	:	Tomographic astigmatism
TCRP	:	Total corneal refractive power
TCT	:	Thinnest corneal thickness
TL	:	Thinnest location
TNP	:	True net power
TransPRK	:	Transepithelial photorefractive keratectomy
TZ	:	Transitional zone
UDVA	:	Uncorrected distance visual acuity
VA	:	Visual axis
VK	:	Vertex keratoscope
WFG	:	Wavefront-guided
WFO	:	Wavefront-optimized
WTR	:	With-the-rule
ZC	:	Zernike coefficient

SECTION 1

Introduction

SECTION OUTLINE

1. Corneal Optics and Geometry
2. Measuring Corneal Geometry
3. Screening Guidelines

Corneal Optics and Geometry

THE OPTICAL SYSTEM OF THE HUMAN EYE

The human eye has an optical system which is composed of: (1) four main noncoaxial optical elements (anterior and posterior corneal and lens surfaces); (2) the pupil; and (3) the retina, which is aplanatic to compensate for the native spherical aberration (SA) and coma through its nonplanar geometry. The optical surfaces are aligned almost coaxially; however, the deviations from a perfect optical alignment results in a range of axes and their interrelationships (Fig. 1.1). This guides us to the following definitions:

- *The visual axis (VA)*: It is the line connecting the fixation point with the foveola, passing through the two nodal points of the eye, but not necessarily through the pupil center.
- *The optical axis (OA)*: It is the axis connecting the center of curvatures of the optical surfaces of the eye. It can be recognized by the Purkinje images I, II, III, and IV, namely of the outer corneal surface (I), inner corneal surface (II), anterior surface of the lens (III), and the posterior surface of the lens (IV). If the optical surfaces of the eye were perfectly coaxial, these four images would be coaxial, which is seldom observed.
- *The principle line of sight (LOS)*: It is the ray from the fixation point reaching the foveola via the center of the entrance pupil (EP).
- *The pupillary axis (PA)*: It is the normal line to the corneal surface that passes through the center of the EP and the center of curvature of the anterior corneal surface.
- *The achromatic axis*: It is defined as the axis connecting the center of the EP with the nodal points.
- *The vertex keratoscope (VK) normal*: It is the axis that is perpendicular to the plane of the capturing machine (originally, the keratoscope) and intersecting with

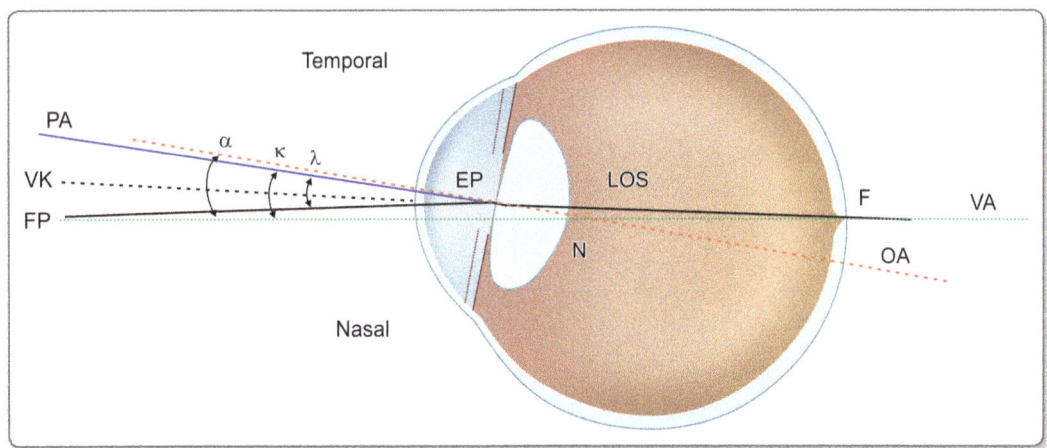

Fig. 1.1: Optical system of the eye (superior view of the right eye). Surfaces, angles, and axes. [EP: entrance pupil (the opening within the dotted line); F: foveola; FP: focal point; LOS: line of sight; N: nodular point; OA: optical axis; PA: pupillary axis; VA: visual axis; VK: video keratoscope axis]

anterior corneal surface at corneal apex (corneal vertex). Therefore, corneal apex is not necessarily the highest point of anterior corneal slope and not necessarily the anatomical center of the cornea.

- *Angle kappa (measured in degrees)*: It is the angle between PA and VA. Measuring angle kappa is very important in refractive surgery in terms of laser ablation centration and multifocal intraocular lens (MFIOLs) implantation. Large angle kappa has an adverse clinical impact on the visual outcomes after laser vision correction (LVC), particularly hypermetropic treatment and astigmatic treatment when the magnitude of astigmatism is more than 1 diopter (D). Pupil-offset technique is recommended in such cases. In addition, large angle causes photic phenomenon and decreased effectiveness of the MFIOL. MFIOL implantation is contraindicated when angle kappa is larger than 400–500 μm.

Normal distribution in angle kappa was studied by using Orbscan II (Placido-based) and the Synoptophore. It was found that values of angle kappa measured by the Orbscan II were almost as twice as when measured by the Synoptophore. Based on Orbscan II, Hashemi and associates determined an average value of angle kappa of 5.46 ± 1.33° in Iranian adults with insignificant intergender difference. In another study, Gharaee and associates determined an average value of 4.96 ± 1.38° in total, an average horizontal angle kappa of –0.02 ± 0.49 mm, and an average vertical angle kappa of –0.09 ± 0.32 mm.

In addition, studies reporting normative angle kappa values in different conditions found that angle kappa was significantly larger in exotropes than in esotropes or controls, and tended to be larger in the left eye than in the right eye. Moreover, there was a positive correlation between angle kappa and positive refractive errors, which can be explained by the negative correlation with the axial length of the globe.

Unlike Placido-based topographers, Scheimpflug-based tomographers cannot measure angle kappa. This raises the need to find a way to estimate this angle in Scheimpflug-based topographers. However, the VA can roughly be considered as passing in between the center of the EP and the corneal apex, and might be half the distance. Therefore, in Scheimpflug-based devices, angle kappa can roughly be half values of X and Y coordinates of the EP center.

- *Angle alpha (measured in degrees)*: The angle formed at the first nodal point by OA and VA.
- *Angle lambda (measured in degrees)*: The angle between PA and LOS.
- *Chord μ (measured in mm)*: It is the chord length of angle kappa in polar coordinates relative to the center of the EP.

The refractive power of the human eye comes mainly from the cornea and the crystalline lens. In emmetropia, corneal power ranges in between 39 D and 48 D (average 43.05 D), while the power of the crystalline lens ranges from 15 D to 24 D (average 19.11 D). The refractive media in the human eye are: tear film (n = 1.336), cornea (n = 1.376), aqueous humor (n = 1.336), crystalline lens (n = 1.406), and vitreous humor (1.336), where "n" is the refractive index (RI) of the media measured relatively to air (n = 1.000). The dioptric power of these media is determined by the radius of curvature, the RI, and the distance between various interfaces.

CORNEAL GEOMETRY

The cornea has two surfaces separated by corneal substance. The anterior surface is coated with the tear film, and together forms one refractive surface separating air from corneal substance. The posterior surface separates corneal substance from aqueous humor. The cornea is not a part of a perfect sphere. The shape of both surfaces is defined as: an aspheric prolate, toric, and asymmetric conoidal shape (Figs. 1.2 and 1.3). Each of the previous expressions will be explained in detail in the following paragraphs.

Corneal Dimensions

Corneal dimensions include diameters, meridians, radii of curvature, corneal zones, corneal thickness, corneal shape, corneal power, and geometric landmarks.

- *Diameters*: The sclerocorneal junction (base of the cornea) is an *ellipse*. The vertical corneal diameter is 10.6 mm on average, whereas the average horizontal corneal diameter is 11.7 mm.
- *Meridians*: The normal adult cornea has two meridians that are 90° apart. Due to the elliptical base of the cornea at the sclerocorneal junction, the vertical diameter is

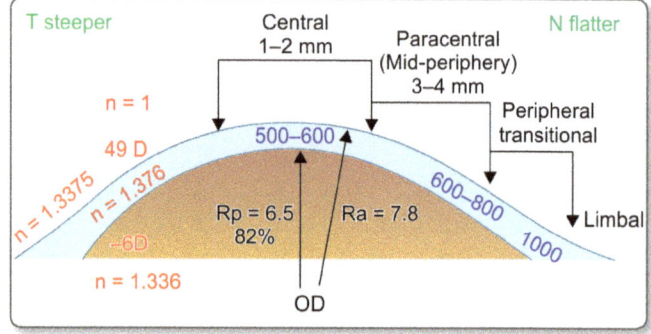

Fig. 1.2: Corneal geometry of the right eye (OD). (n: refractive index; N: nasal; Ra: radius of curvature of the anterior corneal surface; Rp: radius of curvature of the posterior corneal surface; T: temporal)

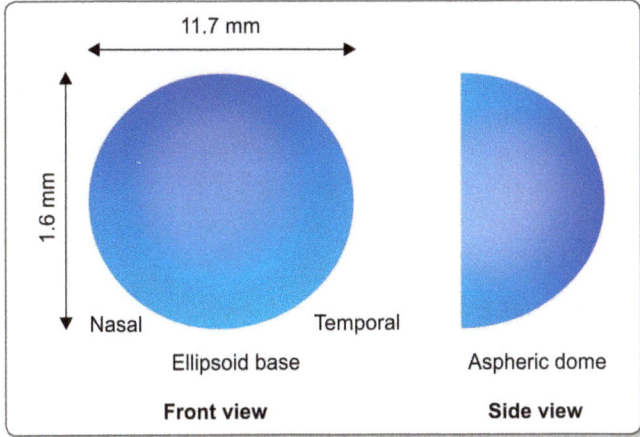

Fig. 1.3: Corneal shape (left eye).

generally shorter than the horizontal one, meaning that the vertical meridian is steeper (smaller radius of curvature) than the horizontal one (greater radius of curvature). Due to this difference, corneal shape is considered as *toric*. This toricity is responsible for corneal astigmatism. In younger eyes, this toricity is represented as with-the-rule (WTR) astigmatism, where the vertical meridian is steeper than the horizontal one. This reverses with age, causing against-the-rule (ATR) astigmatism.

- *Radius of curvature*: The cornea has two surfaces, anterior with an approximate radius of 7.8 mm, and posterior with an approximate radius of 6.5 mm. These two radii are for the central (axial) zone of the cornea. The radii increase while moving to the periphery, indicating a flatter corneal periphery. The normal cornea flattens progressively from center to periphery by 2–4 D, with the nasal area flattening more than the temporal area, and this is shown on the curvature map as the nasal side becoming blue (flat) more quickly (Fig. 1.4). The normal average anterior/posterior radii ratio is 1.21 in virgin nonoperated corneas. This ratio is altered by keratorefractive surgeries which is a major source of error in intraocular lens (IOL) measurements after these surgeries.
- *Corneal thickness*: Due to the difference in radius between the two corneal surfaces, the cornea is thinner in the central zone than at periphery. There are two important values in corneal thickness, the central corneal thickness (CCT) and thinnest corneal thickness (TCT). Both will be discussed later in this chapter.

Corneal Zones

Clinically, the cornea is divided into zones that surround fixation (corneal vertex or apex) and blend into one another:

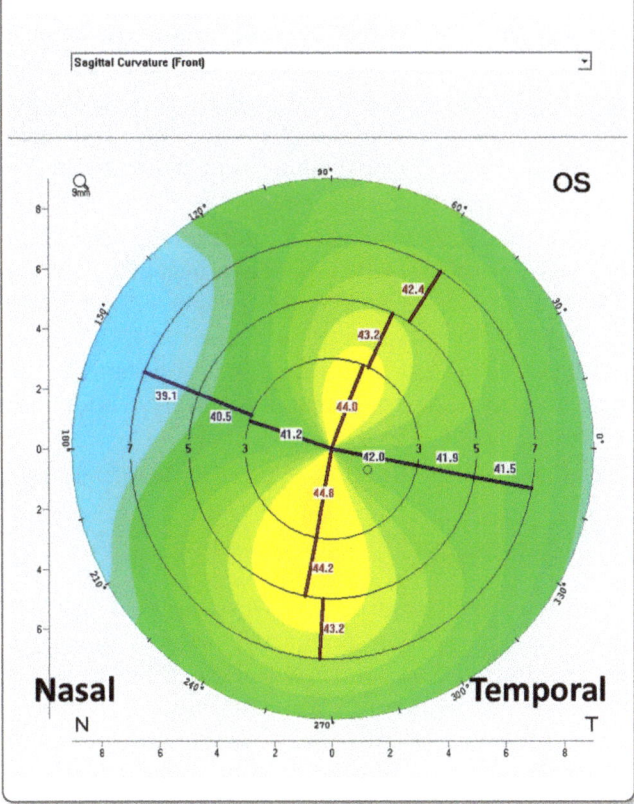

Fig. 1.4: Nasal temporal asymmetry in a normal cornea.

- *The central zone (central 3 mm)*: It overlies the pupil and is responsible for high definition vision. The central part is almost spherical and is also called the apical or axial zone.
- *The paracentral zone (3–6 mm)*: It has a doughnut shape with an outer diameter of 6 mm. It represents an area of progressive flattening toward the third zone.
- The central and paracentral zones are responsible for the refractive power of the cornea, and are used for contact lens fitting.
- *The peripheral zone (6–9 mm)*: It is also known as the *transitional zone*. This zone is asymmetrically flatter than the central zone. The nasal and superior segments are flatter than the temporal and inferior ones.
- *The limbal zone (>9 mm)*: It is adjacent to the sclera and is the area where the cornea steepens prior to merging with the sclera at the limbal sulcus.

Being steeper in the center and flatter at periphery gives the cornea what is known as a "prolate" aspheric shape.

Corneal Shape

Corneal shape is "conoidal" (Fig. 1.3). It is a composition of toricity, asphericity, and asymmetry. From a meridional viewpoint, the cornea is "toric", which is the source of corneal astigmatism. From the zonal viewpoint, the cornea is "aspheric" because the radius of curvature differs from the center toward the periphery. From a sectorial viewpoint, the cornea is asymmetric because the nasal sector is usually flatter than the temporal sector as shown in Figure 1.4.

Corneal asphericity is expressed by "Q-value". The cornea is prolate (steeper in the center), oblate (flatter in the center) or spheric when Q-value is negative, positive, or zero, respectively. The average Q-value in the normal population is approximately –0.27 (–0.10 to –0.30). An abnormal Q-value means abnormal corneal asphericity, the origin of corneal SA. The Q-value at which no SA is found is –0.53 on average.

Corneal shape is discussed in detail in Chapter 9.

Corneal Power

The anterior corneal surface with its associated tear film layer plays a role of a convex refractive surface. Due to both its convexity and separation between two different media: (1) air (smaller RI; n = 1.000) and (2) corneal substance (larger RI; n = 1.376), it encounters the most powerful refractive surface in the optical system of the eye. The refractive power of the central (apical or axial) zone of the anterior corneal surface is approximately 49 D.

On the other hand, although the posterior surface of the cornea is convex, it acts as a negative concave surface because it separates corneal substance (higher RI; n = 1.376) from aqueous humor (lower RI; n = 1.336). The refractive power of the posterior corneal surface is approximately –6 D.

Moreover, corneal epithelium has an impact on corneal power. The shape of the epithelial layer is responsible for about 0.40 D of astigmatism. The mean Q-value is –0.20 ± 0.13 (0.06 to –0.60) with epithelium and –0.26 ± 0.23 (0.07 to –1.51) without epithelium. In other words, the cornea is more prolate without the epithelium, which means that the epithelial layer forms a negative lens (thinner in the center) as shown in Figures 1.5A and B. This fact has a clinical impact on LVC procedures, especially in surface ablation techniques. This fact is more important in cases

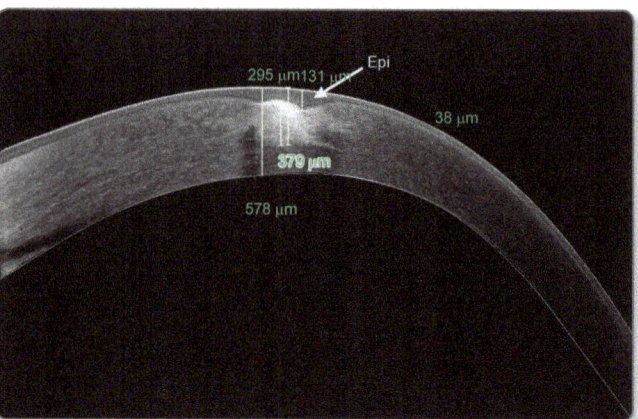

Fig. 1.6: Remodeling characteristic of the epithelium (Epi). It reduces corneal irregularities.

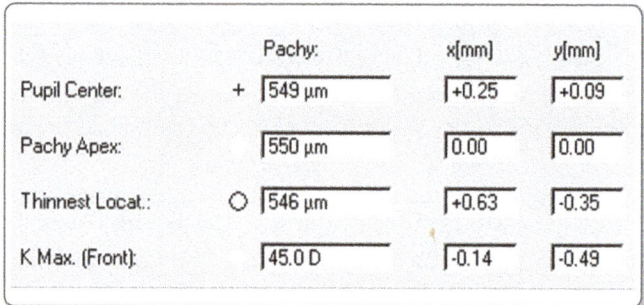

Fig. 1.7: Geometrical landmarks.

with irregular corneal surface because the epithelium has a remodeling (filling) feature, which masks the real corneal power and a significant portion of the underlying corneal irregularities as shown in Figure 1.6. Moreover, the remodeling feature of the epithelium affects refractive results after surface ablation, characterized by undercorrection after both myopic and hypermetropic corrections. The epithelium forms a positive convex lens or a negative concave lens after myopic or hypermetropic correction, respectively.

There are different methods to measure corneal power. They are discussed in Chapter 5.

Geometrical Landmarks

There are virtual landmarks of clinical importance in the cornea. They are corneal apex, thinnest location (TL), mean K-reading (Km), and maximum K-reading (Kmax) (Fig. 1.7).

- *Corneal apex*: As mentioned before, it is the point at which VK normal intersects with the anterior corneal surface; therefore, it is also known as vertex normal. Assumably, it represents Purkinje-Sanson reflex I. However, since the Pentacam does not include a Placido disk, the device considers the point which is confronting the fixation target as corneal apex, which is not true in

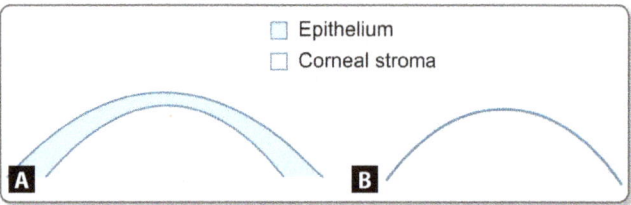

Figs. 1.5A and B: The effect of corneal epithelium on corneal shape. The cornea is more prolate without the epithelium.

most cases. The computer considers this point as the origin of coordinates, X for the horizontal and Y for the vertical axes (Chapter 4). The direction of X is from patient's right to their left, and the direction of Y is from the bottom up. All other landmarks are measured from the corneal apex. Therefore, the X and Y coordinates of this point have a value of 0.00. Corneal thickness at this point is usually referred to as CCT. Depending on the technology used for measuring corneal thickness, the average CCT ranges from 534 μm to 575 μm.

- *Thinnest location*: It is the location of the thinnest point in the measured cornea. Corneal thickness at this point is usually referred to as TCT. In an international multicenter study based on the Pentacam HR (OCULUS Optikgeräte GmbH, Wetzlar, Germany), Feng and associates reported an average TCT of 536 μm overall. Values less than 469 μm or 435 μm (−2 or −3 SD, respectively) would be expected in less than 2.5% or 0.15% of normal corneas, respectively. The X-coordinate averaged 0.44 mm temporally, and the Y-coordinate averaged 0.29 mm inferiorly in relation with corneal apex. Y-coordinates more than 1.00 mm inferiorly were found in less than 0.5% of normal corneas.
- *Mean K-reading*: It is the arithmetic average of the central Sim-Ks on the anterior corneal surface. Based on Placido-disk devices, normal Km is less than 47.2 D, while based on Holladay report (Pentacam), normal Km is less than 48 D.
- *Maximum K-reading*: It is the Kmax on the anterior corneal surface measured by the anterior sagittal curvature map. Interestingly, at this point in time, there is no normative data for Kmax.

Measuring Corneal Geometry

INTRODUCTION

Corneal geometry is measured by "topography" and "tomography". Topography is a term given to the data generated from the anterior corneal surface by the curvature-based devices (topographers), while tomography is a term given to the data generated from both corneal surfaces in addition to corneal thickness mapping by using the elevation-based devices (tomographers).

CURVATURE-BASED DEVICES (TOPOGRAPHERS)

Anterior surface acts as an almost transparent convex mirror; it reflects part of the incident light. Many devices have been developed to assess the anterior surface by measuring the reflected light. These noncontact devices use a light target (in different shapes) and a microscope or other optical systems. The instruments are either quantitative or qualitative, and either reflection-based or projection-based.

Keratometry

Keratometry is a quantitative reflection-based measurement. The keratometer measures corneal radius on a ring in 15° around corneal apex (at 3.2 mm diameter as shown in Figure 2.1) by measuring the size of the reflected image (mires), and converting the image size into corneal radius using a mathematical relationship:

$$r = 2aY/y$$

where
r: anterior corneal radius in mm
a: distance from mire to cornea (75 mm in keratometer)
Y: image size in mm
y: mire size (64 mm in keratometer)

Fig. 2.1: Sim-K measurement.

The keratometer converts corneal radius "r" (measured in mm) into refracting power "RP" (in diopters) using a keratometric refractive index (1.3375) and the relationship:

$$RP = 337.5/r$$

Although the theory of measuring corneal reflex may appear simple, it is not, since eye movement, decentration, or tear film disturbance may affect the data. Video topographers can freeze the reflected corneal image, and perform the measurements once the image is captured on the video or computer screen, allowing greater precision.

Keratoscopy or Photokeratoscopy

The keratometer can obtain measurements from only a small central area (approximately 6%) of the anterior corneal surface, and therefore, does not show corneal asymmetry. Therefore, there was a need for additional imaging modalities which can generate qualitative information about the shape of the entire cornea, hence the keratoscope and the photokeratoscope (illuminated keratoscope) were developed.

The keratoscope and the photokeratoscope are based on Placido disk. They are qualitative reflection-based devices and can obtain measurements from almost 60–70% of the total anterior corneal surface. In the photokeratoscope, the Placido disk is a series of concentric rings (10 or 12 rings) or a cone with illuminated rings lining the internal surface of the instrument (Fig. 2.2). Depending on the changes in the shape of the reflected rings and the spaces in between, the shape of the anterior surface of the cornea can be imagined; for instance, small, narrow, and closely spaced rings suggest steep regions with small radius of curvature (Figs. 2.3A to D).

The use of the photokeratoscope is being abandoned; several computerized topographers—allowing both qualitative and quantitative measurements—are being used.

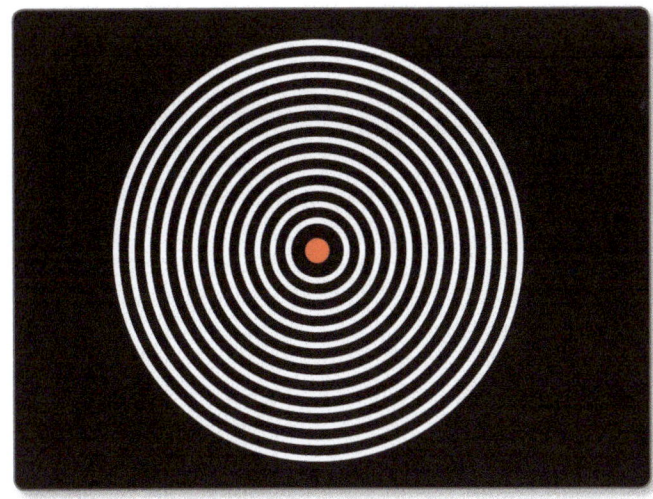

Fig. 2.2: Placido disk.

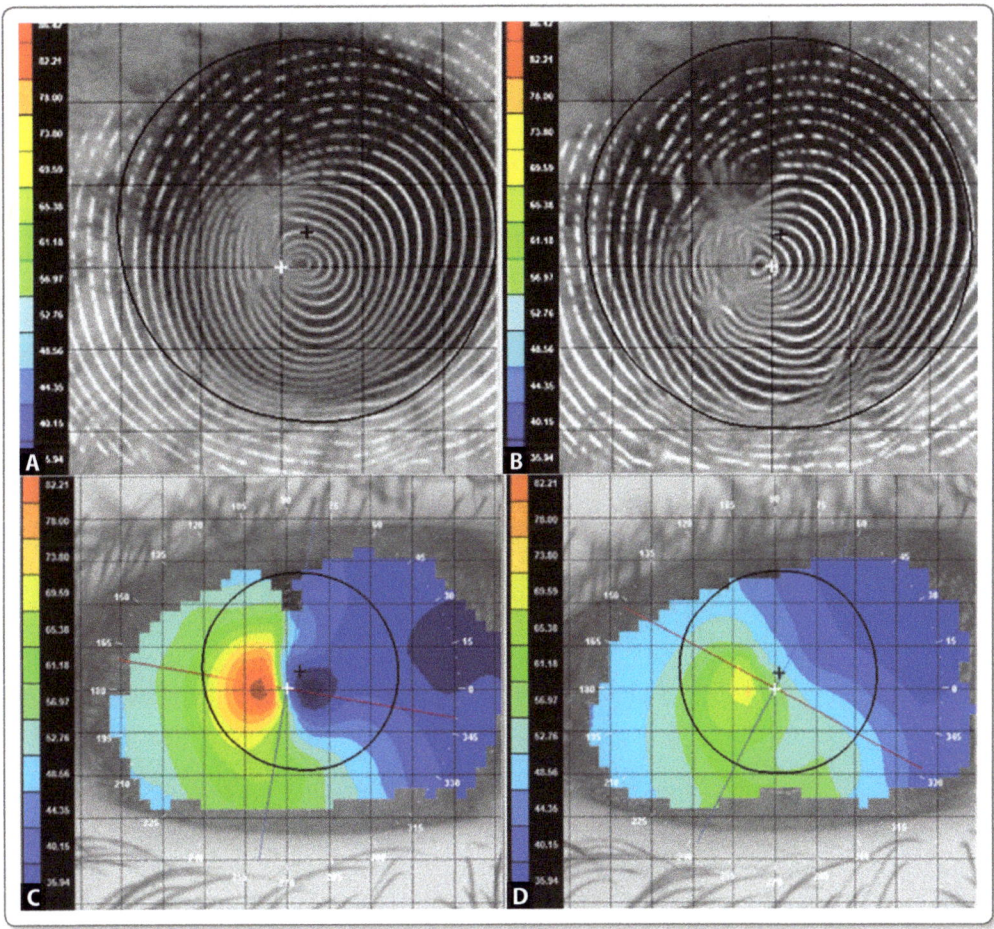

Figs. 2.3A to D: Interpretation of Placido rings' shape into color-coded maps.

Computerized Videokeratoscopy

This is one of the modern topographers. The modern topographers are based on projecting (not reflecting) images.

Basically, a projection-based topographer consists of a Placido disk or cone (small or large) which projects a mire of concentric light rings, a video camera that captures the reflected rings from the tear film layer, and a software to analyze the data (Fig. 2.4). The computer evaluates the distance between the concentric rings (dark and light areas) in a variable number of points. The shorter the distance, the higher the corneal power, and vice versa. After analyzing the data, they are plotted by the computer as a color map.

The Placido cone may be large or small according to the manufacturer. The larger the cone, the more the rings and the wider the area to be estimated. The mires of most systems exclude the very central cornea and paralimbal area.

The reproducibility and validity of videokeratography measurements are mainly dependent on the accuracy of manual adjustment in the focal plane.

Maps Generated by Topographers

Topographers generate three types of maps: (1) the sagittal (axial) curvature map, (2) the tangential (instantaneous or local) curvature map, and (3) the elevation map, but all are for the anterior corneal surface. The topographer directly measures the curvature maps, from which it indirectly calculates (reconstruct) the elevation map. The principle of these maps will be discussed in details in Section 2.

Limitations of Curvature-based Topography

Data obtained by the Placido-based devices has the following restrictions:
- They provide information about the first layer over the cornea, namely tear film layer. This is why tear film disturbance, ocular surface disease (OSD), and using lubricants may cause variable and unreliable measurements.
- They provide no information about the posterior corneal surface. Therefore, early ectatic changes cannot be detected.
- They provide no information about corneal thickness profiles.
- The evaluated area is almost the central 60–70% of the anterior corneal surface, peripheral pathology is, therefore, missing, such as pellucid marginal degeneration (PMD) and peripheral keratoconus (KC).
- The elevation map is calculated (reconstructed) from the curvature map. Any errors in measuring the latter will affect the former. Moreover, the sagittal map is based on a reference axis known as videokeratoscope (VK) normal. It is a misleading axis in cases of large angle kappa and misalignment. The tangential map has a deferent principle and is affected to a less extent.

ELEVATION-BASED DEVICES (TOMOGRAPHERS)

The tomographers obtain information from both corneal surfaces in addition to full thickness profile of the cornea. Moreover, they give information about the anterior chamber and the lens. Contrary to topographers, the tomographers directly measure the elevation maps of both corneal surfaces and indirectly calculate (reconstruct) the curvature map for both surfaces as well.

The tomographer projects a slit light through the cornea to gather information from all media and surfaces that it goes through.

There are two types of tomographers with two different principles:
1. *Scanning-slit devices*: Scanning-slit technology produces multiple slit-lamp images of the anterior segment using

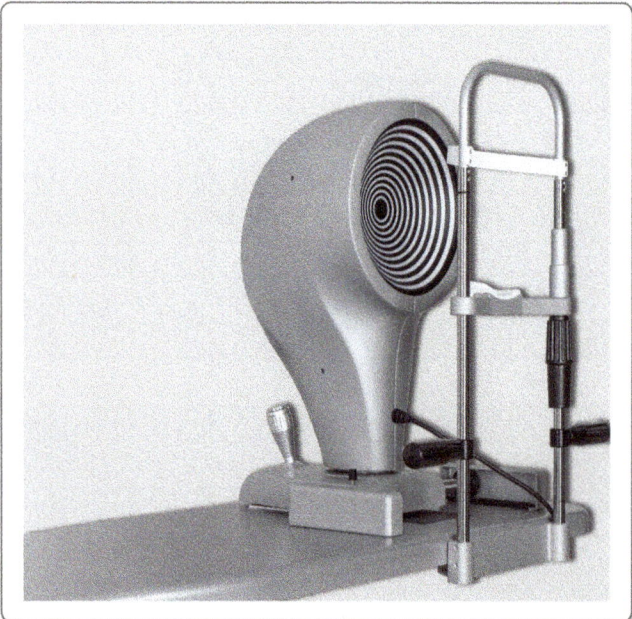

Fig. 2.4: Topographer: Computerized videokeratoscope. Central stable camera and central fixation target within a projection Placido disk.

Chapter 2: Measuring Corneal Geometry

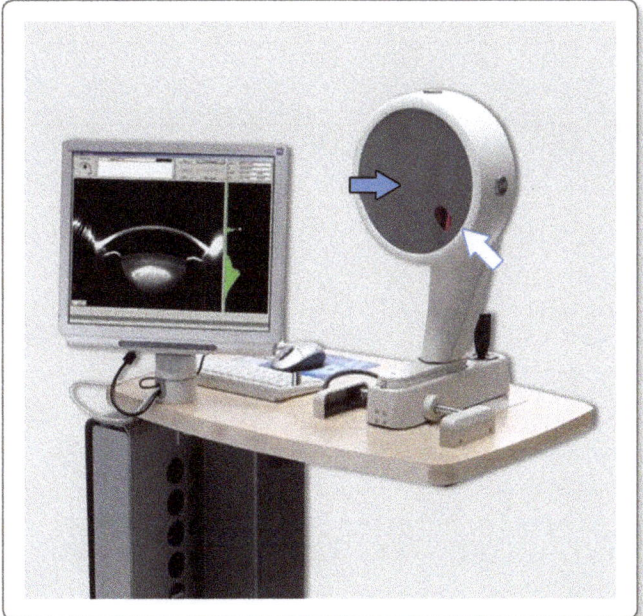

Fig. 2.5: Tomographer: Scheimpflug-based device. Lateral rotating Scheimpflug camera and central fixation target.

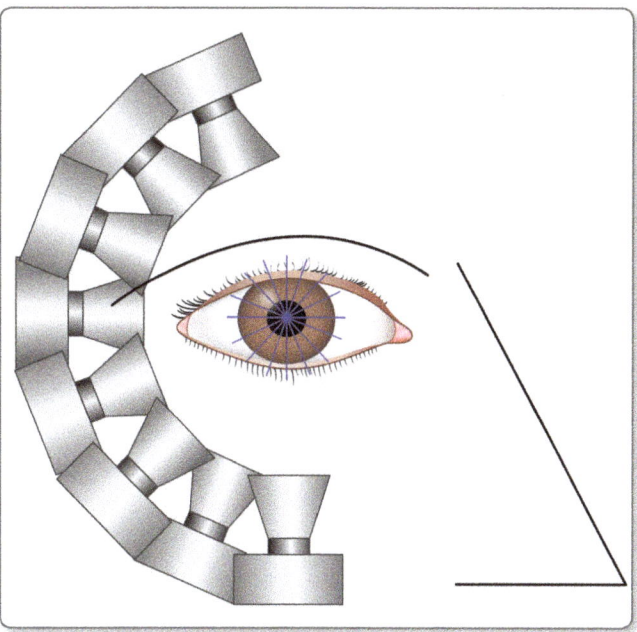

Fig. 2.6: Field of the lateral rotating Scheimpflug camera.

a camera moving horizontally. The Orbscan (Bausch and Lomb) tomographer works with this principle.

2. *Scheimpflug-based devices*: They use the Scheimpflug camera, which is based on the Scheimpflug principle by which an obliquely tilted object can be placed in maximum depth of focus with minimal image distortion. The Pentacam (OCULUS Optikgeräte GmbH, Wetzlar, Germany), Sirius (Costruzione Strumenti Oftalmici, Italy), Galilei (Ophthalmic Systems AG, Switzerland), and Tomey (Tomey Corporation, Japan) systems use this technology. This book focuses on Pentacam HR.

The Scheimpflug system consists of a rotational central slit light that coincides with a fixation target, and a lateral rotational Scheimpflug camera (Figs. 2.5 and 2.6). The rotational measuring procedure generates Scheimpflug images in three dimensions, with the dot matrix fine-meshed in the center due to the rotation. The Pentacam HR calculates a three-dimensional model of the anterior eye segment from 138,000 true elevation points.

The Scheimpflug principle can be understood by looking at Figures 2.7 and 2.8. Figure 2.7 illustrates the image in the conventional camera. The three planes (the picture plane, the objective plane, and the film plane) are parallel. Figure 2.8 illustrates the Scheimpflug camera. The Scheimpflug law states: To get a higher depth of focus, move the three planes, provided that the picture plane, the objective plane, and the film plane have to intersect in one line or one point. Advantages of the Scheimpflug camera include higher depth of focus and sharp picture, but distorted.

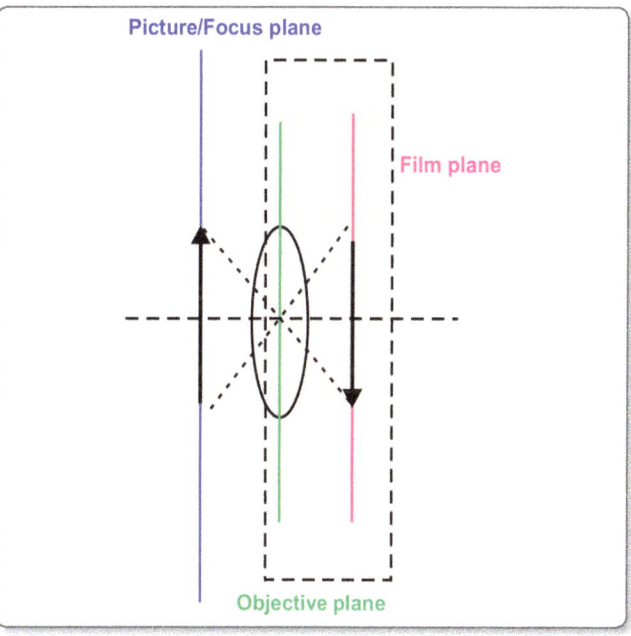

Fig. 2.7: Principle of imaging in the conventional camera.

TOPOGRAPHY VERSUS TOMOGRAPHY

Both technologies have advantages and disadvantages. Table 2.1 is a comparison between the two technologies.
- Topography provides information from the anterior cornea surface, while tomography measures both.
- Corneal thickness map and profiles are not obtained by topography.

Table 2.1: A comparison between topography and tomography.

Topography	Tomography
Anterior surface	Both surfaces
No pachymetry map and thickness profiles	Pachymetry map and thickness profiles
Better in scar and haze	Less accurate in scar and haze
Measures angle kappa	Does not
Very much affected by tear film and ocular surface disease (OSD)	Less affected
Both are affected by large angle kappa and misalignment	
More sensitive in detecting misalignment	Misalignment may be missed

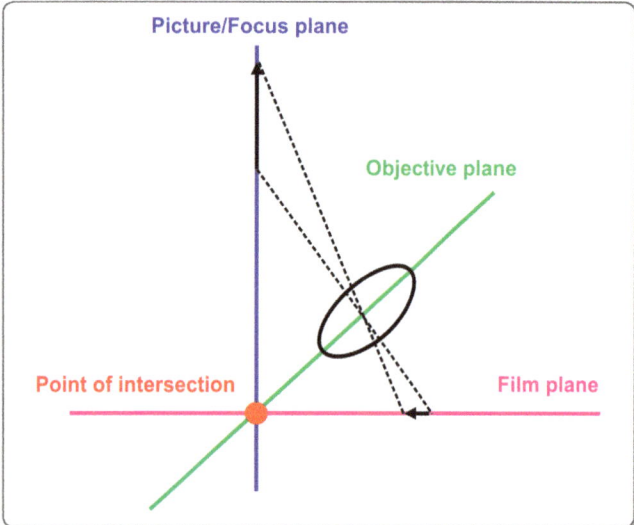

Fig. 2.8: Principle of imaging in the lateral rotating Scheimpflug camera.

- Since the Placido-based technology is reflection-based, it is much more accurate than tomography in describing the anterior corneal surface in case of scars and stromal haze. That is because in tomography, light suffers from scattering and provides misleading information as the cornea will appear thinner and flatter in case of haze. This is why, topography is essential for some types of customized laser vision correction.
- Topography can measure angles kappa and lambda, while tomography cannot.
- Topography is very much affected by tear film disturbance and OSD, while tomography is less affected.
- Maps generated by both technologies are affected by abnormal angle kappa and misalignment during taking the capture. However, Placido-based technology is more sensitive in detecting misalignment than the Scheimpflug technology.

HYBRID DEVICES (TOPO-TOMOGRAPHERS)

Some devices implement both Placido and Scheimpflug technologies in order to gain the advantages of both systems and overcome the disadvantages. These devices are Orbscan, Sirius, Galilei, and Tomey. In these devices, the anterior curvature map is directly measured by the Placido disk, while the elevation maps are directly measured by the Scheimpflug camera.

CHAPTER 3

Screening Guidelines

INTRODUCTION

Before capturing an eye, standard settings should be adjusted for the following reasons:
- To display the captures in a standard form that will make it easy to compare the captures in different visits and with other captures in other centers.
- To validate the accuracy and reliability of the capture.
- To avoid over- or underestimation.
- To avoid factors generating false positives and false negatives.

These settings are related to the diameter of the display, color scale, reference body diameter and mode in addition to special precautions in preparing the eye for acquisition.

THE FOUR-COMPOSITE MAP

The four-composite map is the main map to be studied. There are different types of this map as shown in Figure 3.1, however, the standard map in clinical practice is the "four maps refractive" (Fig. 3.2). Chapter 4 is devoted to explain this map in detail. In this chapter, settings of the map will be discussed.

GENERAL SETTINGS

It is recommended to use the general settings shown in Figure 3.3.
- *Radius of curvature*: To be presented as horizontal/vertical rather than flat/steep. This is easier to recognize with-the-rule (WTR) astigmatism (vertical in red) from against-the-rule (ATR) astigmatism (vertical in blue).
- *Axis of astigmatism*: To be the flat (blue) rather than the steep (red) because the flat axis is the axis of a correcting minus cylindrical lens; therefore, it is easier to compare it with the manifest astigmatism in the minus cylindrical equation.
- The box of "show sign of astigmatism" should be left blank because in many instances the sign will be misleading.
- Store 9 mm zone setting. This is discussed below in "maps overlay".
- *Shape factor presentation*: To be presented as asphericity (Q-value). Q-value is the standard expression used to describe the overall slope of the cornea.
- *Eccentricity calculation zone*: To be measured in 6 mm ring if the "peripheral mm-rings" option was chosen, or in 20° ring if the "sagittal angle" option was chosen, however, both are the same. The 6 mm (or the 20°) ring is the standard because it is the functional optical zone in the cornea.
- *Elevation reference shape*: To be stored in sphere, float, and optimize shift mode with a manual calculation diameter of 8 mm. This is discussed below in "reference shape".
- *Anterior chamber depth range*: To be presented as "internal (endothelium)". This means that anterior chamber depth (ACD) will be measure from corneal endothelium to anterior surface of the lens without considering corneal thickness, which is considered if "external (epithelium)" is used. The internal ACD is important for phakic intraocular lens (IOL) implantation and glaucoma workup.
- *Color map appearance*: To be presented in black dots rather than white area mode because missing data will be recognized easily. This is discussed below in "maps overlay".

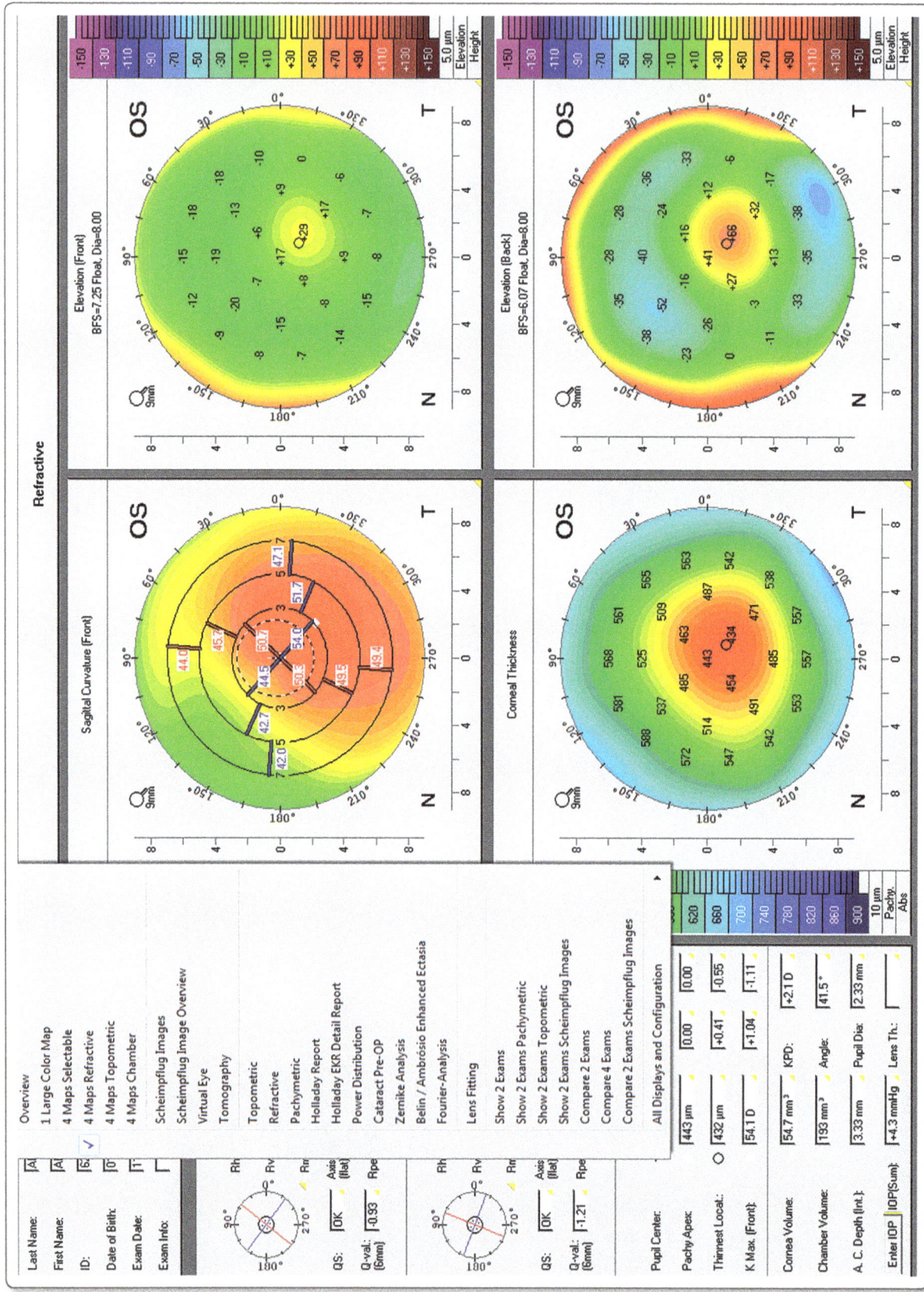

Fig. 3.1: List of maps and displays in the Pentacam HR.

Chapter 3: Screening Guidelines 15

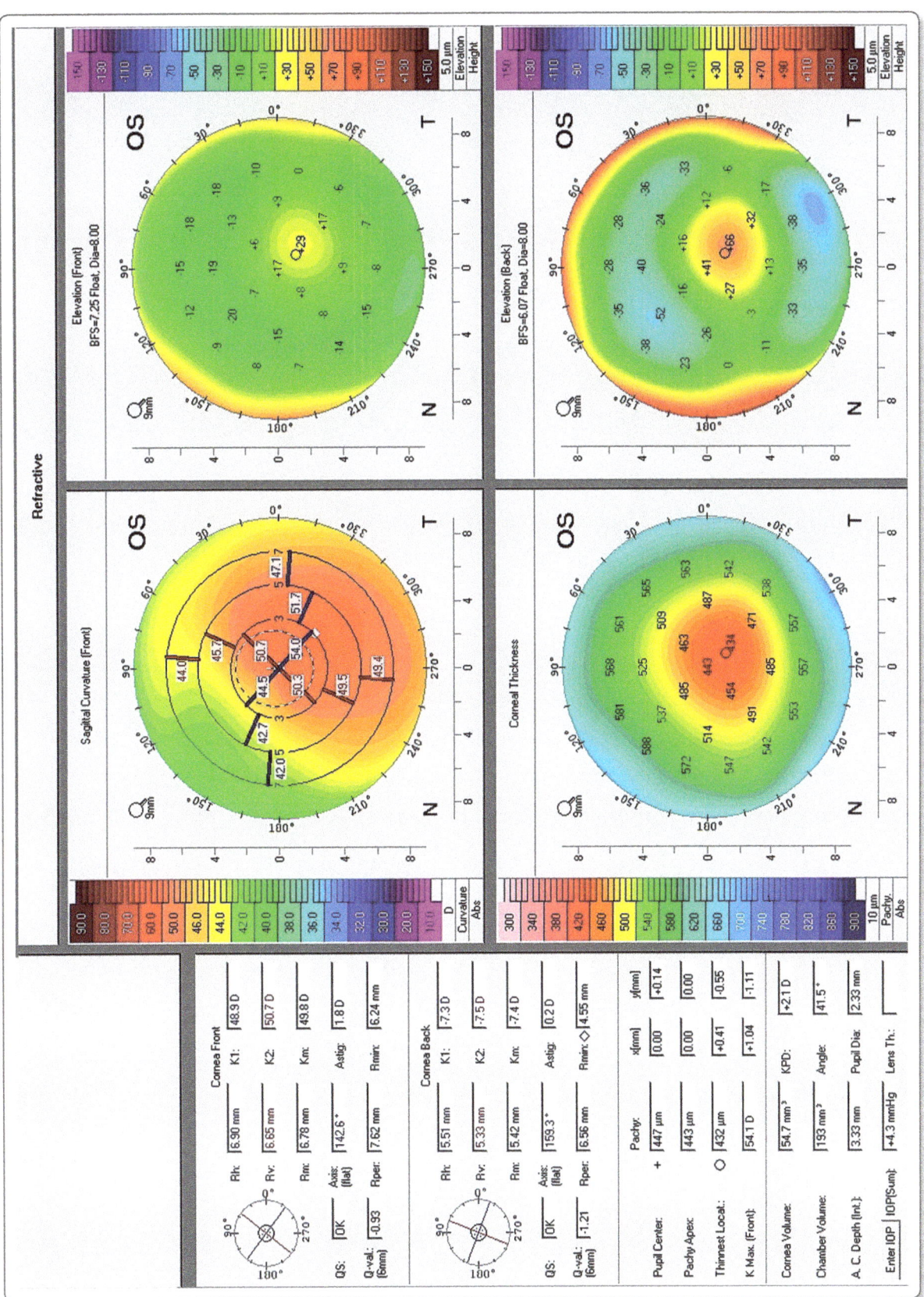

Fig. 3.2: The "four maps refractive" display. This is the standard map in clinical practice.

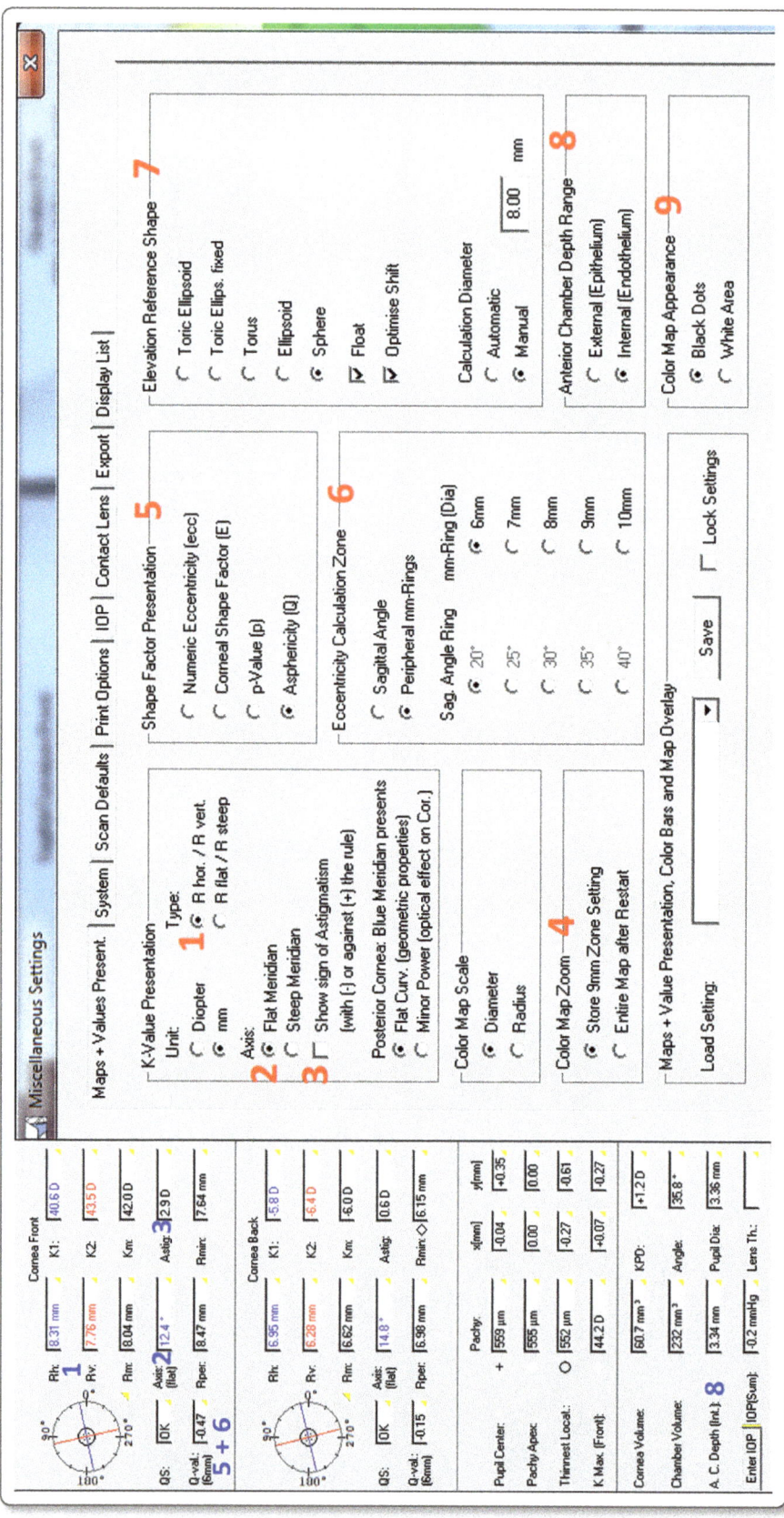

Fig. 3.3: General settings that are recommended in Pentacam HR.

COLOR SCALE

There are two types of color scale: (1) the normalized and (2) the absolute scales. In the normalized scale, the computer provides color contour maps based on the average dioptric value of the measured cornea. The disadvantage is that the color of two maps cannot be compared directly and have to be interpreted based on the values. In the absolute (standardized) scale, the computer displays all corneas on the same scale, making comparison between corneas possible. Additionally, the color increments of the curvature map can be chosen to be in 0.25 D, 0.5 D, 1 D, or 1.5 D scales. In general, using fine scale exaggerate irregularities while using coarse scale may hide them as shown in Figures 3.4 to 3.6. It is recommended to use the 1 D scale with the sagittal map and the 1.5 D scale with the tangential map to avoid over- and underestimation. The same can be said for elevation and pachymetry maps. For the elevation maps and pachymetry map, it is recommended to use the 5 μm and the 10 μm scales, respectively (Fig. 3.7).

Additionally, there are different sets of color scales in the Pentacam software: Oculus, Holladay Primary, American Style, Atlas (fixed), Belin Intuitive, Smolek/Klyce USS, Ambrosio2, and TMS. These sets of colors differ in color coding but not in the displayed values. Belin and Ambrosio recommend Belin Intuitive for the curvature map and the elevation maps, and Ambrosio2 for the pachymetry map. However, readers can choose the color set that they are satisfied with, but in all cases, it is strongly advised to use the absolute color scale, the 1 D scale for the curvature map, the 1.5 D scale for the tangential map, the 5 μm scale for the pachymetry map, the 10 μm scale for the elevation maps, and the 61 colors option.

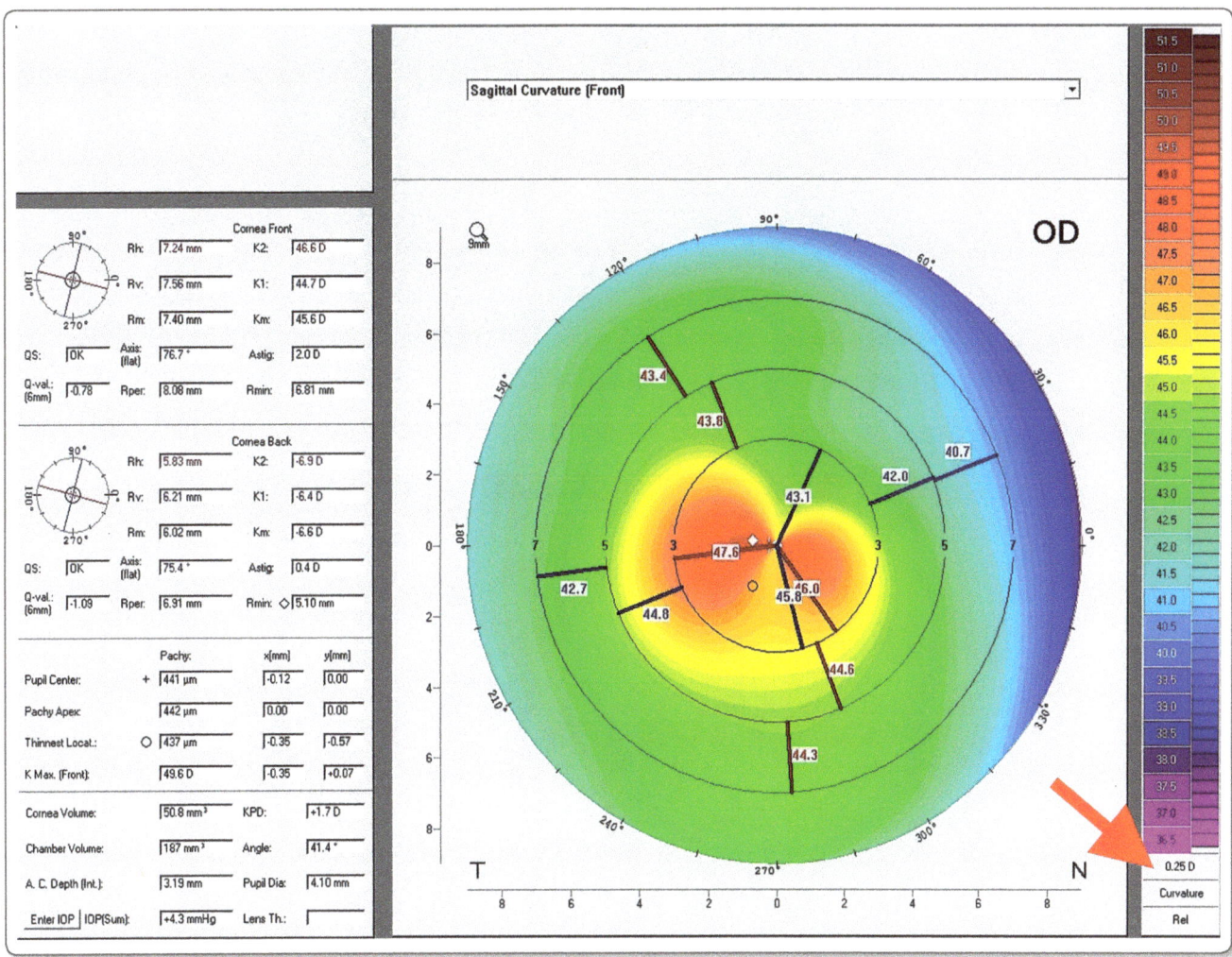

Fig. 3.4: The curvature map in the 0.25 D color scale. This scale is very fine and exaggerates colors but not values.

Section 1: *Introduction*

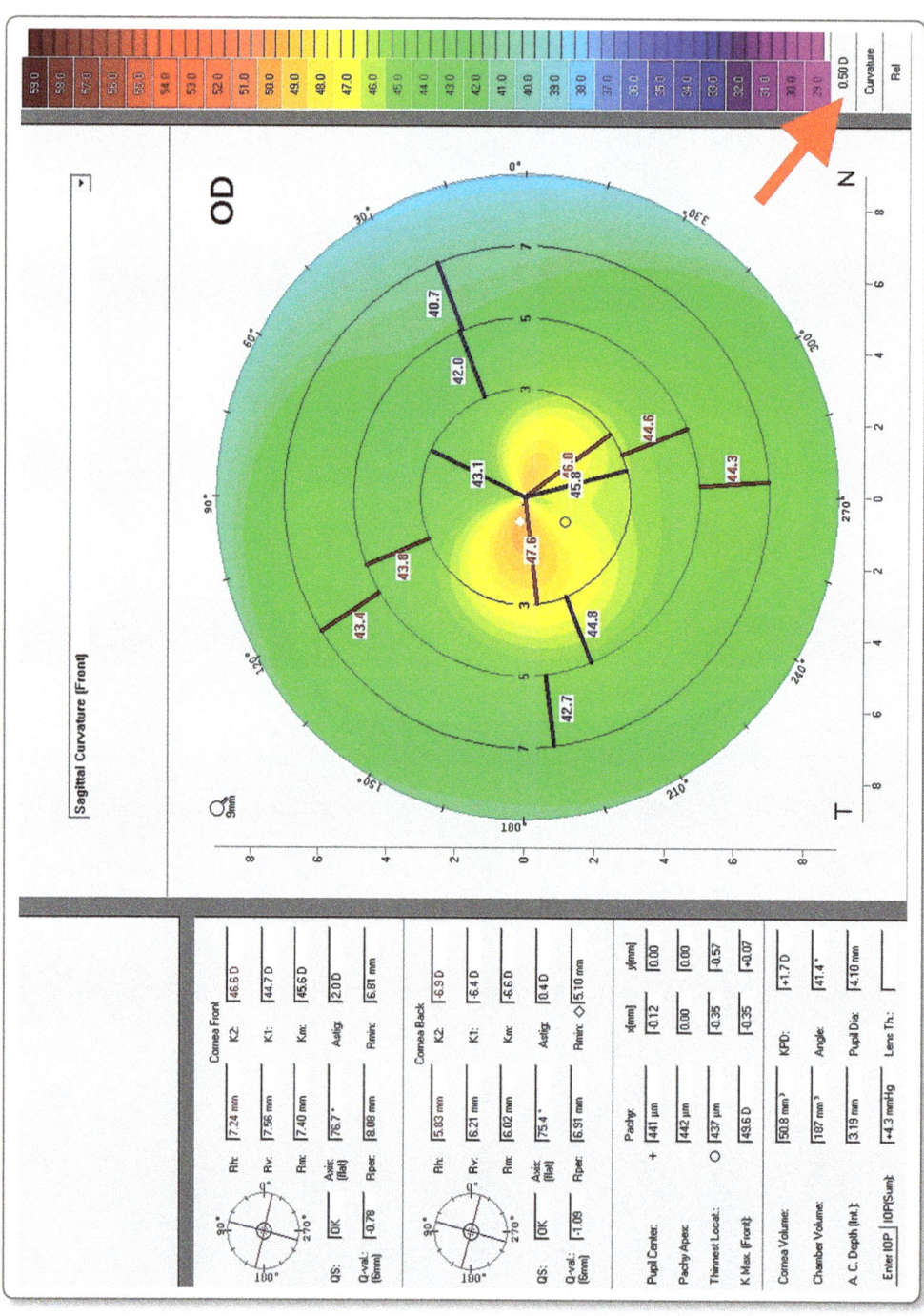

Fig. 3.5: The curvature map in the 0.5 D color scale. This scale is fine and exaggerates colors but not values.

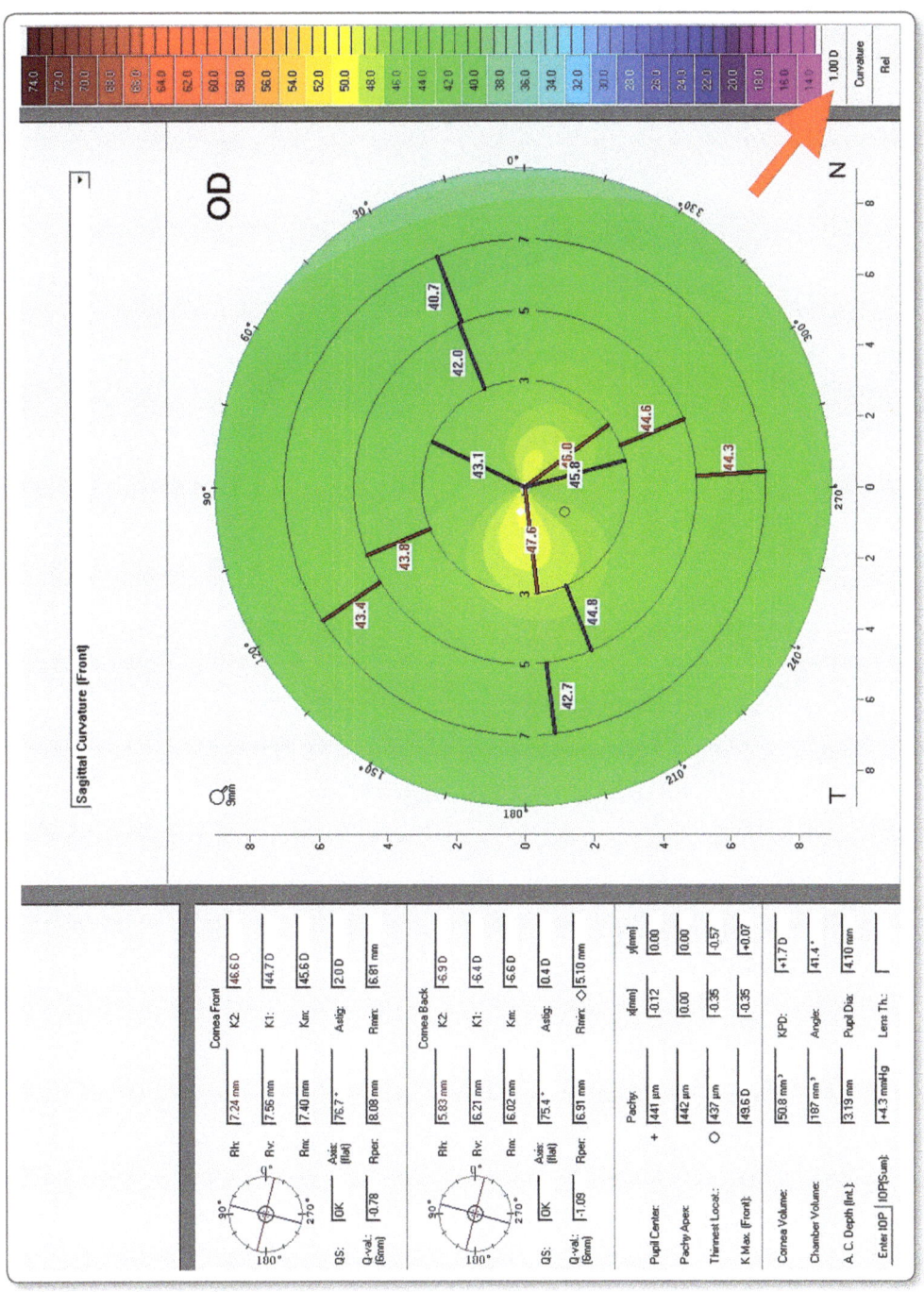

Fig. 3.6: The curvature map in the 1.00 D color scale. This scale is neutral, i.e. neither coarse to hide nor fine to exaggerate the details.

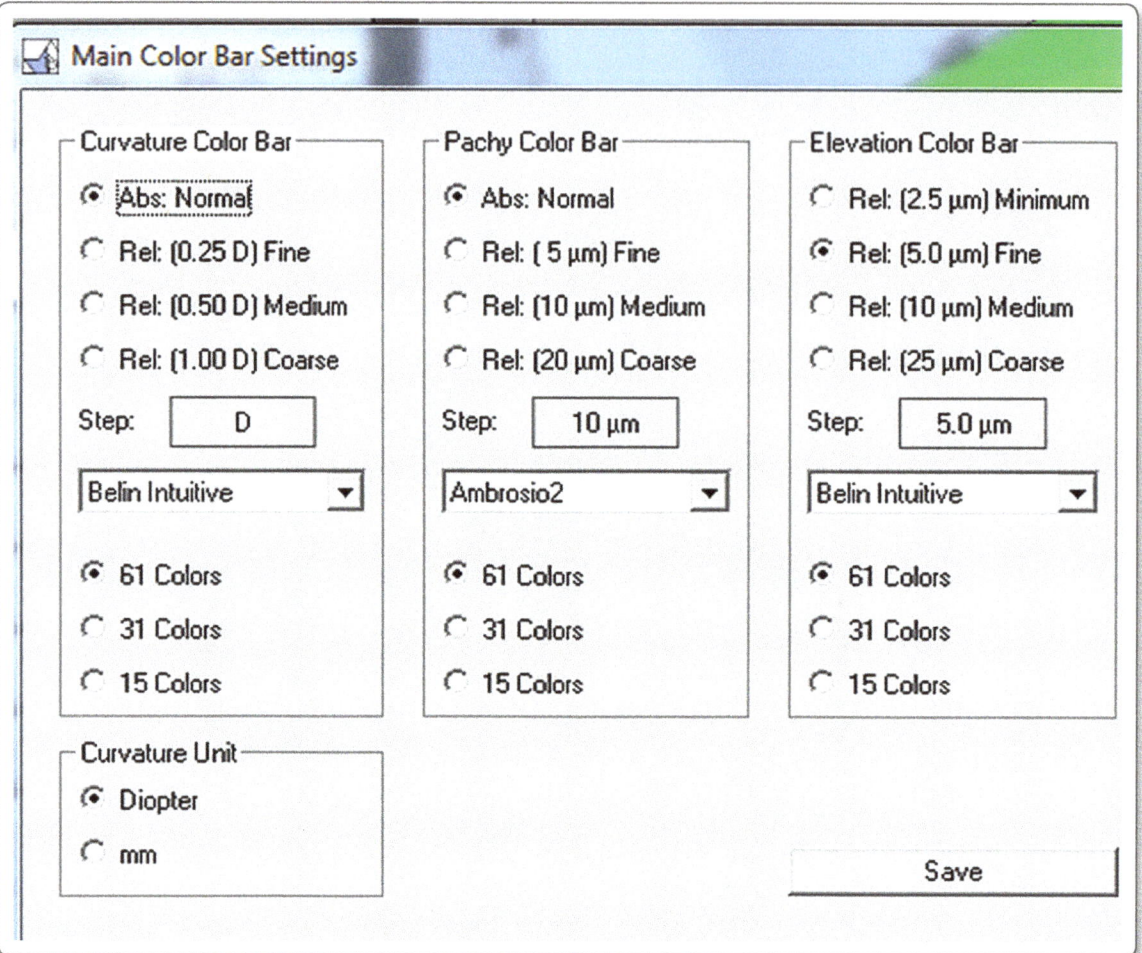

Fig. 3.7: Color scales for the curvature, pachymetry, and elevation maps.

MAPS OVERLAY

Map overlay is the components that should appear on the map for the complementary study.

Curvature Map Overlay

Figure 3.8 shows the overlay of the curvature map.
- *Apex position*: This is the position of the cornea vertex.
- Thinnest location.
- *Minimum radius position front*: It is the position of maximum K-readings (Kmax) on anterior corneal surface. It is usually encountered in the center of an island of high K-readings known as "hot spot" (Fig. 3.9: red arrow). If it is very peripheral, it might be an artifact due to a peripheral scar, lid interference of the capture, or tear film disturbance (Fig. 3.10).
- Pupil center and pupil edge are important to check for misalignment. Pupil edge is important to study power gradient along the pupil in customized laser vision correction.
- Nasal/temporal and OD/OS.
- *Maximum diameter 9 mm*: The 9 mm display is important to check the quality of the capture. In case of missing data, the computer will extrapolate the areas of missing data either in black dots (Fig. 3.11) or as white blank areas (Fig. 3.12). As mentioned earlier in the general settings, the black dot option is easier to recognize. If there were extrapolated areas on the full diameter map

Chapter 3: Screening Guidelines **21**

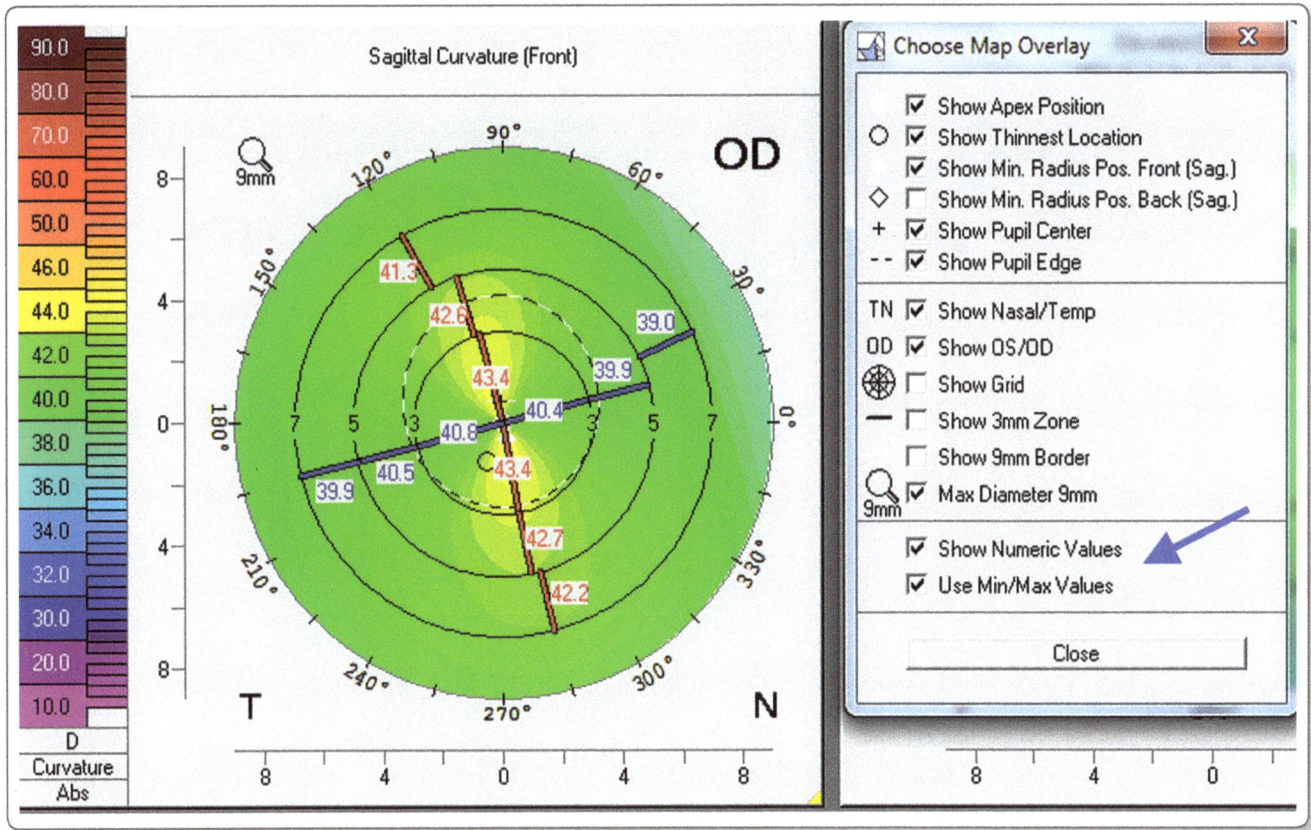

Fig. 3.8: Overlay for the anterior sagittal curvature map.

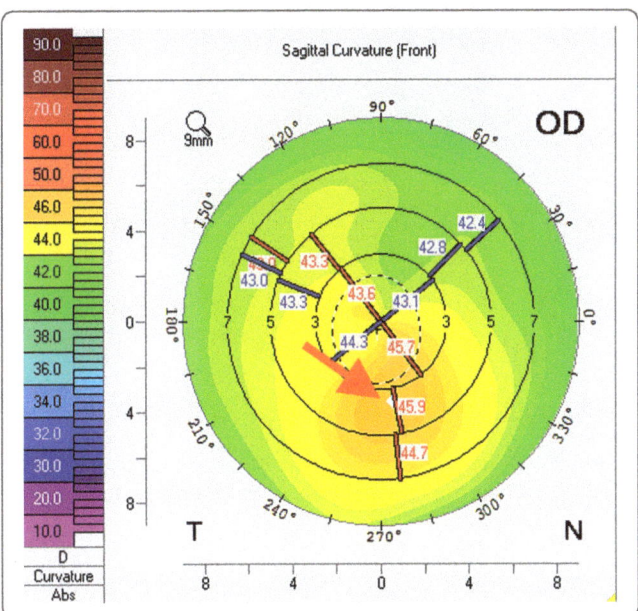

Fig. 3.9: Kmax symbol within the center of the hot spot.

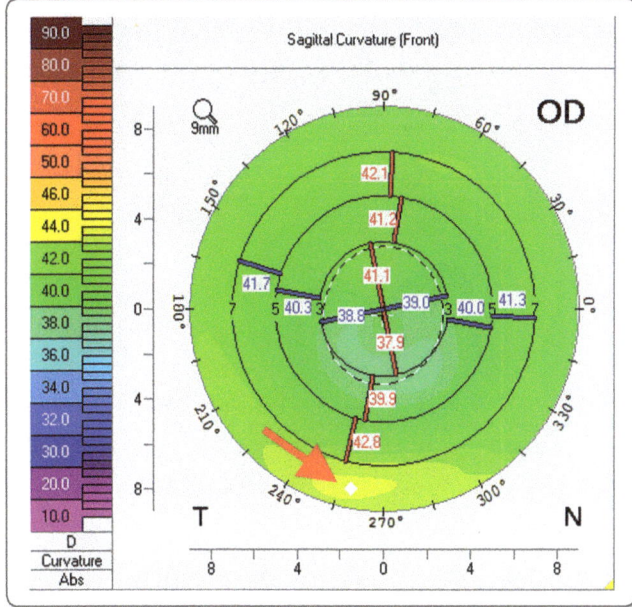

Fig. 3.10: A very peripheral Kmax symbol indicating an artifact. The capture should be repeated.

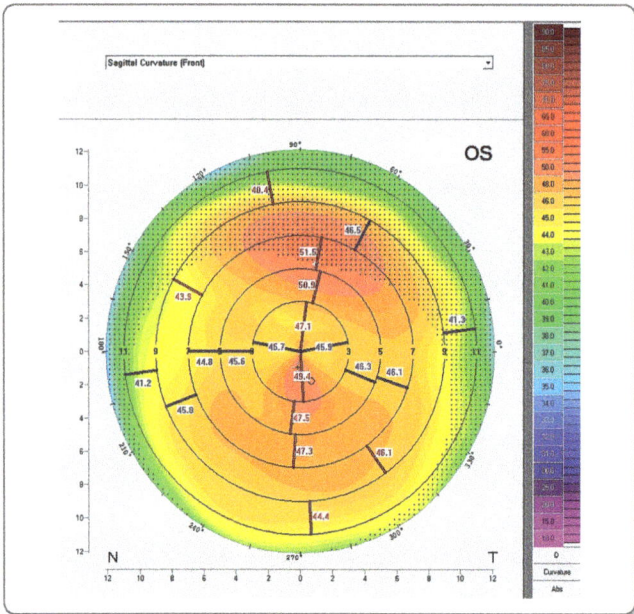

Fig. 3.11: Extrapolated data displayed as black-dotted areas at corneal periphery.

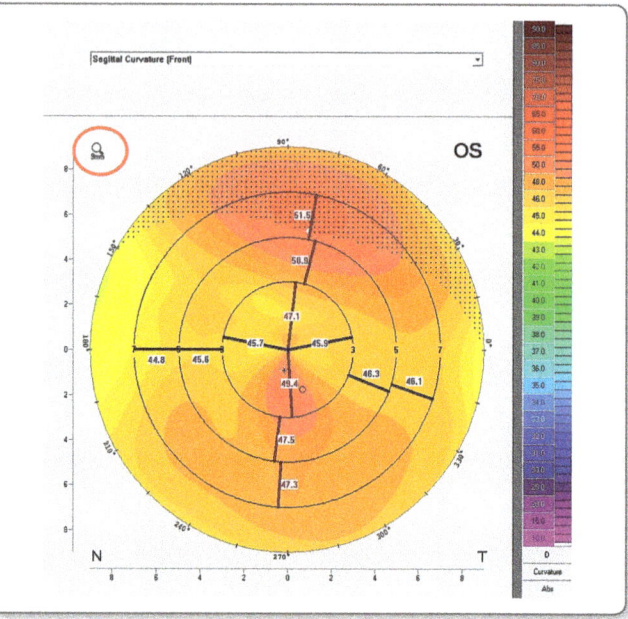

Fig. 3.13: Extrapolated data in the 9 mm display (red circle).

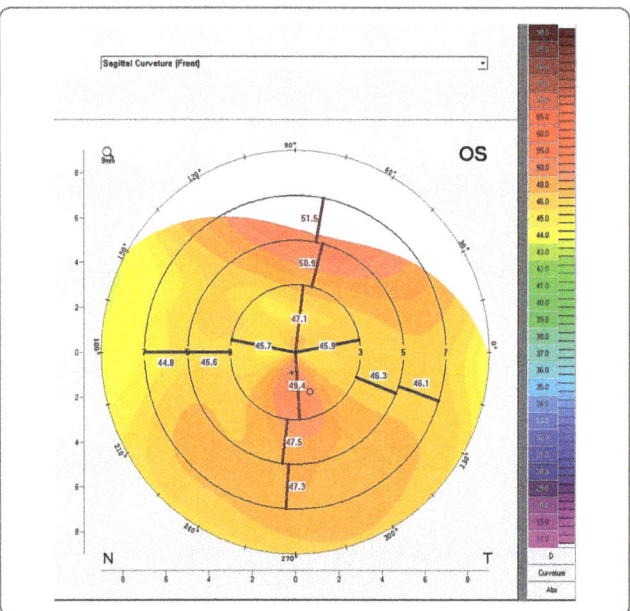

Fig. 3.12: Extrapolated data displayed as blank white areas at corneal periphery.

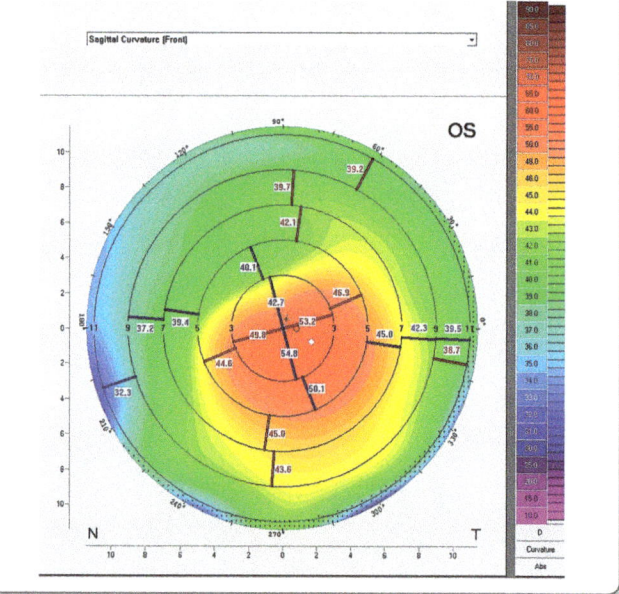

Fig. 3.14: Mild peripheral extrapolation on the full display. It disappears on the 9 mm display in the next figure.

(see Figure 3.11), and they do not disappear on the 9 mm magnified display (Fig. 3.13: red circle), the capture cannot be accepted. Figures 3.14 and 3.15 represent a case of extrapolation that disappears on the 9 mm magnified display.

- *Numeric values and minimum/maximum values (Fig. 3.8: blue arrow)*: This represents the distribution of keratometric power of the anterior sagittal map as blue (flat) and red (steep) segments (semimeridians). This is important for predicting corneal irregularities, and

Chapter 3: Screening Guidelines

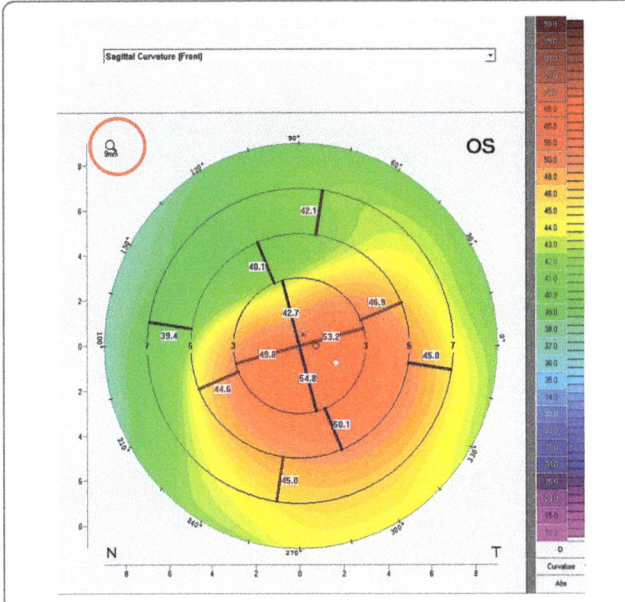

Fig. 3.15: Disappearance of extrapolation on the 9 mm display. See the previous figure.

studying and classifying the patterns. This is discussed in Chapter 5 in detail.

Elevation Maps Overlay

Figure 3.16 shows the overlay of the elevation maps displayed in the best fit sphere float mode and 8 mm diameter (see reference shape below).
- The symbol of the thinnest location (red arrows) is important to study the corresponding values on the elevation maps. This will be discussed in Chapter 6 in detail.
- Nasal/temporal and OD/OS.
- Maximum diameter 9 mm.
- Full numeric values should be displayed (blue arrow).

Thickness Map Overlay

Figure 3.17 shows the overlay of the thickness map.
- Thinnest location.
- Nasal/temporal and OD/OS.
- Maximum diameter 9 mm.
- Full numeric values should be displayed (red arrow).

REFERENCE BODY SHAPE

It is recommended to use the best fit sphere in float mode and 8 mm diameter as shown in Figures 3.18 and 3.19.

Using a smaller diameter will underestimate irregularities (false negatives), while using a larger diameter will overestimate them (false positives), as shown in Figures 3.20 and 3.21, respectively.

PREPARING THE EYE FOR THE CAPTURE

Before capturing the eye, exclude all sources of false positives and false negatives:
- *Contact lenses*: They should be stopped at least 1 week before eye examination.
- *Misalignment*: The patient should be fully educated about how the device works and what is required from them during the capture.
- *Tear film disturbance*: Both dryness and excess tears have a bad effect on the capture. If the patient is frequently blinking, an anesthesia drop must *not* be used because it will alter the integrity of the epithelium, tear film, and corneal surface. The patient should be treated properly and recaptured *later*.
- *Corneal opacities or previous surgeries*: They should be excluded by careful history taking and detailed slit lamp biomicroscopy examination.
- *Bad exposure to the camera*: This can be due to small eyes, deep set-eyes, nasal bridge, long lashes, or tight headscarves. Special face positions can overcome the anatomical reasons, while the headscarves should be loosened backward.

CHECKING THE QUALITY OF THE CAPTURE

Before printing the capture and sending it to the physician, the technician should follow a five-step checklist to be sure of a good, valid, and reliable capture.

1. *Qs*: It should be white OK.
2. *Km*: Three captures should be done in the session. The Km is compared. If more than 0.3 D difference is found between the captures, they should be repeated. The capture with the median number should be adopted. Example 1: three captures with Km 45.3 D, 45.8 D, and 45 D, the captures should be repeated. Example 2: three captures with Km 43.4 D, 43.7 D, and 43.5 D, the captures are accepted and the one with 43.5 D is adopted as the main capture for this visit. This is important especially in observing progression of ectatic corneal diseases (ECDs) and comparing pre- with postoperative results. Please note that the variation in Km will be very wide in people

Section 1: *Introduction*

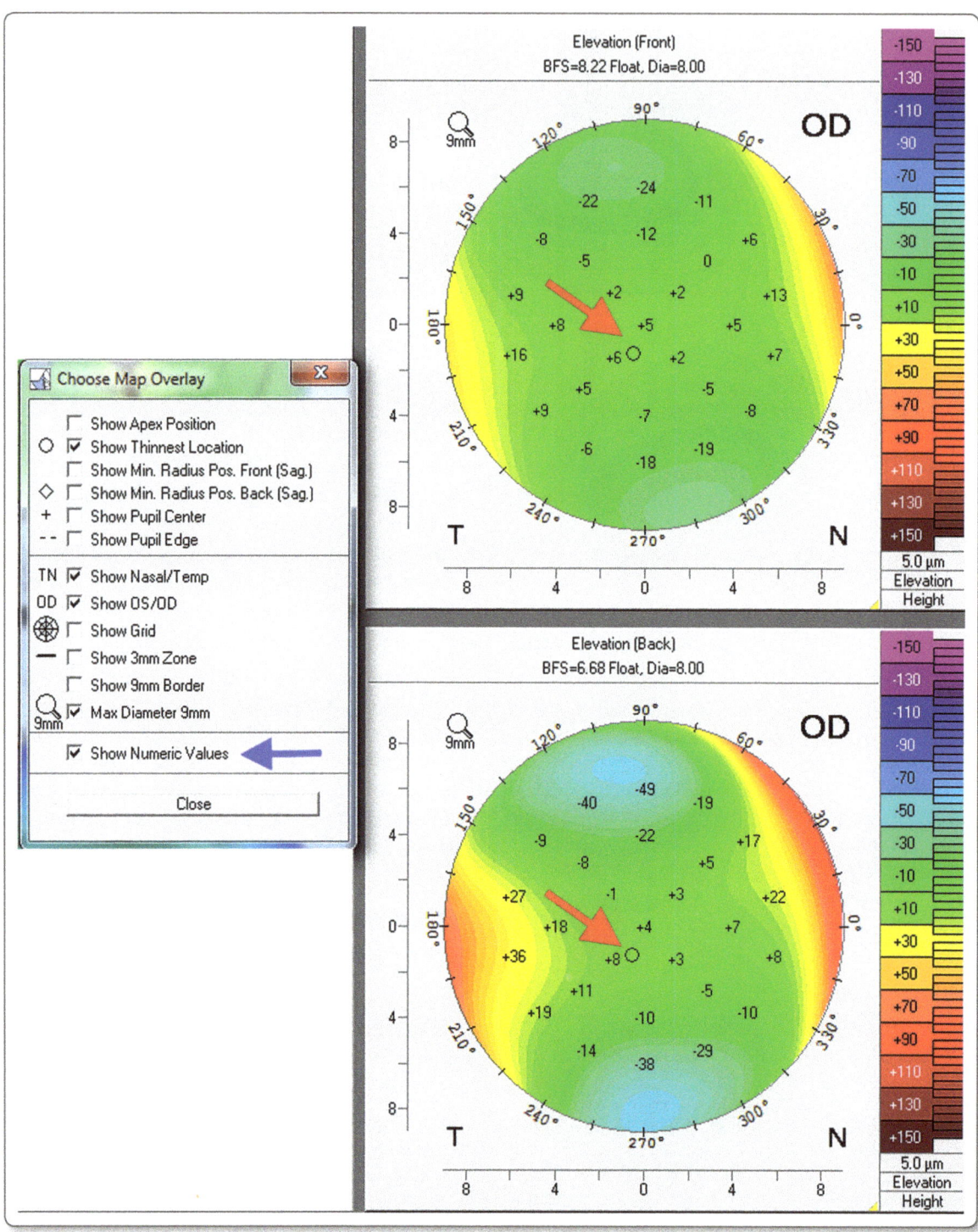

Fig. 3.16: Overlay for the elevation maps.

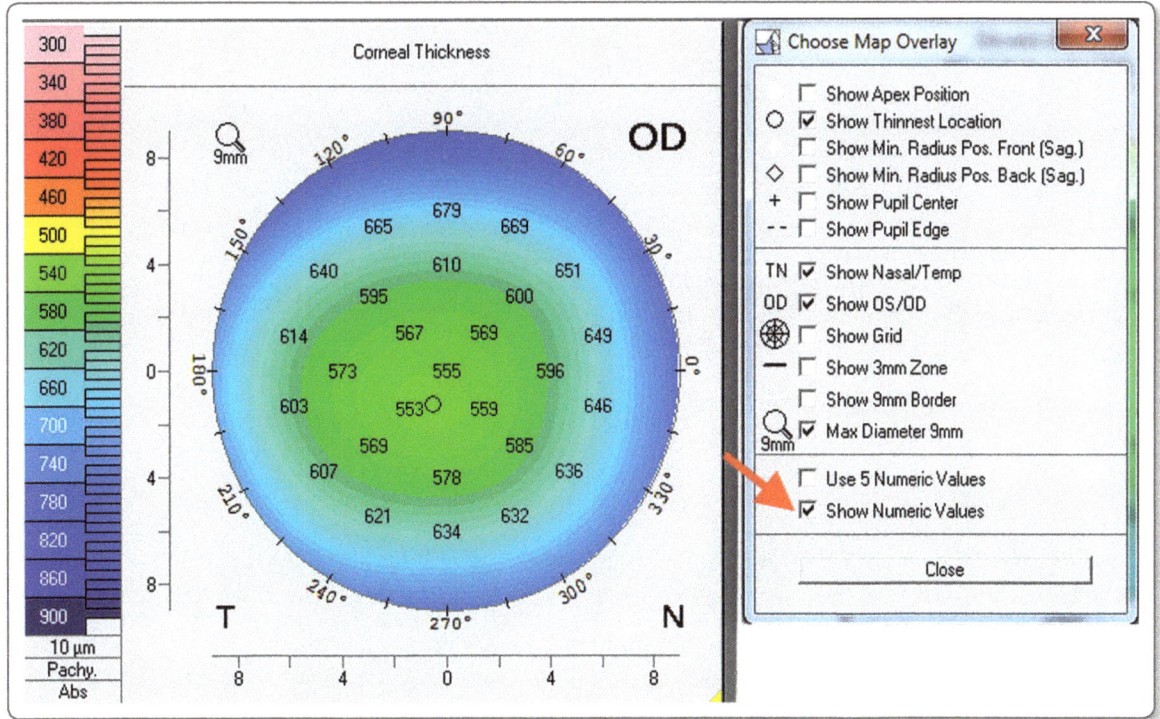

Fig. 3.17: Overlay for the corneal thickness map.

with ECDs, hence, the need to be patient in capturing the eye of the patient.

3. *Kmax*: Check the symbol on the curvature map. If it is very peripheral, recapture the cornea; if it is repeatedly peripheral, check lid position on Scheimpflug images; if there is no lid interference, tell the physician to check tear film and look for blepharitis or corneal scars.
4. *Pupil and thinnest location coordinates*: If X and/or Y of pupil center and/or thinnest location *in the capture* is >0.2 mm, repeat the capture.
5. *Intereye asymmetry*: If there is a difference *between the two eyes* >0.1 mm in X and/or Y of pupil center and/or thinnest location, repeat the capture.

SPECIFIC SETTINGS FOR HOLLADAY REPORT

Figure 3.22 shows the general settings for Holladay report. These settings are automatically set by default. Figure 3.23 is corneal thickness map overlay. Figure 3.24 is the overly for the five other maps.

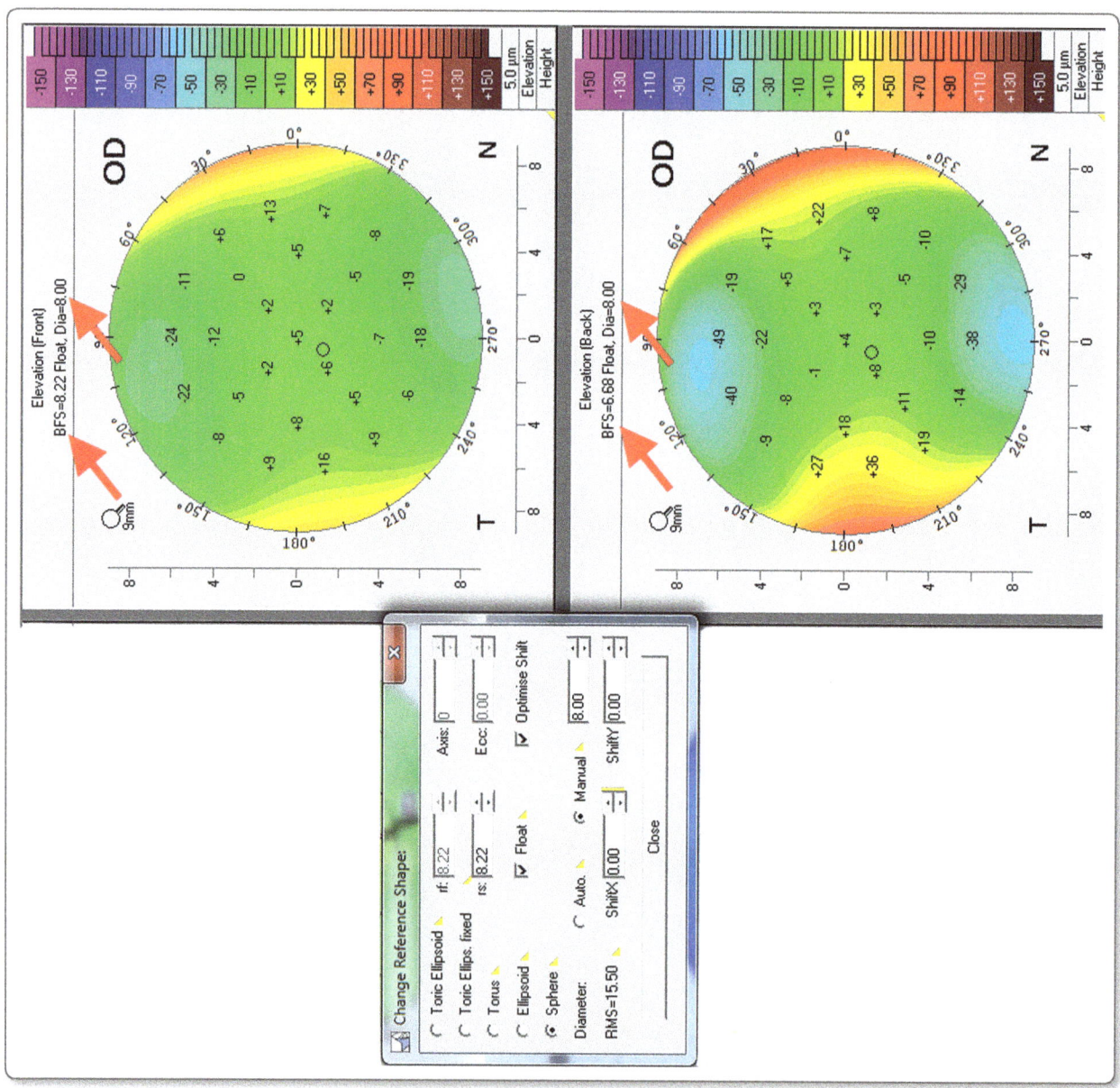

Fig. 3.18: The standard 8 mm zonal diameter for the best fit sphere (BFS) reference surface.

Chapter 3: Screening Guidelines

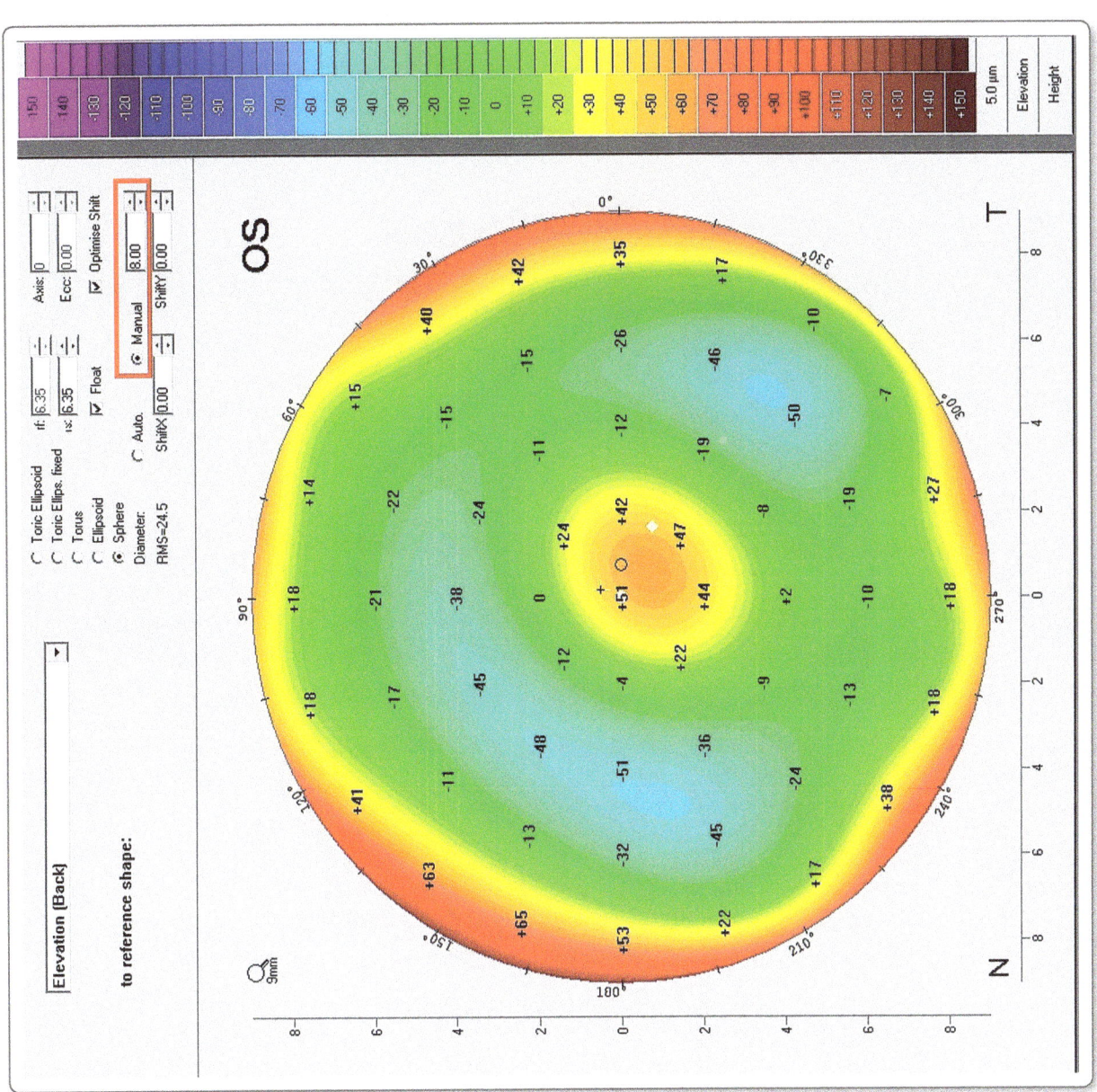

Fig. 3.19: Posterior elevation map with the standard 8 mm best fit sphere (BFS).

Section 1: Introduction

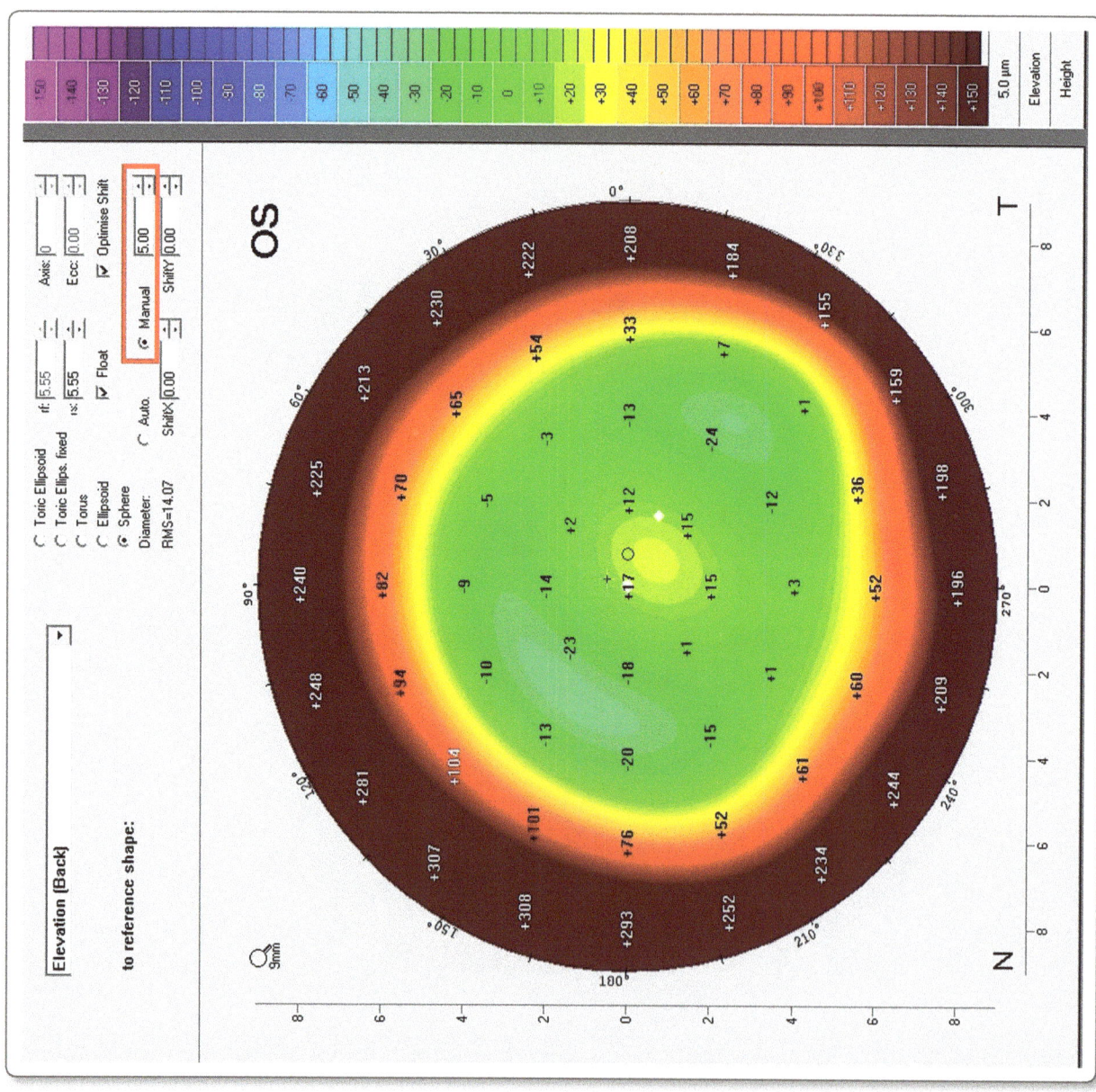

Fig. 3.20: Same posterior elevation map with 5 mm best fit sphere (BFS). Values are underestimated.

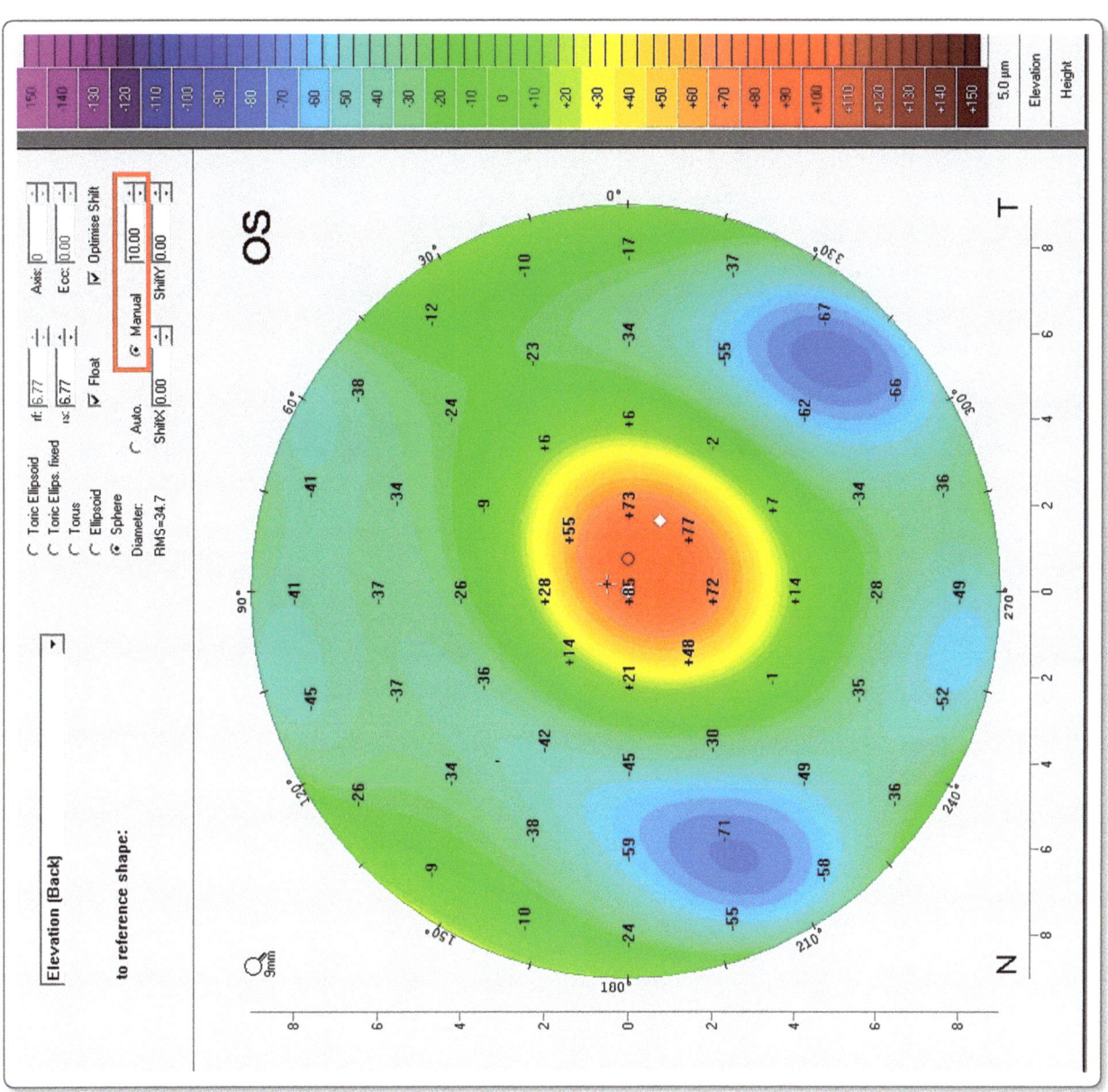

Fig. 3.21: Same posterior elevation map with 10 mm best fit sphere (BFS). Values are overestimated.

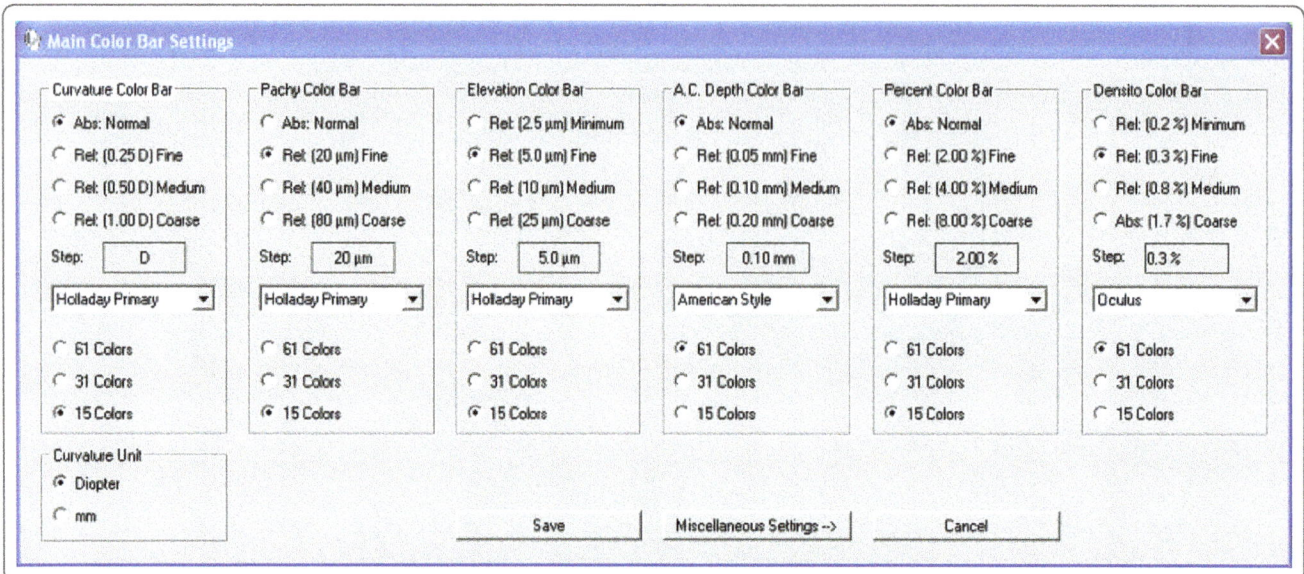

Fig. 3.22: General settings for Holladay report.

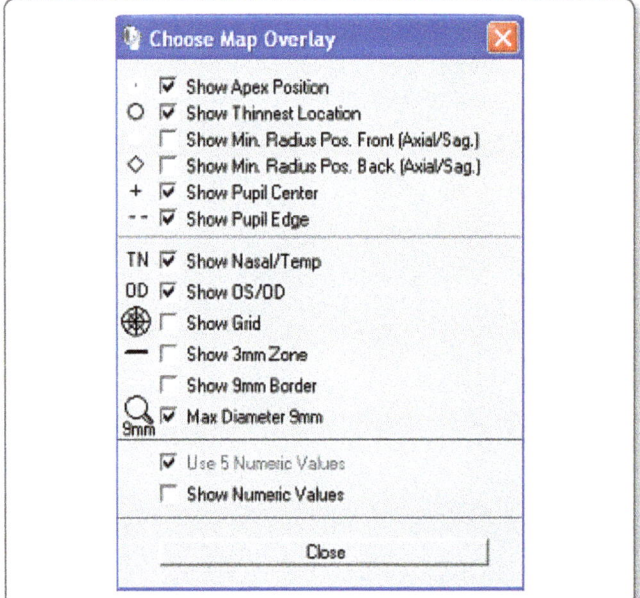

Fig. 3.23: Overlay for corneal thickness map in Holladay report.

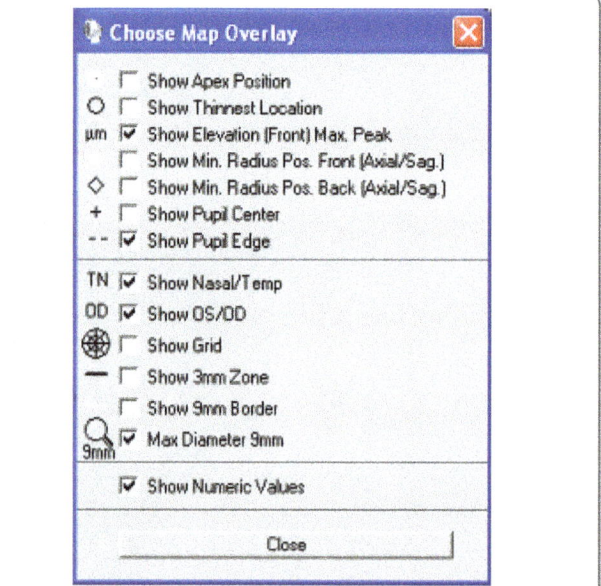

Fig. 3.24: Overlay for all the maps, except thickness map, in Holladay report.

SECTION 2

Corneal Maps and Profiles

SECTION OUTLINE

4. Overview
5. Corneal Power Maps
6. Elevation Maps
7. Belin/Ambrosio Enhanced Ectasia
8. Corneal Thickness Maps and Profiles
9. Geometric Tomography and Corneal Topometry

CHAPTER 4

Overview

INTRODUCTION

The four-composite map consists of corneal parameters displayed on the left side and four maps displayed on the right side of the display. Corneal parameters are for cornea front (anterior corneal surface), cornea back (posterior corneal surface), parameters of thickness, and miscellaneous. For refractive surgery screening and keratoconus management, the "four maps refractive" option should be chosen. In this option, the four maps on the right side are: anterior sagittal curvature map, anterior and posterior elevation maps and the pachymetry (thickness) map. Full evaluation of the four-composite map in *both* eyes is mandatory before making a decision.

CORNEAL PARAMETERS (FIG. 4.1)

Cornea Front (Anterior Surface)

- *Qs*: Quality specification. It specifies the quality of the tomographic capture; it should be "OK", otherwise there are some missed information which were virtually reproduced (extrapolated) by the computer, and therefore, the capture should be repeated. However, since the Pentacam is not Placido-based, its sensitivity to misalignment is relatively not high; in some instances, there is misalignment and Qs is OK (Chapter 16).
- *Q-value*: Q-value in the central 6 mm zone. It represents the asphericity of the anterior surface of the cornea.
- *K1*: The anterior flat simulated keratometer (Sim-K1) on a ring in 15° (at 3.2 mm) around corneal apex.
- *Rh*: Horizontal radius of anterior corneal curvature of the central Sim Ks. If it is in blue, the cornea has with-the-rule (WTR) astigmatism. If it is in red, the cornea has against-the-rule (ATR) astigmatism.

- *K2*: The anterior steep simulated keratometer (Sim-K2) on a ring in 15° (at 3.2 mm) around corneal apex.
- *Rv*: Vertical radius of anterior corneal curvature of the central Sim-Ks. If it is in red, the cornea has WTR astigmatism. If it is in blue, the cornea has WTR astigmatism.
- *Km*: The arithmetic mean (average) of the central Sim-Ks. It is discussed in Chapter 1.
- *Rm*: The arithmetic mean (average) radius of anterior corneal curvature of the central Sim-Ks.

  N.B: Km is important in screening and for decision making in laser vision correction (LVC) for the following reasons:
  - It is one of the factors to check the quality of the capture, as mentioned in Chapter 3.
  - In Placido-based devices, Km more than 47.2 D is suspicious. In Scheimpflug-based devices, Km more than 48 D is suspicious.
  - It is usually used to choose the size of the suction ring and determine hinge width in laser in situ keratomileusis (LASIK).
  - It is affected by myopic correction. Each −1 D of spherical equivalent (SE) correction reduces Km roughly by 0.8 D; postoperative Km is recommended to be more than 33 D to avoid positive spherical aberration.
  - It is affected by hypermetropic correction. Each +1 D of SE correction increases Km roughly by 1.25 D; postoperative Km is recommended to be less than 50 D to avoid negative spherical aberration.
- *Astigmatism*: The absolute amount of anterior corneal astigmatism related to the Sim Ks. This astigmatism does not reflect the true corneal astigmatism because

it does not take into consideration the posterior surface and corneal thickness, it uses the keratometric index (n = 1.3375) rather than the real corneal index (n = 1.376), and it is limited to the 3.2 mm central ring.

- *Axis*: The axis of the flat or steep meridian of the Sim-Ks of the anterior corneal surface. The flat axis is usually used because it is consistent with the axis of a corrective minus cylindrical lens.
- *Rmin*: The minimum (steepest) radius of the anterior sagittal curvature (see Kmax below).
- *Rper*: Average radius of anterior sagittal curvature between the 7 mm and 9 mm zones around the anterior corneal apex.

Cornea Back (Posterior Surface)

The posterior corneal surface has the same parameters of the anterior surface, but related to the posterior surface. However, it should be noted that the posterior surface plays a role of a concave refractive surface although it is convex. This is because the incident light passes from a medium of higher refractive index (RI) (stroma = 1.375) to a medium of lower RI (aqueous humor = 1.336). This is why, the Sim-Ks of the posterior surface are negative.

Corneal Landmarks

Corneal landmarks are displayed with the corresponding X and Y coordinates (Fig. 4.2).
- *Pachy apex*: It represents corneal thickness from epithelium to endothelium at the anterior corneal apex position. The X and Y coordinates of this point is 0.00 because it is the origin of X and Y of the other landmarks.
- *Pupil center*: It is the position of the entrance pupil center. The X and Y coordinates are important to get an idea about angle kappa as mentioned in Chapter 1, and to check the accuracy of the capture as mentioned in Chapter 3. The position of pupil center differs according to pupil mydriasis or miosis; pupil center is usually shifted up to 0.7 mm superior-temporally when dilated.
- *Thinnest location*: The thinnest location (TL) is the thinnest point in the measured cornea (Chapter 1). It is important for decision making in LVC and management of ectatic corneal diseases (ECDs). Additionally, the

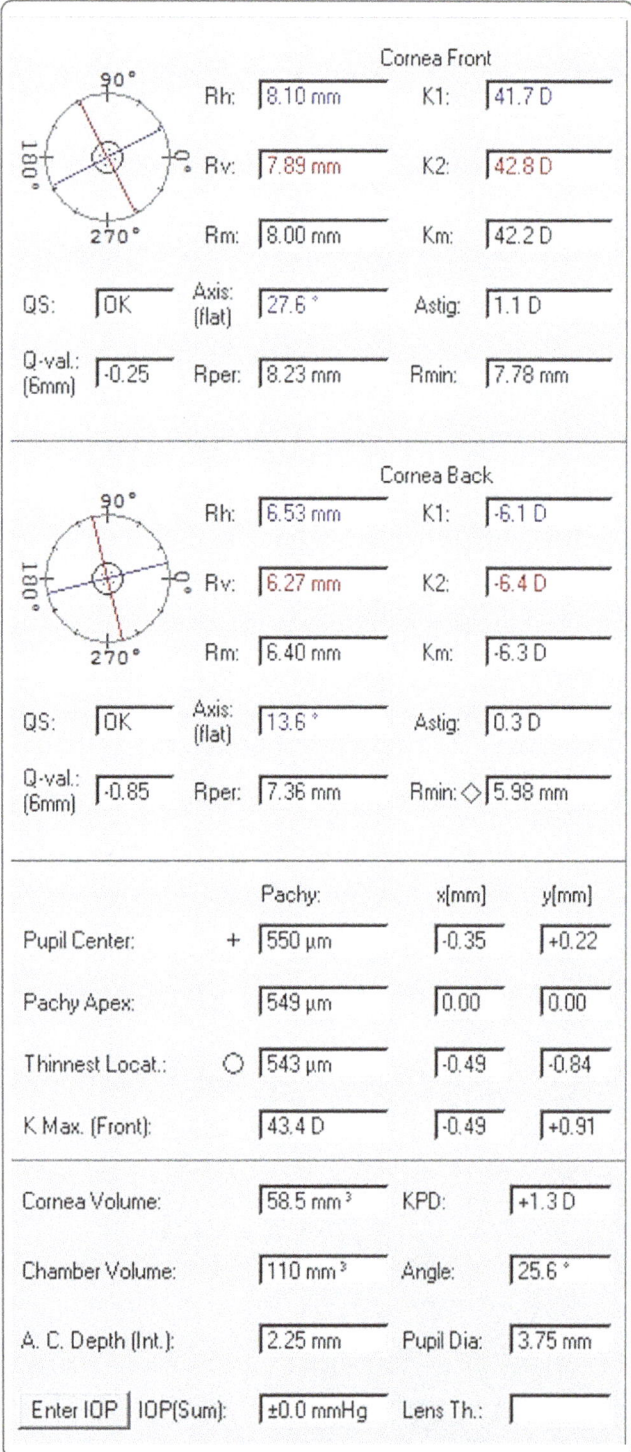

Fig. 4.1: Corneal parameters.

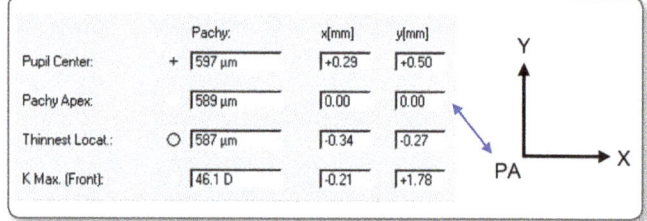

Fig. 4.2: Corneal landmarks.

thickness at the TL is one of the two cardinal factors in observing progression (Chapter 21).

- *Kmax (front)*: This is the steepest radius of curvature of the anterior corneal surface displayed in keratometric dioptric power. Since there is no normative data yet, its location is more important than the value itself. Kmax is important for three reasons:
  1. As mentioned in Chapter 3, when the Kmax is peripheral, the quality of the capture should be questioned.
  2. In LVC, if the difference between Kmax and K2 is > 1 D, postoperative-induced irregularities are most likely to occur, especially in hypermetropic corrections.
  3. In ECDs, Kmax is one of the two cardinal factors in observing progression (Chapter 21).

Miscellaneous

- *Cornea volume*: The volume of the cornea in a 10-mm zone around the anterior corneal apex.
- *KPD*: The keratometric power deviation. It displays the difference between the anterior sagittal power map and the true net power map in the apex position. The normal value is <+0.75 D. It is suspicious between +0.75 D and +1.5 D, and abnormal if >1.5 D, such as in ECDs and postsurgeries.
- *Anterior chamber volume (ACV)*: The volume in mm^3 of the anterior chamber (AC) from endothelium down to iris and anterior surface of the lens evaluated in a 12-mm zone around the anterior corneal apex.
- *Anterior chamber angle (ACA)*: The smaller of both chamber angles in the horizon position (180°) calculated from the three-dimensional (3D) model.
- *Anterior chamber depth (internal/external)*: The AC depth, related to the anterior corneal apex position, measured from epithelium (external) or endothelium (internal). *N.B*: Intraocular lens (IOL) power calculation formulas usually require the ACD measured from the epithelium (external).

  N.B: ACV of less than 100 mm^3, ACA of less than 24°, or ACD of less than 2.1 mm may indicate the risk of an angle closure glaucoma. On the other hand, if phakic intraocular lens (PIOL) implantation is indicated, ACD (internal) should be more than 3.0 mm for anterior chamber PIOLs and more than 2.8 mm for posterior chamber PIOLs, and the ACA should be more than 30° for both types.
- *Pupil diameter*: The mean pupil diameter during the measurements under the illumination circumstances (photopic, mesopic, or scotopic according to the amount of illumination). Mesopic pupil diameter is important for decision making in LVC (selection of optical zone).
- *Intraocular pressure (IOP)*: When measuring IOP by Goldmann Applanation Tonometer, the IOP should be corrected with reference to central corneal thickness based on the selected correction table. There are several correction tables that can be selected from the settings.
- *Lens thickness*: The thickness of the crystalline lens based on the anterior corneal apex. This value is displayed only if the pupil was dilated wide enough to detect the posterior crystalline lens surface.

Corneal Power Maps

INTRODUCTION

There are several maps measuring corneal power differing from one another by considering or not considering four factors.

FACTORS AFFECTING CORNEAL POWER MEASUREMENT

Factor 1: The Refractive Effect

Refraction of a spherical surface suffers from spherical aberration (SA) due to the difference in incidence angles of light rays between the central and peripheral zones of the spherical surface. The shape of corneal surfaces is conoidal, which is a composition of toricity, asphericity, and asymmetry. Mathematically, asphericity can be described by eccentricity, corneal shape value (E), p-value, and Q-value. Q-value is the standard value used in this regard. The normal range of Q-value is (+0.40, −0.80), and the average range in normal population is −0.10 to −0.30 with an average of −0.27. If Q = 0, the shape is spheric (Fig. 5.1). If Q > 0, the shape is oblate (Fig. 5.2). If Q is between 0 and −1.0, the shape is prolate (Fig. 5.3). If Q < −1.0 (e.g. −1.2), the shape is hyperprolate (Fig. 5.4). The value at which no SA is found is −0.53 (Fig. 5.5). Any corneal asphericity deviating from Q = −0.53 means SA in the wavefront measurements. The SA is positive, when Q is more than −0.53 (more positive), and negative, when Q is less than −0.53. Q-value and SA are discussed in detail in Chapter 9.

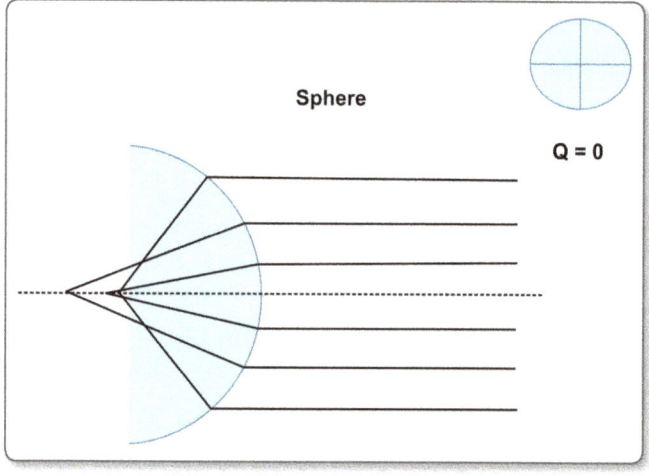

Fig. 5.1: Spherical corneal shape.

Factor 2: Inclusion of the Anterior and Posterior Corneal Surfaces

The keratometer measures the refractive power of the anterior corneal surface and represents it as the refractive power of the cornea. This is not accurate because both surfaces contribute to the total corneal power. Moreover, in nonoperated corneas, the average ratio of posterior/anterior radii is 82.2%, indicating a steeper posterior corneal surface. This is equal to anterior/posterior radii = 1.21. It is called the Gullstrand ratio. This ratio will no longer be accurate after keratorefractive procedures. This is why, the autorefractometer will give wrong readings after corneal

Chapter 5: Corneal Power Maps

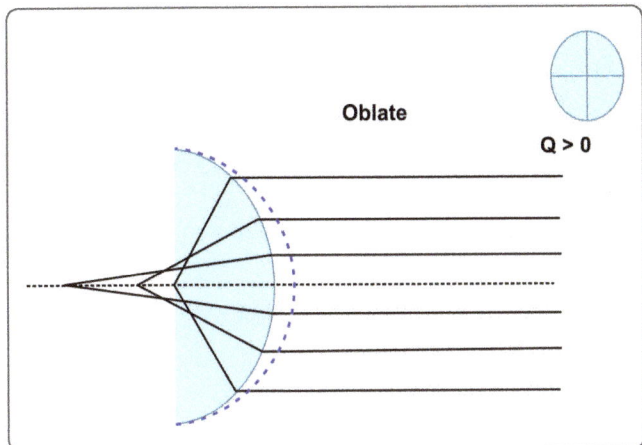

Fig. 5.2: Oblate corneal shape.

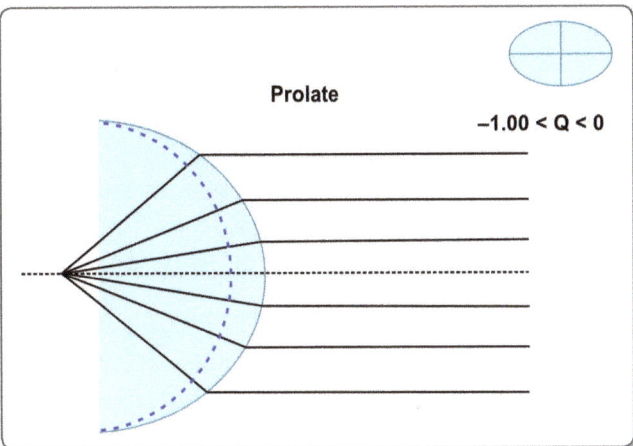

Fig. 5.3: Prolate corneal shape.

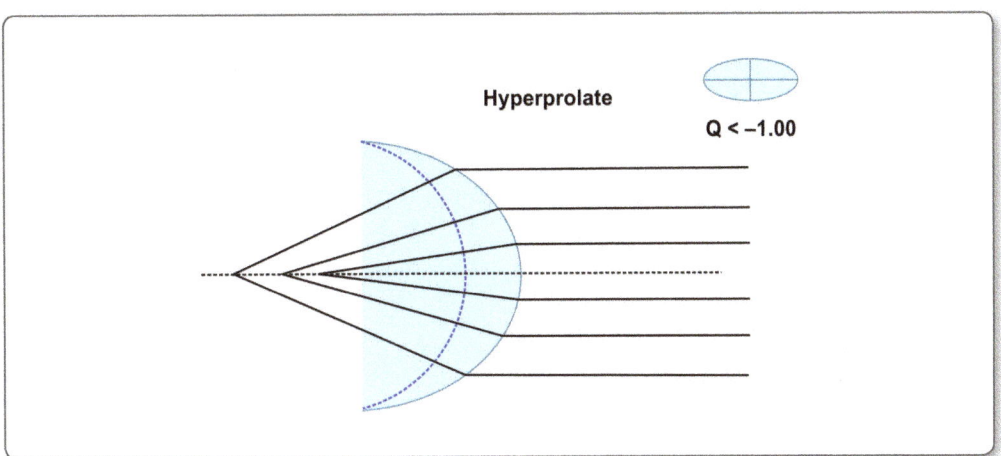

Fig. 5.4: Hyperprolate corneal shape.

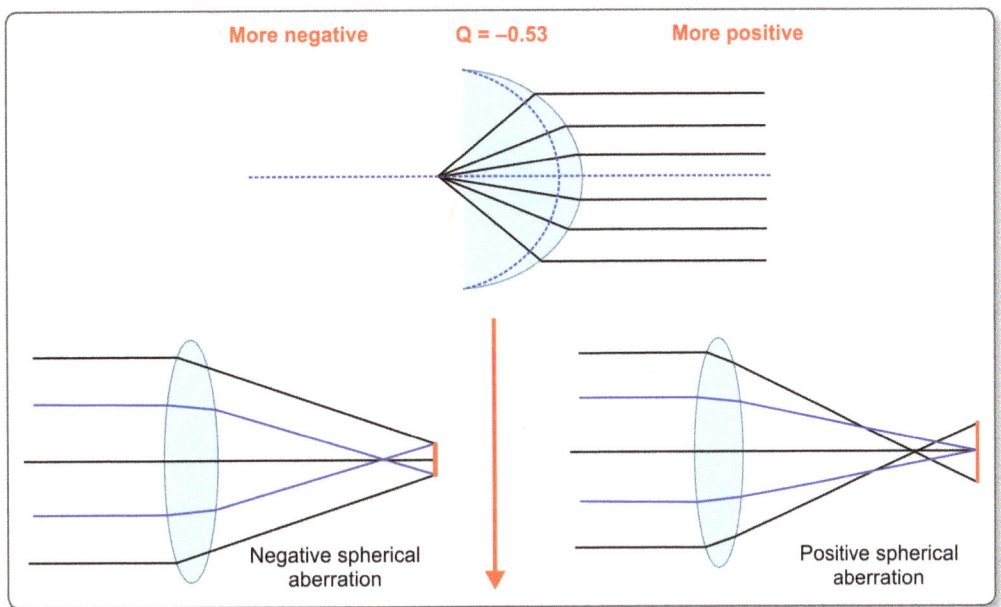

Fig. 5.5: Q-value and spherical aberration. When Q = –0.53, SA = 0.

surgeries because this device is calibrated based on the Gullstrand ratio.

Factor 3: The Refractive Index

Most topographers and keratometers use a refractive index (RI) of 1.3375 for calculating corneal power. This index is known as the keratometric calibration index. The true RI of corneal tissue is 1.376. However, most intraocular lens (IOL) power calculation formulas use n = 1.3375 to calculate the desired "K-reading", and perform an empirical correction to obtain the correct IOL power in normal eyes. Moreover, after keratorefractive procedures, the measured K-readings are no longer reliable due to changes in the posterior/anterior ratio (see Factor 2). In such cases, the measured K-readings must first be converted into equivalent K-readings before they can be put into formulas that are based on the RI of 1.3375.

Factor 4: Location of the Principal Planes

Since the cornea has two difference surfaces separated by corneal thickness, the cornea has two different optical principle planes. In other words, corneal thickness contributes to corneal power.

MAPS MEASURING CORNEAL POWER (TABLE 5.1)

The Anterior Sagittal (Axial) Curvature Map (Fig. 5.6)

This map measures the power of the anterior corneal surface using the sagittal principle, the keratometric RI (1.3375), and

Table 5.1: Principle of measurements of corneal power maps.

Map	Refractive effect	Both surfaces	True refractive index = 1.376	Corneal thickness
Sagittal	–	–	–	–
Tangential	–	–	–	–
Refractive power	Yes	–	–	–
True net power	–	Yes	Yes	–
Equivalent K power	Yes	Yes	Yes	–
Total corneal refractive power	Yes	Yes	Yes	Yes

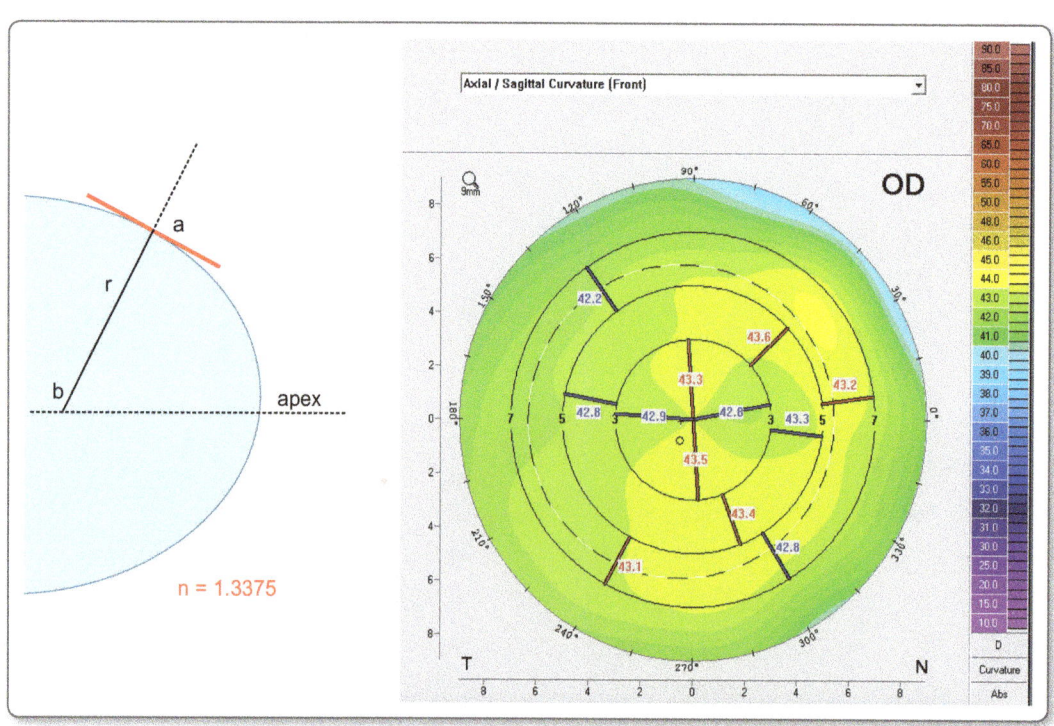

Fig. 5.6: The anterior sagittal (axial) curvature principle and map.

the laws of Gaussian optics by the following keratometric formula:

$$P = (n_2 - n_1)/r$$

where "P" is the power of refraction at the given point measured in diopters, "n_1" is the RI of the medium of incidence, "n_2" is the RI of the medium of refraction, and "r" is the radius of curvature at the given point measured in meters. When applying this law on the cornea, K is used instead of P to express K-readings. Therefore, this map does not take into consideration any of the four factors. However, most of the classic formulas used in IOL calculation are based on the K-readings obtained by this map.

The Anterior Tangential (Local or Instantaneous) Curvature Map (Fig. 5.7)

This map is similar to the sagittal map, but uses the tangential principle in calculating the radius of curvature. This map is more detailed than the sagittal map and less affected by misalignment. When measured by this map, the K-readings are higher than when measured by the sagittal map; therefore, they cannot be used in IOL calculation formulas.

The Refractive Power Map (Fig. 5.8)

This map measures the power of refraction of the anterior surface depending on the keratometric RI (1.3375) and using the Snell's law (ray tracing):

$$Sin_a/Sin_b = n_1 - n_2$$

where "a" is the angle of incidence, "b" is the angle of refraction, "n_1" is the RI of the medium of incidence, and "n_2" is the RI of the medium of refraction.

Therefore, this map takes into consideration only factor 1 and cannot be used in IOL calculation formulas because it depends on Snell's law rather than the keratometric formula. However, this map can give an idea about the SA of the anterior corneal surface when compared with the anterior sagittal map as shown in Figures 5.9A and B.

The True Net Power Map (Fig. 5.10)

This map depends on the sagittal formula and the true RI of the cornea (1.376). It measures corneal power in total by measuring the power of the anterior and posterior corneal surfaces without taking into consideration corneal thickness. Therefore, it considers factors 2 and 3. The formula of the true net power (TNP) is:

$$TNP = (n_2 - n_1)/r_a + (n_3 - n_2)/r_p$$

where $n_1 = 1$ for air, $n_2 = 1.376$ for corneal tissue, $n_3 = 1.336$ for aqueous humor, and "r_a" and "r_p" are the radii of curvature of the anterior and posterior surfaces, respectively, at the given points.

This map cannot be used in IOL calculation formulas because it depends on the true index of corneal tissue rather than the keratometric index.

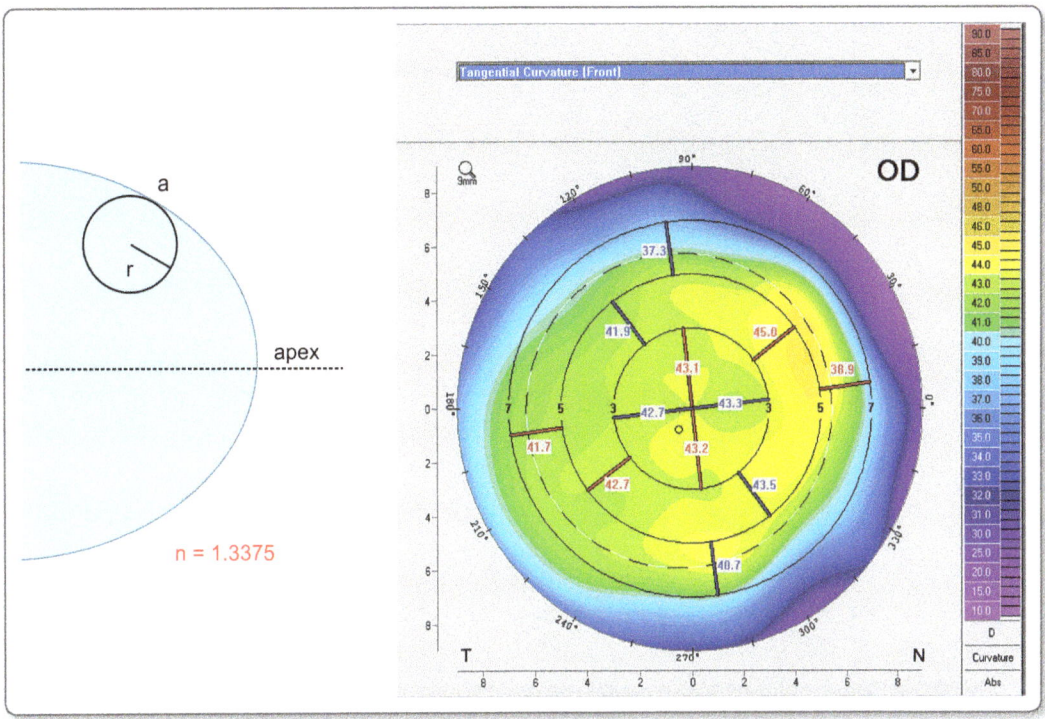

Fig. 5.7: The anterior tangential (instantaneous or local) principle and map.

Section 2: *Corneal Maps and Profiles*

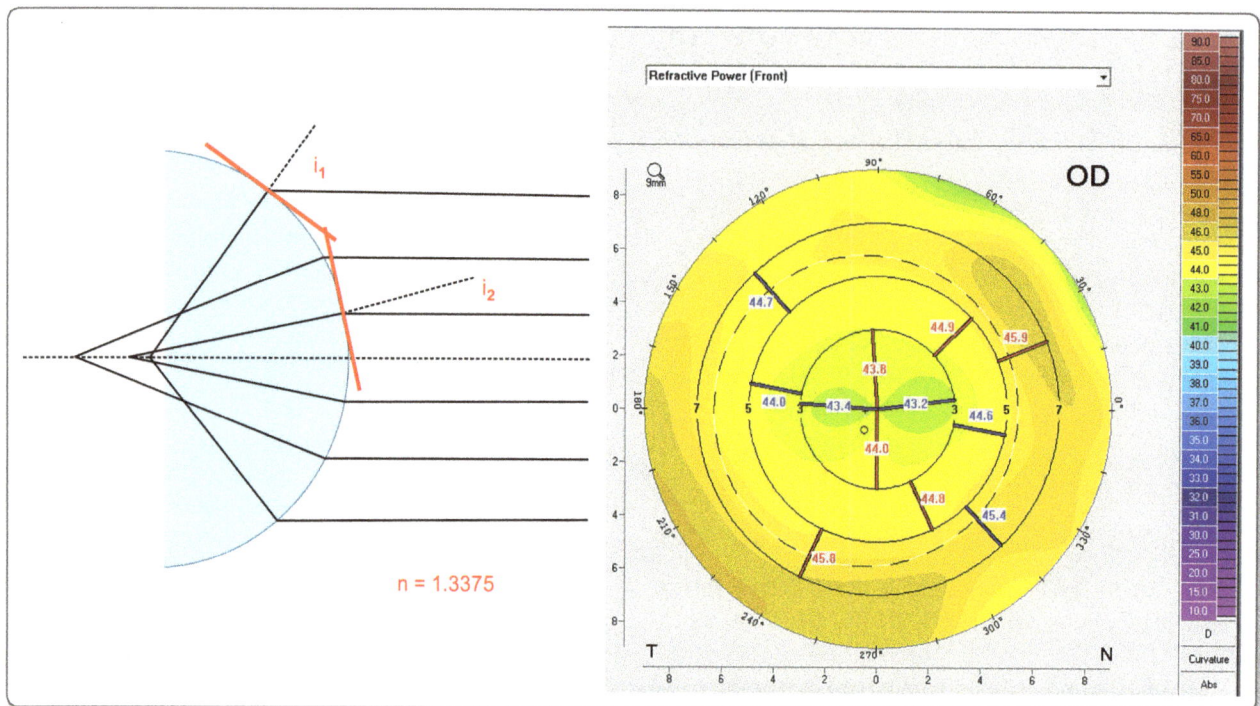

Fig. 5.8: The anterior refractive power principle and map.

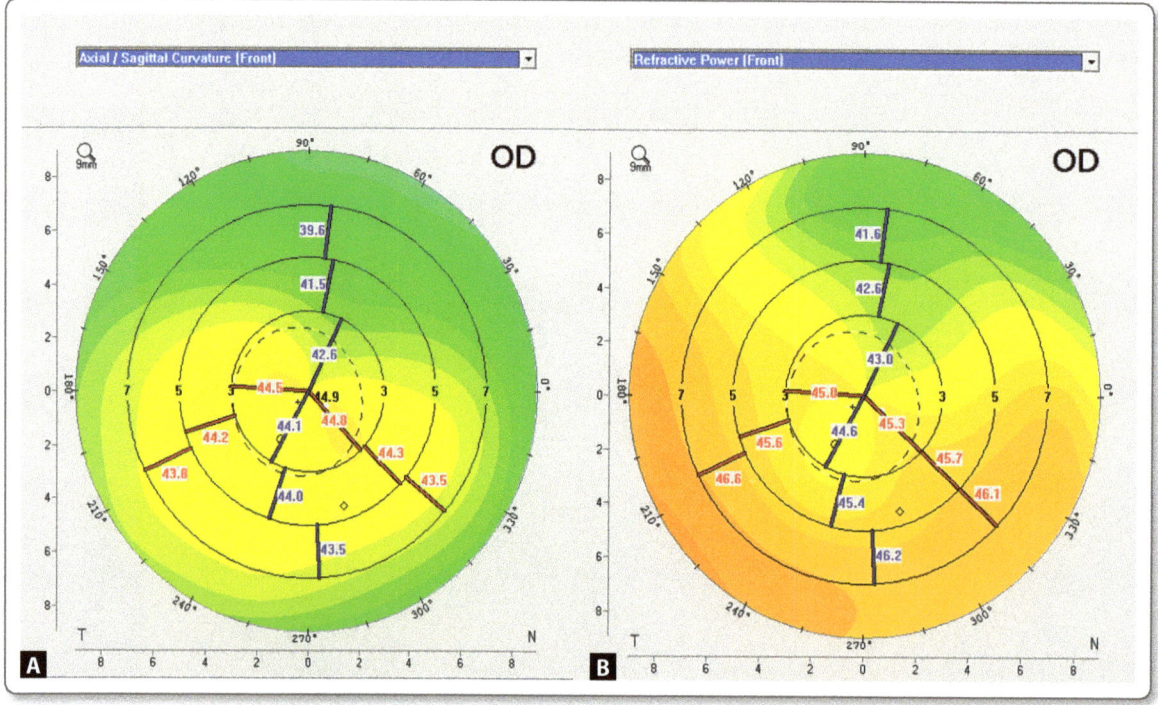

Figs. 5.9A and B: Comparison between the anterior sagittal map and the anterior refractive power map for the same cornea. The latter gives an idea about spherical aberration resulting from the anterior corneal surface.

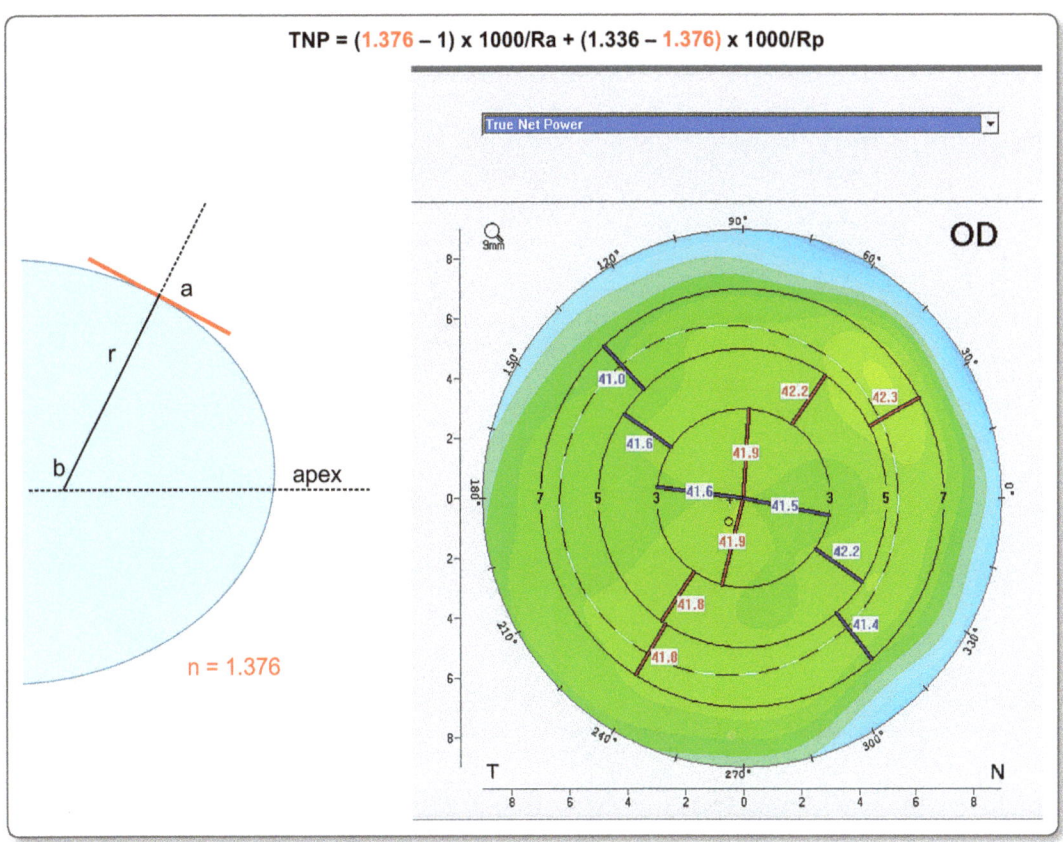

Fig. 5.10: The true net power principle and map.

The Equivalent K-reading Power Map (Fig. 5.11)

As mentioned earlier, Gullstrand ratio in normal population is 82.2%. Keratometers are calibrated based on this fact. Unfortunately, this ratio does not apply on operated corneas and irregular corneas. Keratometers generate wrong readings in such cases. This leads to misinterpretation and is a major factor of miscalculation of IOL for cataract surgery after keratorefractive surgeries.

The equivalent K-reading (EKR) was developed by Jack Holladay to recalculate K-readings as they should have been if the ratio was 82.2%. The EKR map depends on Snell's law and the true RI (1.376). It was designed to consider factors 1 to 3. In addition, its output (equivalent K-readings, or EKR) for untreated eyes are approximate to the corresponding simulated K-reading (Sim-K) values, which are usually derived from the sagittal power map. For these reasons, the output can be used in both the classic formulas in nonoperated eyes and in postkeratorefractive procedures. To validate the EKR method, a study was conducted using the Holladay 2 formula. The study showed that after laser in situ keratomileusis (LASIK), the best correlation with the classic method, with a mean prediction error of -0.06 D $\pm$ 0.56 D, was obtained using a mean zonal EKR for the 4.5-mm zone. For post-RK patients, the mean prediction error was -0.04 D $\pm$ 0.94 D.

The Total Corneal Refractive Power Map (Fig. 5.12)

This map is based on ray tracing principle to calculate the power. It is dependent on the true refractive indices of air, corneal tissue and aqueous humor, the slope of the cornea, and the exact point of refraction, which in turn depends on corneal principle planes and corneal thickness. Therefore, it takes into consideration the four factors.

Although this map represents the truest possible representation of the power of the cornea, its output values cannot be used in the classic IOL formulas, which are based on the keratometric RI (1.3375). However, corneal astigmatism based on this method corresponds better, both in variability and accuracy, with manifest astigmatism than the corneal astigmatism based on anterior corneal power

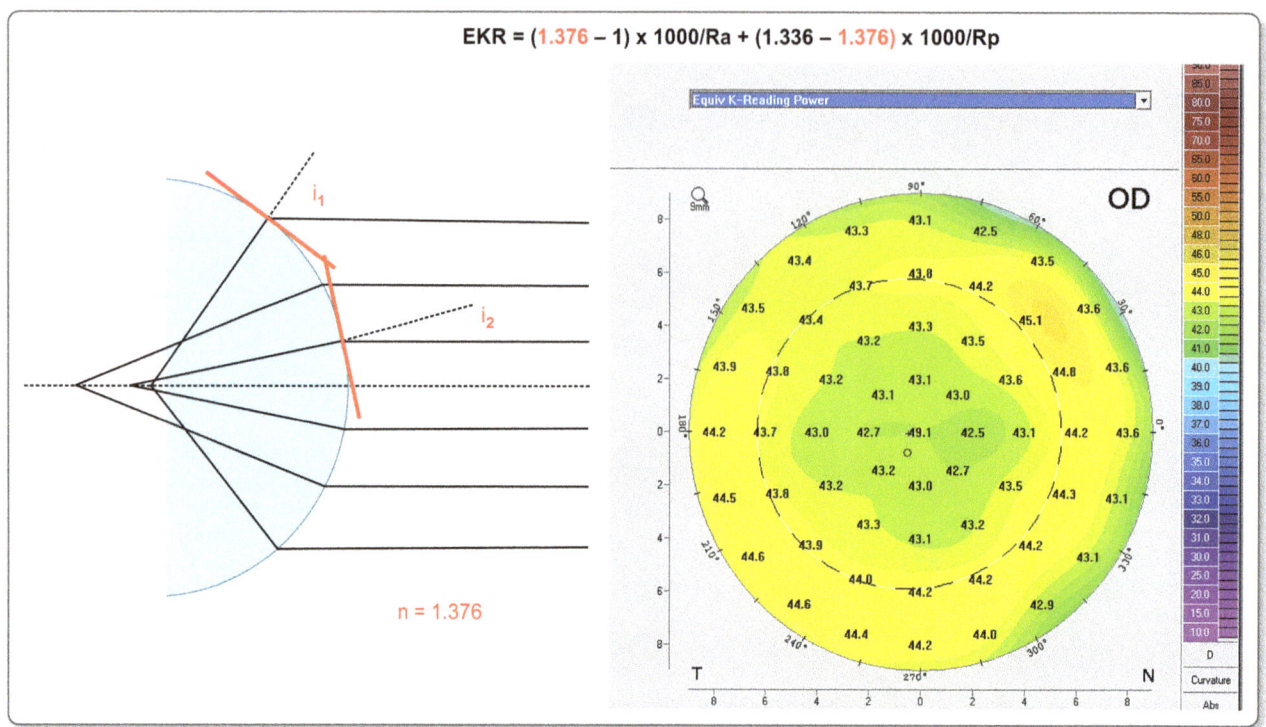

Fig. 5.11: The equivalent K-reading principle and map.

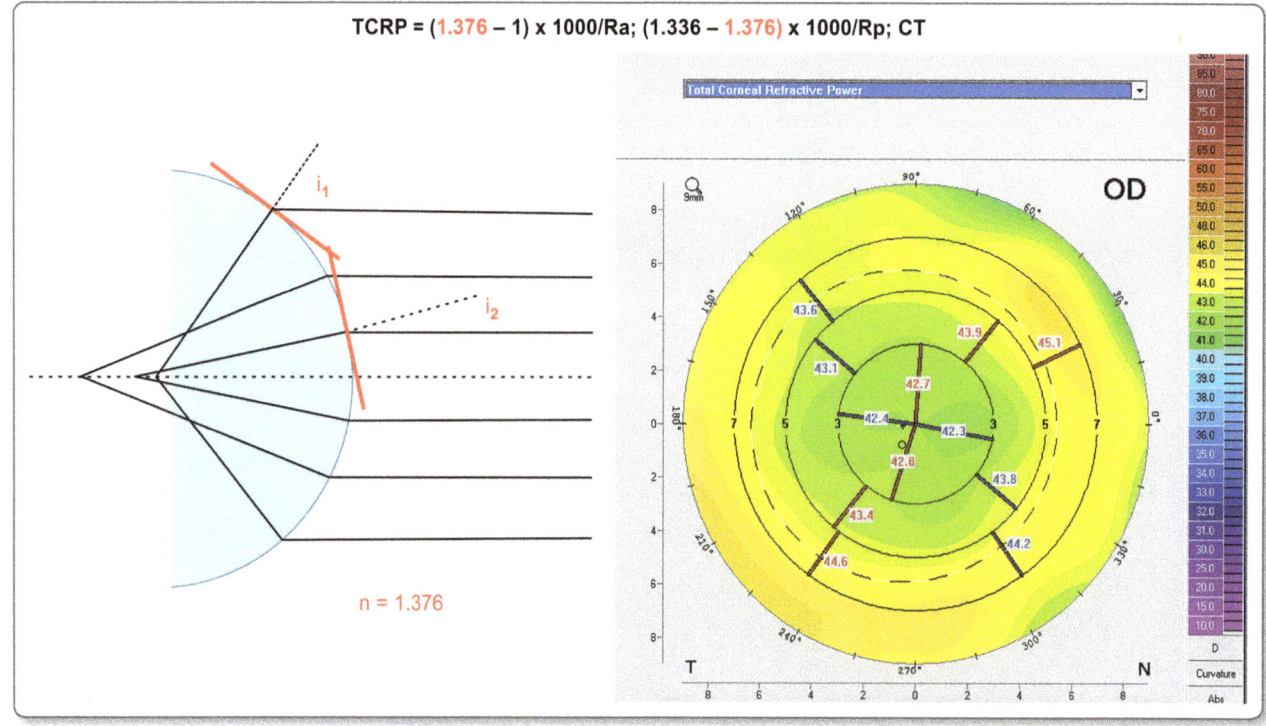

Fig. 5.12: Total corneal refractive principle and map.

measurements (Sim-K astigmatism). This total corneal astigmatism would be fundamental when planning for toric IOL or limbal relaxing incisions or other corneal astigmatic surgery.

In general, the total corneal refractive power (TCRP) can be applied in regular corneas, while the EKR can be applied in irregular corneas.

PATTERNS OF CORNEAL CURVATURE

In spite of the limitations of the anterior sagittal and tangential curvature maps, they are used to describe the patterns of power on the anterior corneal surface, where the sagittal map is used to describe normal and abnormal patterns while the tangential map is specifically used to describe corneal irregularities.

The Reference Axis

As mentioned before, the sagittal method depends on an axis used as a reference in measuring the curvature radii. There are three main axes in this regard (Fig. 5.13): (1) the visual axis, (2) the optical axis, and (3) the VK normal (Chapter 1).

All topographic systems adopt the VK normal, considering that the three axes are identical, which is not true. This misconception leads to invalidity of curvature maps due to misalignment during taking the capture. This leads, of course, to wrong diagnosis and wrong decision of treatment. Misalignment is discussed in detail in Chapter 16.

Patterns of Corneal Curvature Map

To study the patterns properly on the anterior sagittal curvature map, steep and flat segments should be displayed for the following important reasons:
- The overall distribution of the segments gives an idea about the severity of irregularity; the minimal the

segmentation, the more regular the cornea. This is important when indicating toric IOL implantation, in which high segmentation is a contraindication. Figures 5.14 and 5.15 are examples of insignificant and significant segmentation, respectively.
- In case of high segmentation, the captures should be repeated to avoid any false findings.

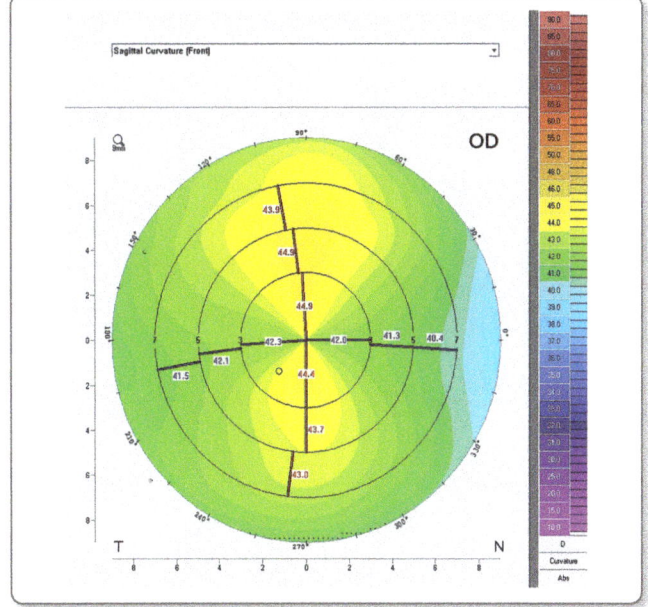

Fig. 5.14: Insignificant segmentation of the steep (red) and flat (blue) semi-meridians.

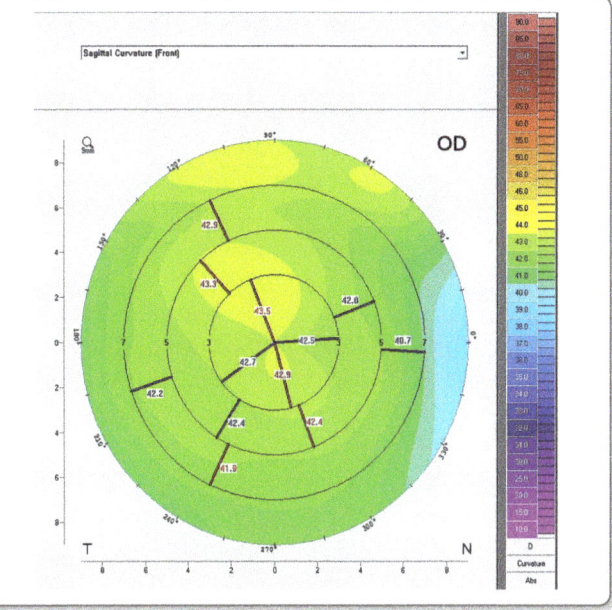

Fig. 5.15: Significant segmentation of the steep (red) and flat (blue) semi-meridians.

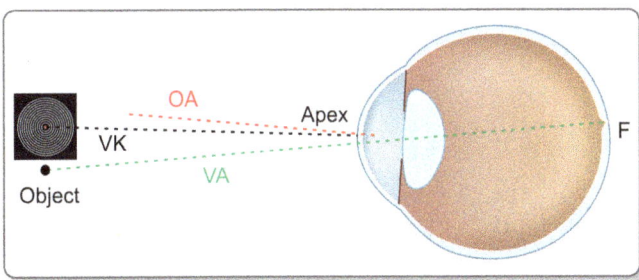

Fig. 5.13: Reference axes in curvature maps. (OA: optical axis; VA: visual axis; VK: video keratoscope)

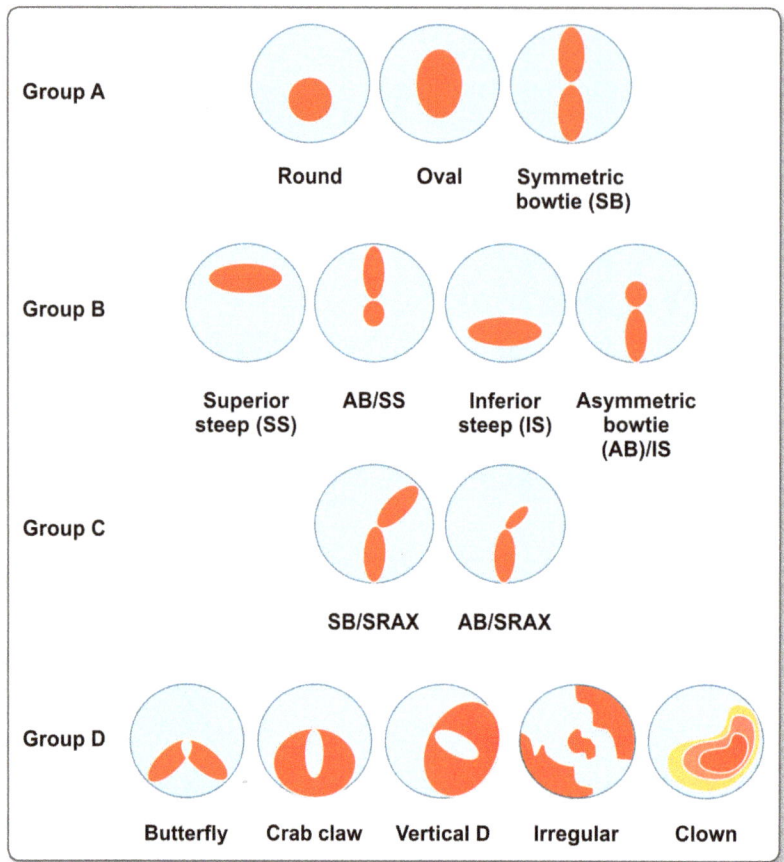

Fig. 5.16: Patterns of the anterior sagittal curvature map.

- The distribution of segments specifies some patterns such as skewed radial axis (SRAX) and the vortex patterns (see below).

Patterns on the anterior sagittal map are classified into four groups (Fig. 5.16):

1. *Group A (symmetric patterns)*: It consists of round, oval, and symmetric bowtie (SB) patterns. They are found in 23%, 21%, and 18% of normal population, respectively. Contrary to the SB pattern, round and oval patterns are encountered in corneas with insignificant astigmatism in the anterior surface (<1 D), but all of them represent a regular anterior surface. Although this group has symmetric patterns, they are not always normal. Group A is considered as *abnormal* when Km is >47.2 D in Placido-based devices, or Km >48 D in Scheimpflug-based devices.

   The SB is oriented vertically (Fig. 5.17), horizontally (Fig. 5.18), or obliquely (Fig. 5.19) in with-the-rule (WTR), against-the-rule (ATR), or oblique astigmatism, respectively. In this regard, it is important to define WTR, ATR, and obliques astigmatism.

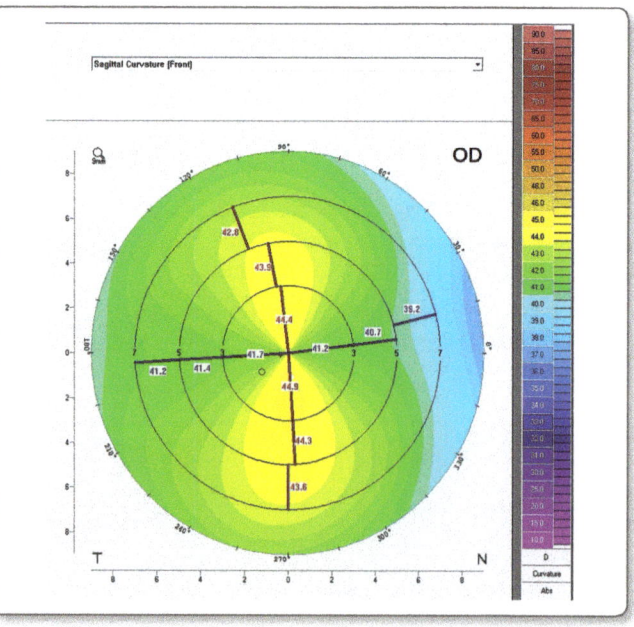

Fig. 5.17: Vertical symmetric bowtie indicating with-the-rule astigmatism.

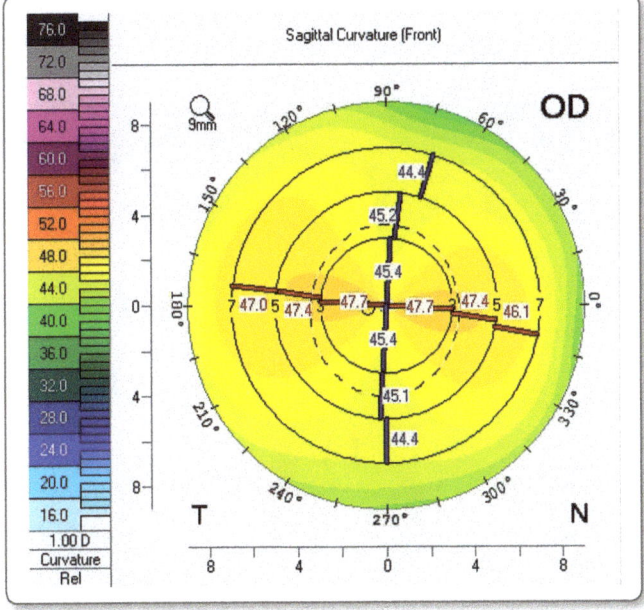

Fig. 5.18: Horizontal symmetric bowtie indicating against-the-rule astigmatism.

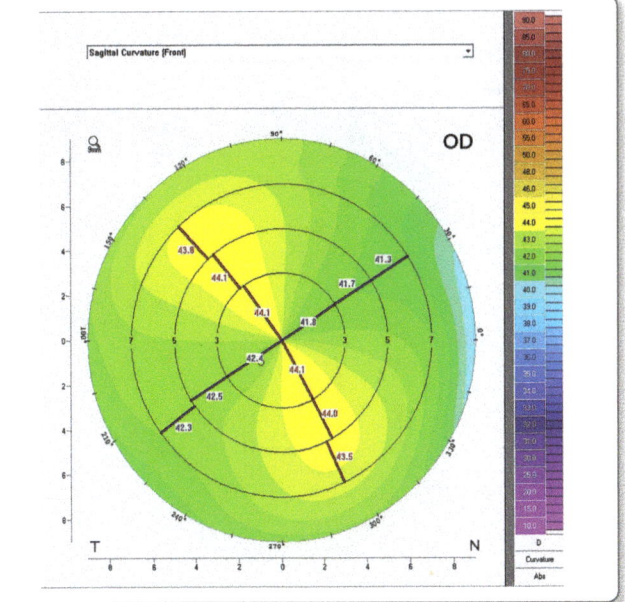

Fig. 5.19: Oblique symmetric bowtie indicating oblique astigmatism.

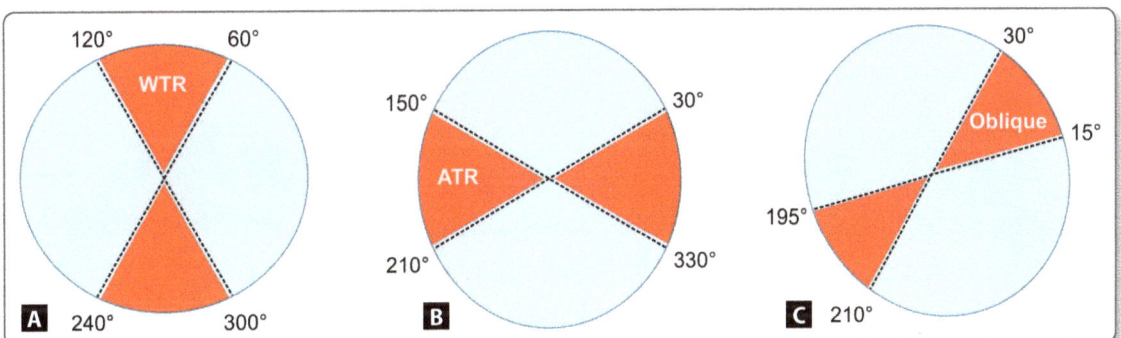

Figs. 5.20A to C: Sectors defining the orientation of corneal astigmatism. (A) With-the-rule; (B) Against-the-rule; and (C) Oblique.

- *With-the-rule astigmatism*: When the meridian of maximum power of refraction is within 90° ± 30° (Fig. 5.20A). In this type, the vertical image formed by this meridian is frontal to the other horizontal one.
- *Against-the-rule astigmatism*: When the meridian of maximum power of refraction is within 180° ± 30° (Fig. 5.20B). In this type, the horizontal image formed by this meridian is frontal to the other vertical one.
- *Oblique astigmatism*: When the two principle meridians are neither vertical nor horizontal (Fig. 5.20C).

2. *Group B (asymmetric patterns)*: It consists of asymmetric bowtie inferior steep (AB/IS) (Fig. 5.21), asymmetric bowtie superior steep (AB/SS) (Fig. 5.22), inferior steep (IS) (Fig. 5.23), and superior steep (SS) (Fig. 5.24) patterns. The AB/SS and the AB/IS are found in 12% and 20% of normal population, respectively. Although this group has asymmetric patterns, they are not always abnormal. Group B is considered as *abnormal* in case of abnormal Km and/or abnormal vertical asymmetry. The vertical asymmetry is defined as the difference between the average inferior (I) and the average superior (S) values at 1.5 mm distance from corneal apex and 30° apart (Fig. 5.25A). The vertical asymmetry is abnormal when I-S is >1.4 D in case of I > S, and when S-I is >2.5 D in case of S > I. Since most of the devices do not show the difference in this way, and to simplify the method of

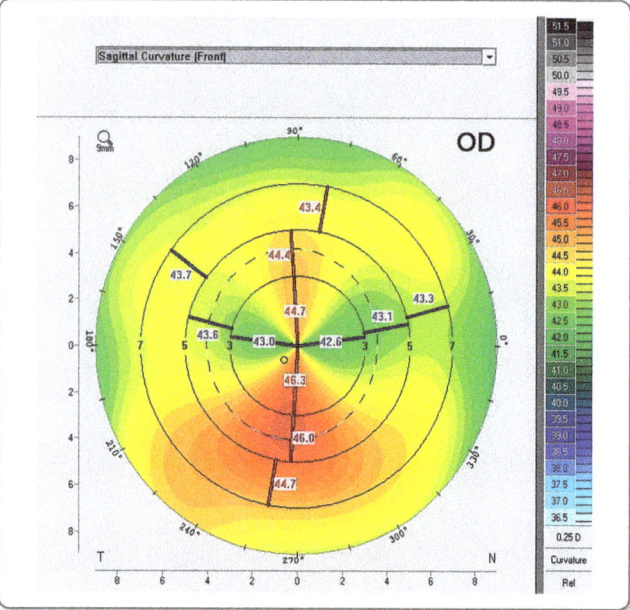

Fig. 5.21: Asymmetric bowtie inferior steep.

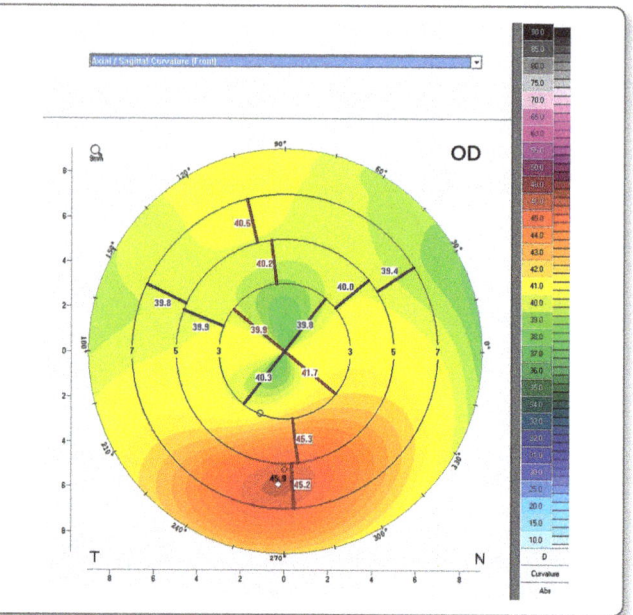

Fig. 5.23: Inferior steep.

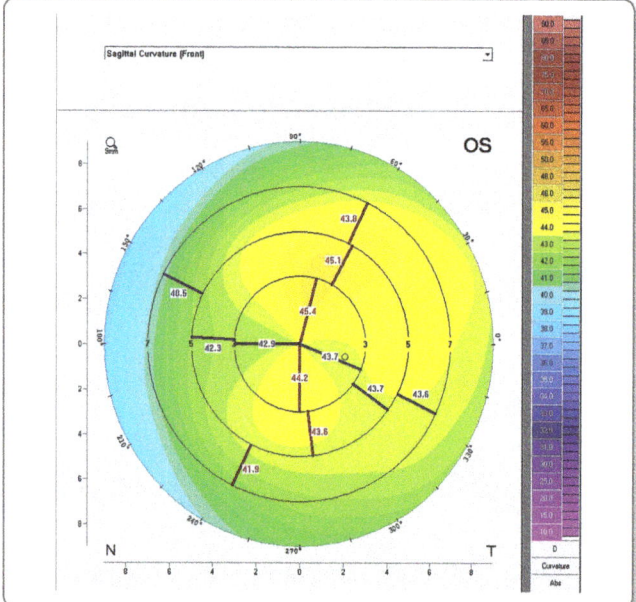

Fig. 5.22: Asymmetric bowtie superior steep.

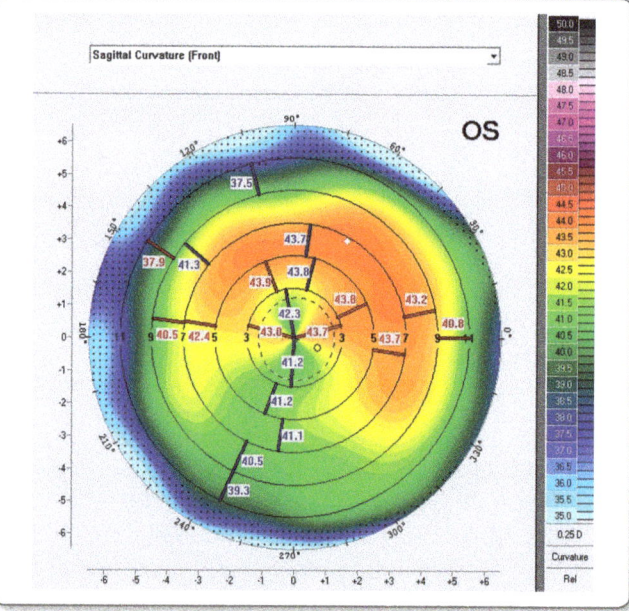

Fig. 5.24: Superior steep.

reading, the difference between the inferior and the superior values on the steep meridian on the second circle of numbers can be considered (Fig. 5.25B).

3. *Group C (angulated patterns)*: It consists of two patterns: (1) symmetric bowtie with skewed radial axis (SB/SRAX) index (Fig. 5.26) and (2) asymmetric bowtie with skewed radial axis (AB/SRAX) index (Fig. 5.27).

Group C is considered as *abnormal* when the angle between the axes of the superior and inferior segments in the innermost circle (3 mm) is more than 21° and the Sim-K astigmatism is significant (≥1 D). In case of insignificant astigmatism, any SRAX can be ignored (Fig. 5.28).

Chapter 5: Corneal Power Maps

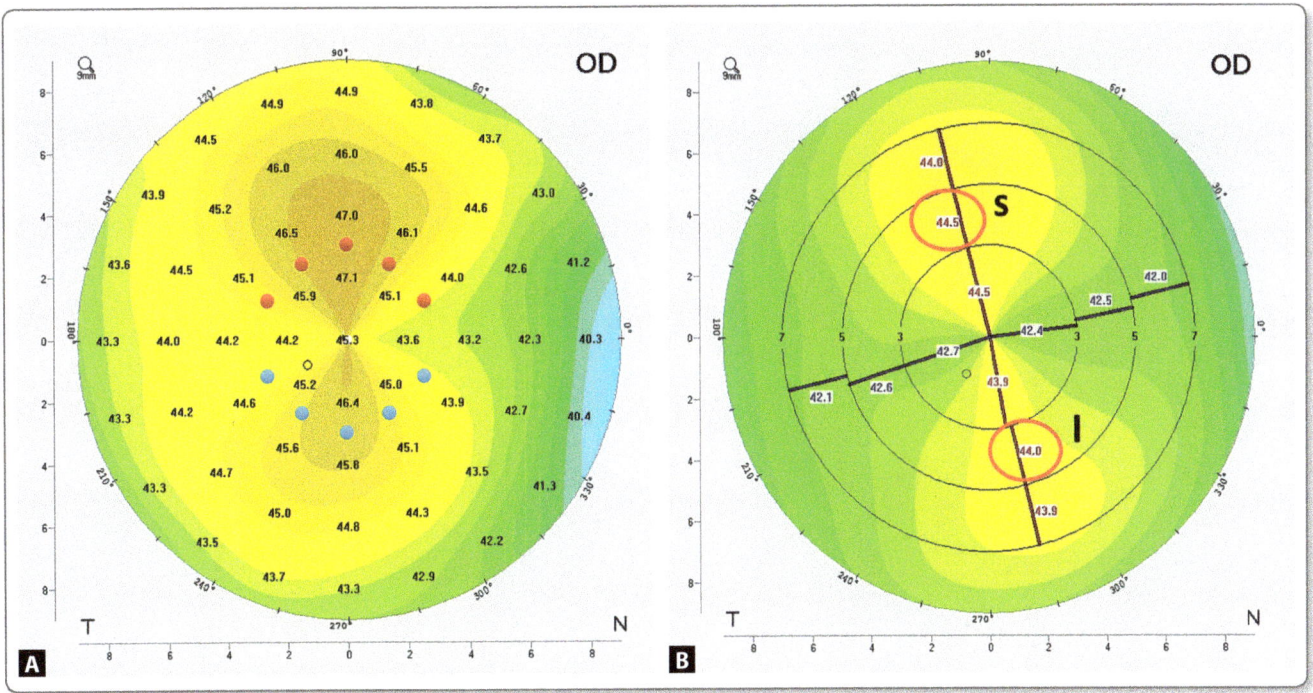

Figs. 5.25A and B: Principle of calculating superior inferior difference. (A) Rabinowitz method; and (B) Simple rough method.

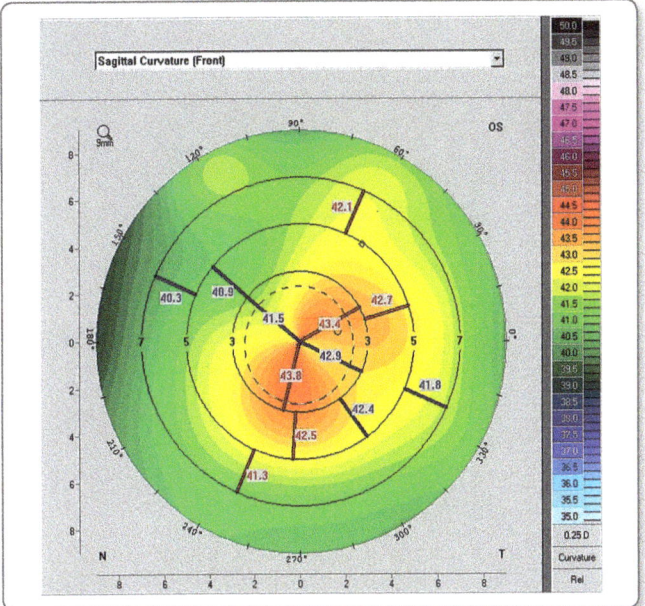

Fig. 5.26: Symmetric bowtie with skewed radial axis index.

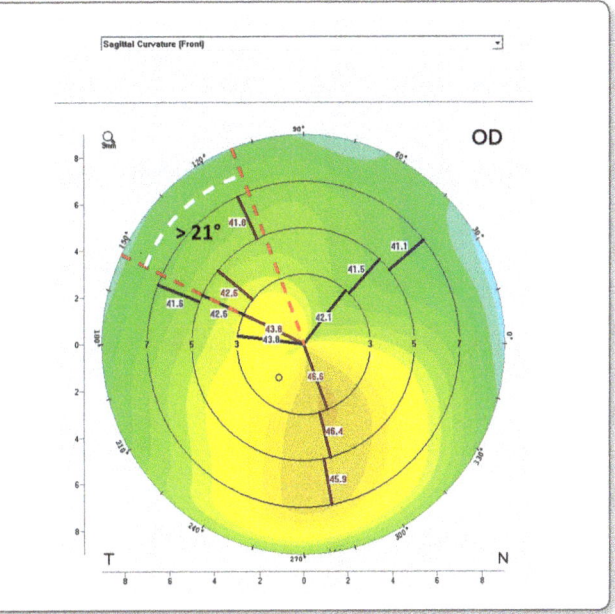

Fig. 5.27: Asymmetric bowtie with skewed radial axis index.

4. *Group D (special shapes)*: It consists of crab-claw (Fig. 5.29), butterfly (Fig. 5.30), vertical D (Fig. 5.31), clown face (Fig. 5.32), vortex (Fig. 5.33), and nonspecific irregular patterns. The nonspecific irregular pattern is found in 7% of the normal population. The other five patterns in this group are always abnormal.

CLINICAL DIFFERENCES BETWEEN SAGITTAL AND TANGENTIAL CURVATURE MAPS

- The tangential map is more susceptible to local curvature changes, because it depends on circles. Therefore, it is

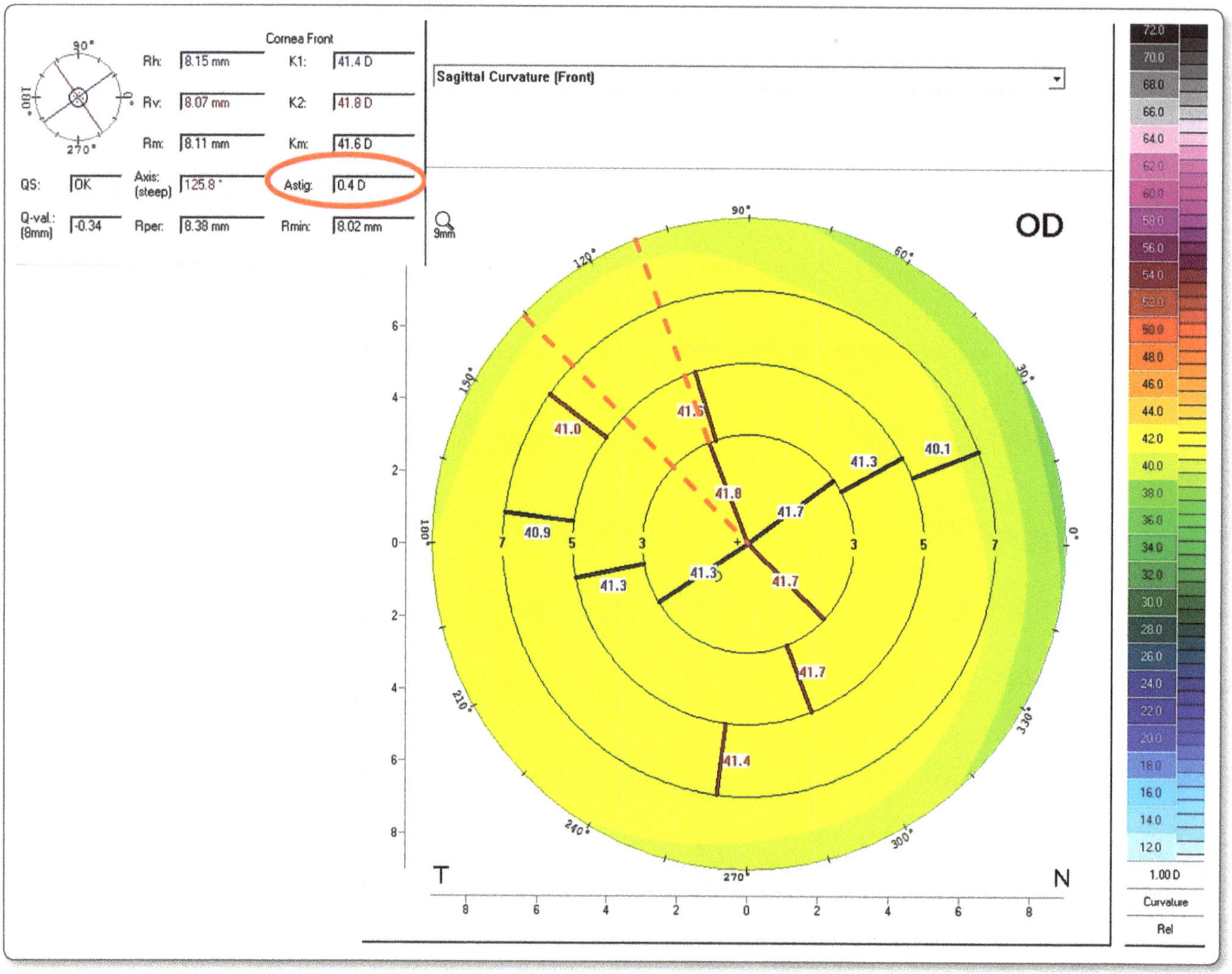

Section 2: *Corneal Maps and Profiles*

Fig. 5.28: Insignificant skewed radial axis index.

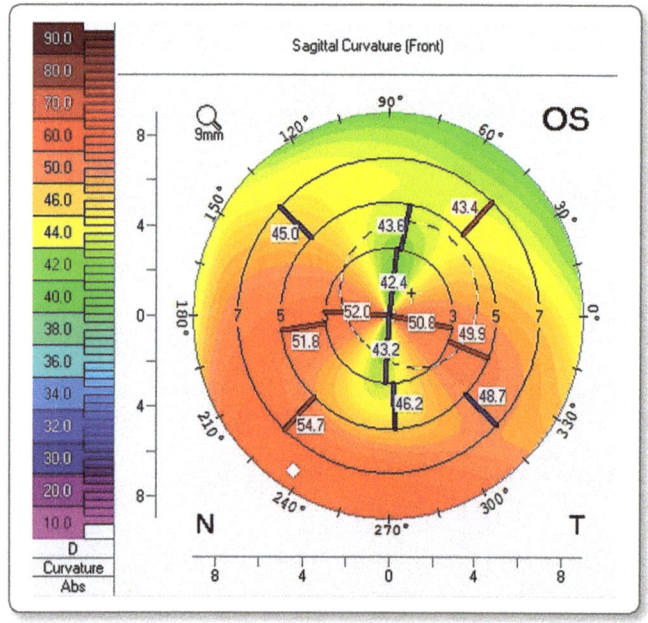

Fig. 5.29: Crab claw.

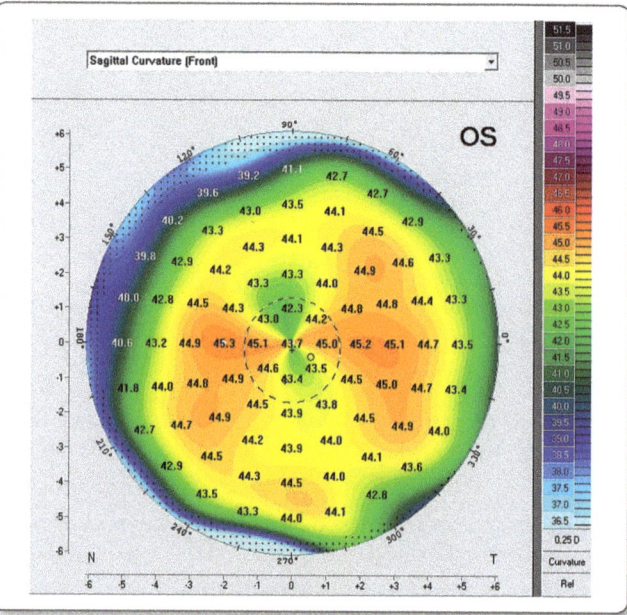

Fig. 5.30: Butterfly.

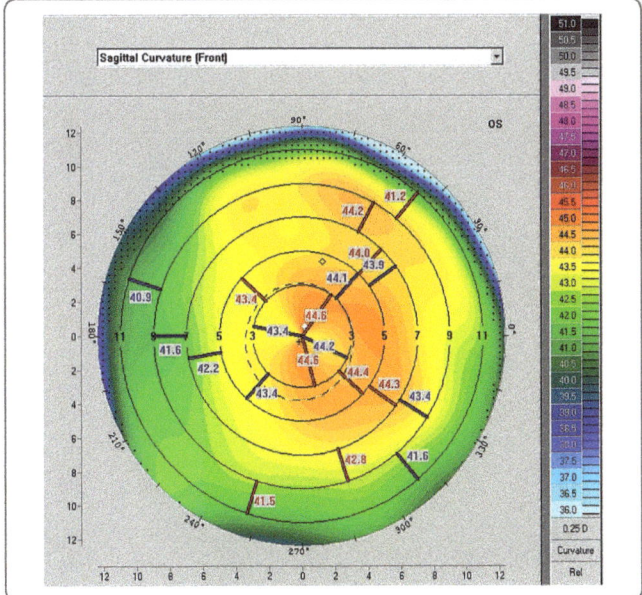

Fig. 5.31: Vertical D.

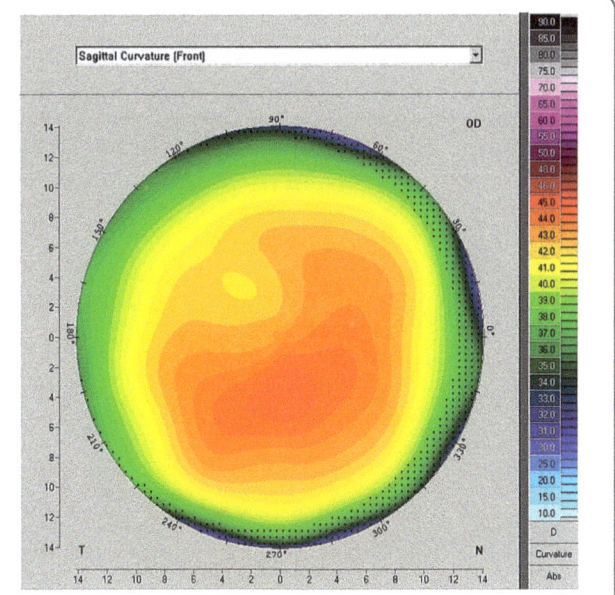

Fig. 5.32: Clown face.

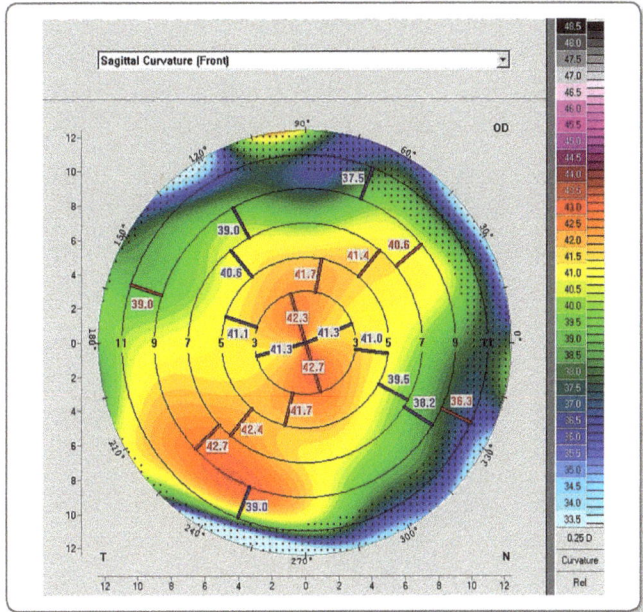

Fig. 5.33: Vortex pattern.

more capable of revealing corneal irregularities. This is clear when comparing Figure 5.34A with Figure 5.34B; they are two maps of the same cornea.

- The tangential map is better in describing the contour of zones. Therefore, it is better used in describing postsurgical corneas (Chapter 22).
- Each point on the tangential map is calculated independently, i.e. there is no reference axis. Therefore,

it is, to some extent, less affected by misalignment during acquisitions.
- Despite all these advantages of the tangential map, the sagittal map is widely adopted.
- K-readings when measured by the tangential map are higher than when measured by the sagittal map for the same corneal surface. Therefore, the tangential map readings cannot be used in IOL calculation formulas.

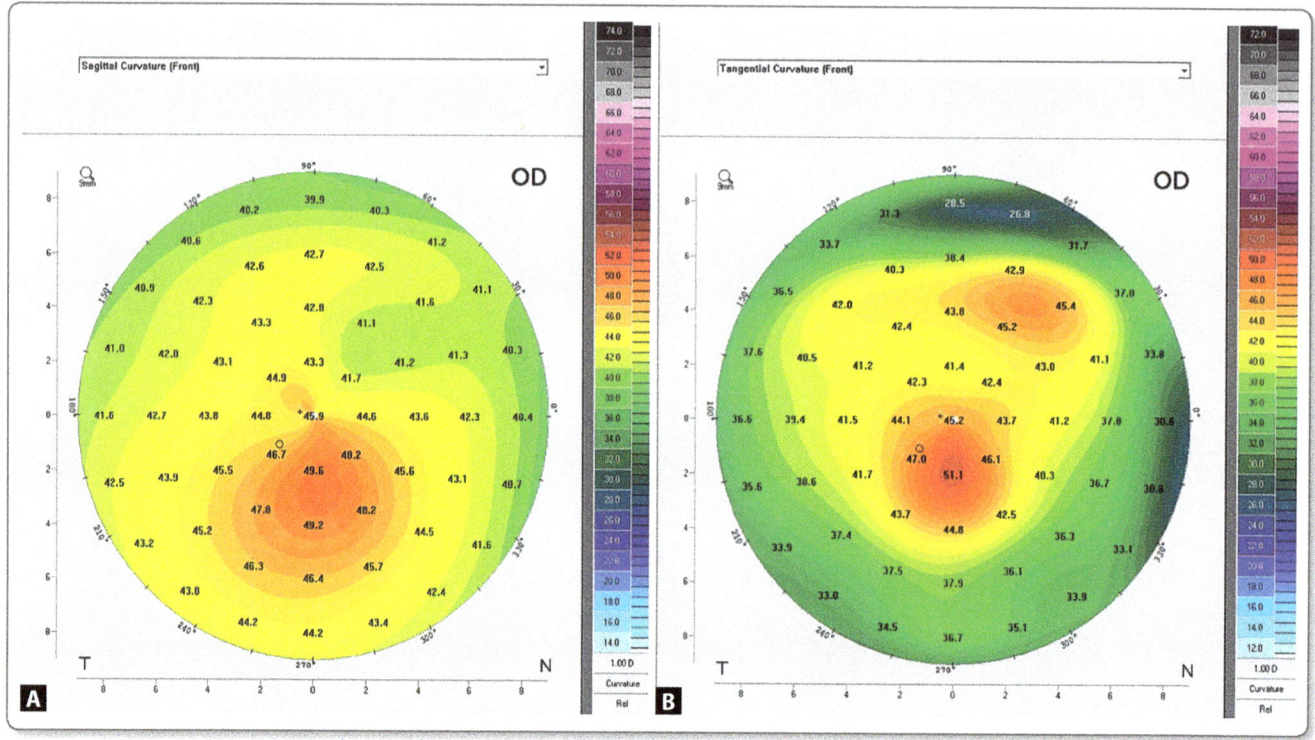

Figs. 5.34A and B: Comparison between the anterior sagittal map and the anterior tangential map for the same cornea.

Elevation Maps

PRINCIPLE OF THE ELEVATION MAPS

The surface of the cornea is mostly similar to the surface of the earth in terms of elevations and depressions. These elevations and depressions should be measured and expressed to have a realistic tomography of the cornea. The main difference between the earth and the cornea is that the former has a reference surface (RS), namely the sea level, to which all elevations (mountains) and depressions (valleys) are related. Because the cornea has no similar natural RS, it is imperative to create an artificial one based on the mean central radii of the examined surface.

THE REFERENCE SURFACE

Principle

The computer of the device builds an RS for each surface being captured (Fig. 6.1). The computer adjusts the RS with the measured surface and considers all points above the RS as elevations, being displayed in positive values and given hot colors, and considers all points below the RS as depressions, being displayed in negative values and given cold colors, all values are in microns. The coincidence points between the RS and the measured surface are displayed as zeros, i.e. exactly like the sea level (Fig. 6.2). In other words, all parts of corneal surface that are below the RS are given negative values and cold colors and vice versa. Therefore, the display will totally depend on the position of the RS in relation with the measured surface.

Position

There are two positions of the RS: (1) the float and (2) the nonfloat modes (Figs. 6.3A and B). In the float mode, the

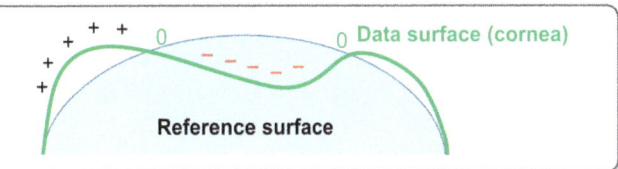

Fig. 6.1: Principle of the elevation map.

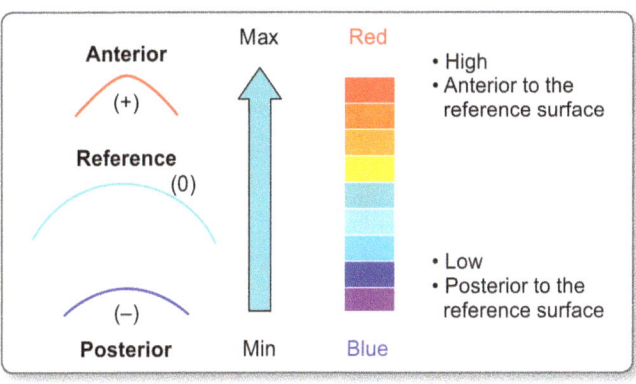

Fig. 6.2: Principle of measurement and color scale of the elevation map.

computer will adjust the position of the RS in relation with the corneal surface based on a principle stating that area a + area b = area c, meaning that the RS will be in a neutral position where all elevations are equal to all depressions. In the nonfloat mode, the RS will touch the apex of the cornea as shown in Figures 6.3A and B. The standard position of the RS is the float mode.

In case of corneal astigmatism, there are a steep and a flat meridian. Since the steep meridian is steeper than the RS, it slopes below it, and is displayed as depression and given cold colors. On the other hand, because the flat meridian is flatter than the RS, it slopes above it, and is displayed as

Section 2: *Corneal Maps and Profiles*

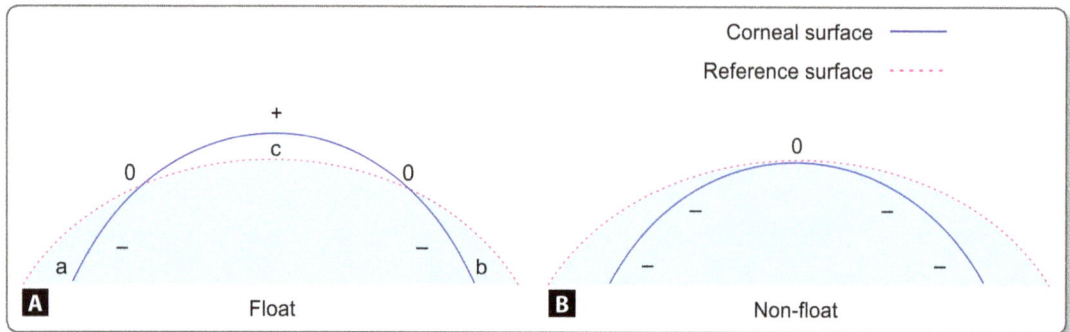

Figs. 6.3A and B: Positions of the reference surface. (A) Float mode; and (B) Nonfloat mode.

elevation and given hot colors (Fig. 6.4). This produces the shape of an "hourglass" regardless of the float or nonfloat modes (Fig. 6.5). The hourglass pattern reflects significant (≥1 D) corneal astigmatism on the measured surface. The hourglass is colored by blue because it corresponds to the steep meridian, which is below the RS as mentioned earlier. This explains the difference between steepness and elevation. Moreover, similar to the symmetric bowtie (SB), the hourglass is oriented vertically in with-the-rule (WTR) astigmatism (Figs. 6.6A and B), horizontally in against-the-rule (ATR) astigmatism (Figs. 6.7A and B), and obliquely in oblique astigmatism (Figs. 6.8A and B). In the last three figures, the steep meridian is plotted in hot colors on the curvature map (because it measures power) and in cold colors on the elevation map (because it measures height in relation with the position of the RF). Note that the hourglass shape is only displayed when using the best fit sphere (BFS) RS as will be discussed below in types.

Parameters

Each RS is specified by two parameters: (1) the radius (blue ellipse) and (2) the diameter (red ellipse) as shown in Figure 6.9. The radius of the RS is chosen by the computer based on the mean central radii of the examined corneal surface. The diameter is the diameter of the used zone of this specific RS. Figures 6.10A and B are an illustration of this concept. In this figure, a spherical RS is demonstrated. As shown in this figure, same corneal surface and same RS in A and B (RS radius = 7.81 mm), but the difference is in the diameter of the studied zone; 8 mm in A and 10 mm in B. As mentioned above, the computer in the float mode will adjust the position of the RS in relation with the corneal surface based on the principle a + b = c. Due to this principle, corneal surface takes a more prominent position in larger diameters and vice versa. Choosing a larger diameter causes false positives because of increased sensitivity and reduced specificity, while choosing smaller diameters causes false

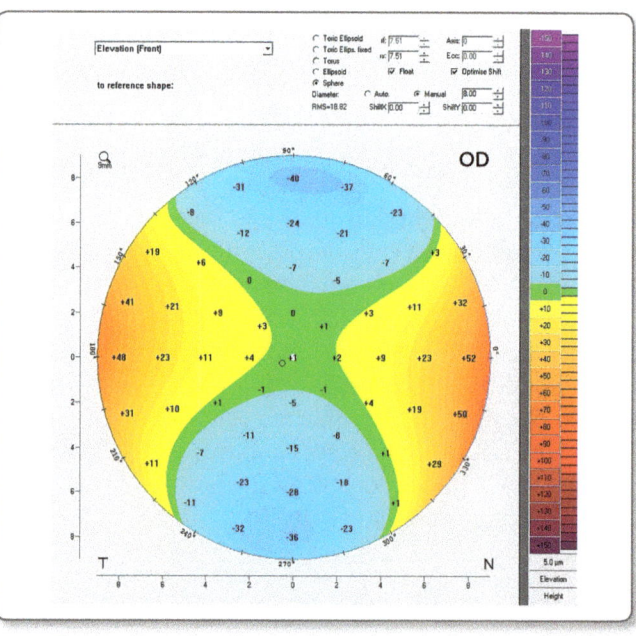

Fig. 6.4: Regular corneal astigmatism in relation with the reference surface.

Fig. 6.5: Hourglass shape indicating corneal astigmatism.

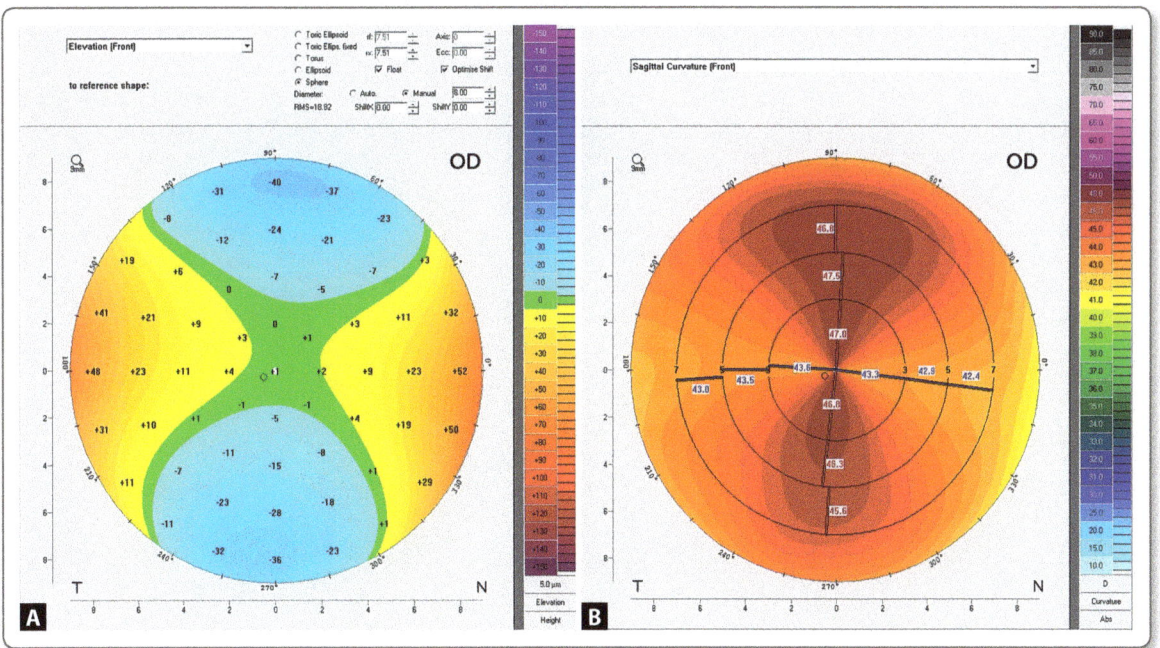

Figs. 6.6A and B: With-the-rule astigmatism on the elevation map (A) and the sagittal map (B).

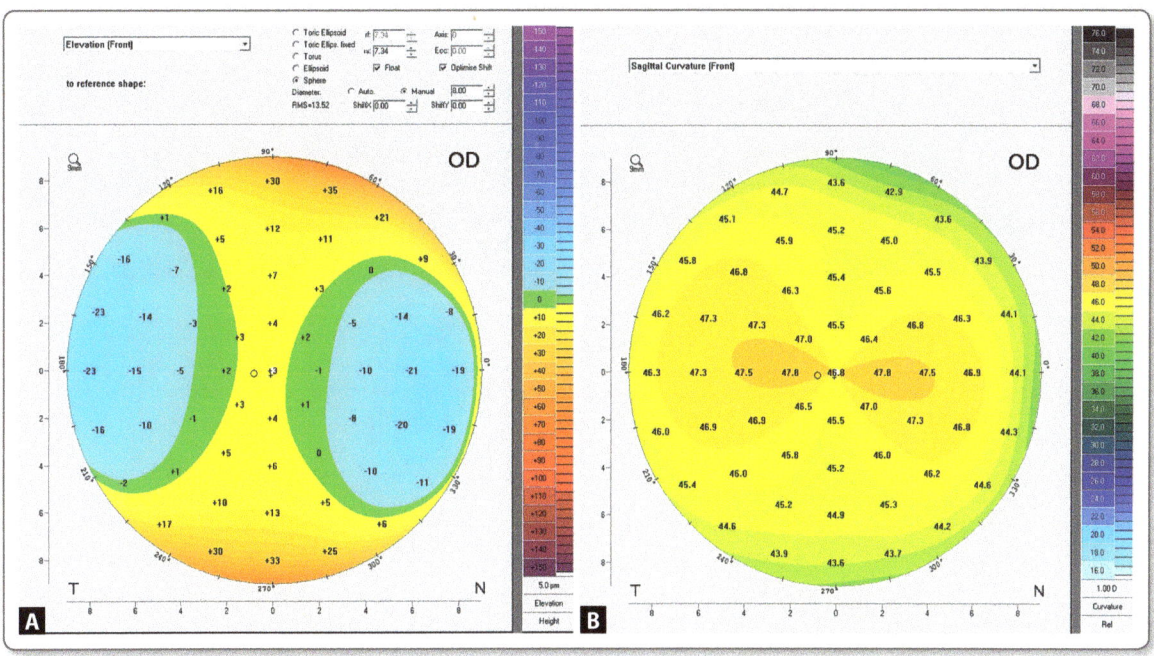

Figs. 6.7A and B: Against-the-rule astigmatism on the elevation map (A) and the sagittal map (B).

negatives (hides the cone) due to reduced sensitivity and increased specificity as shown in Figures 6.11A and B. In this figure, on the left (A), the diameter is 10 mm, and on the right (B), the diameter is 5 mm. Notice the difference in the presentation of the center of the same corneal surface. For these reasons, the recommended standard diameter is 8 mm.

Types

There are three main types or shapes of the RS, sphere, ellipsoid, and toric ellipsoid (Fig. 6.12):

1. *Best fit sphere*: This shape has only one radius (Fig. 6.13A). It is the standard type for highlighting corneal astigmatism, studying the shape of the cornea, and

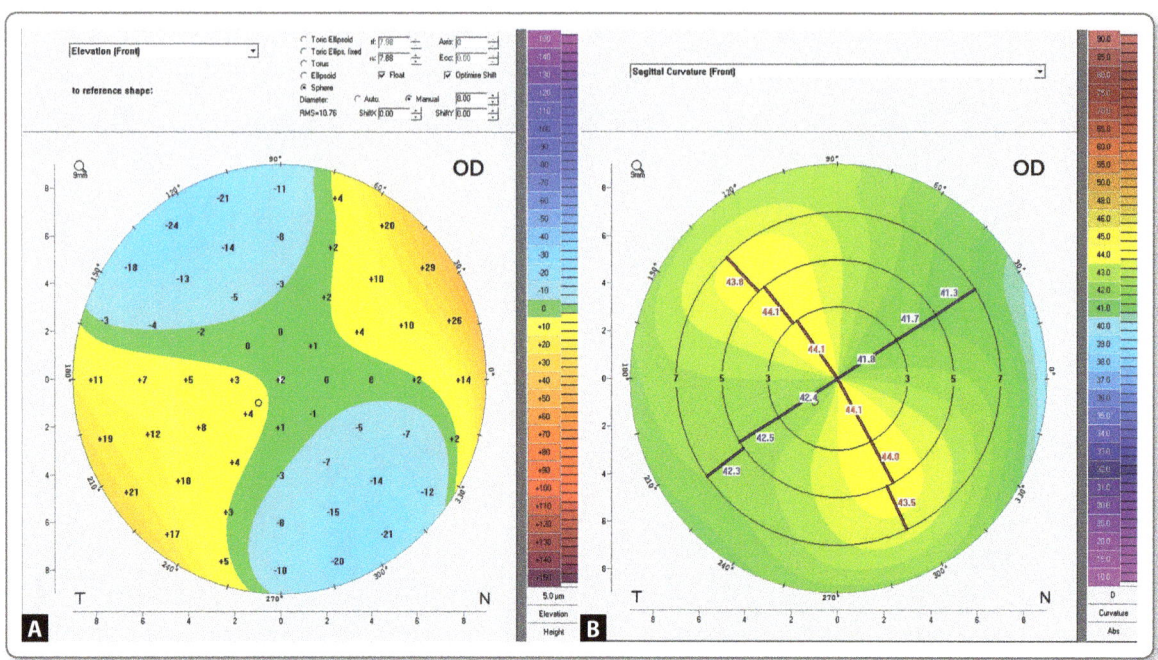

Figs. 6.8A and B: Oblique astigmatism on the elevation map (A) and the sagittal map (B).

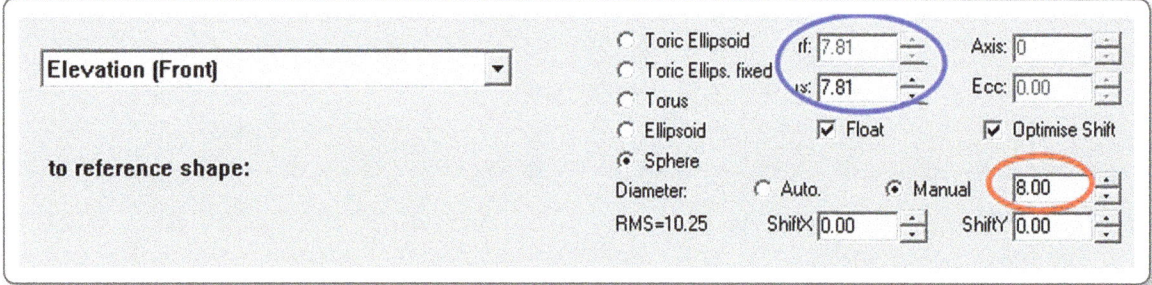

Fig. 6.9: Parameters of the reference surface: radius (blue ellipse) and zonal diameter (red ellipse).

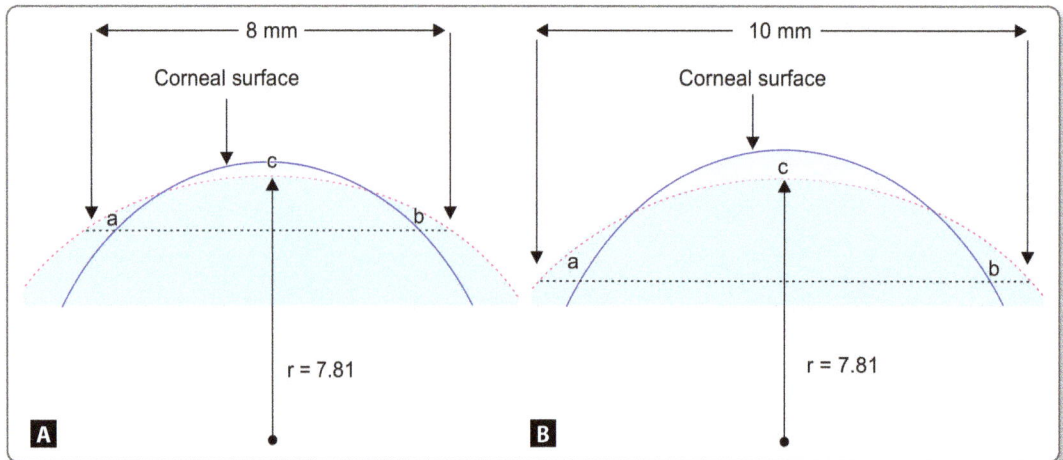

Figs. 6.10A and B: The principle of zonal diameter of the studied area.

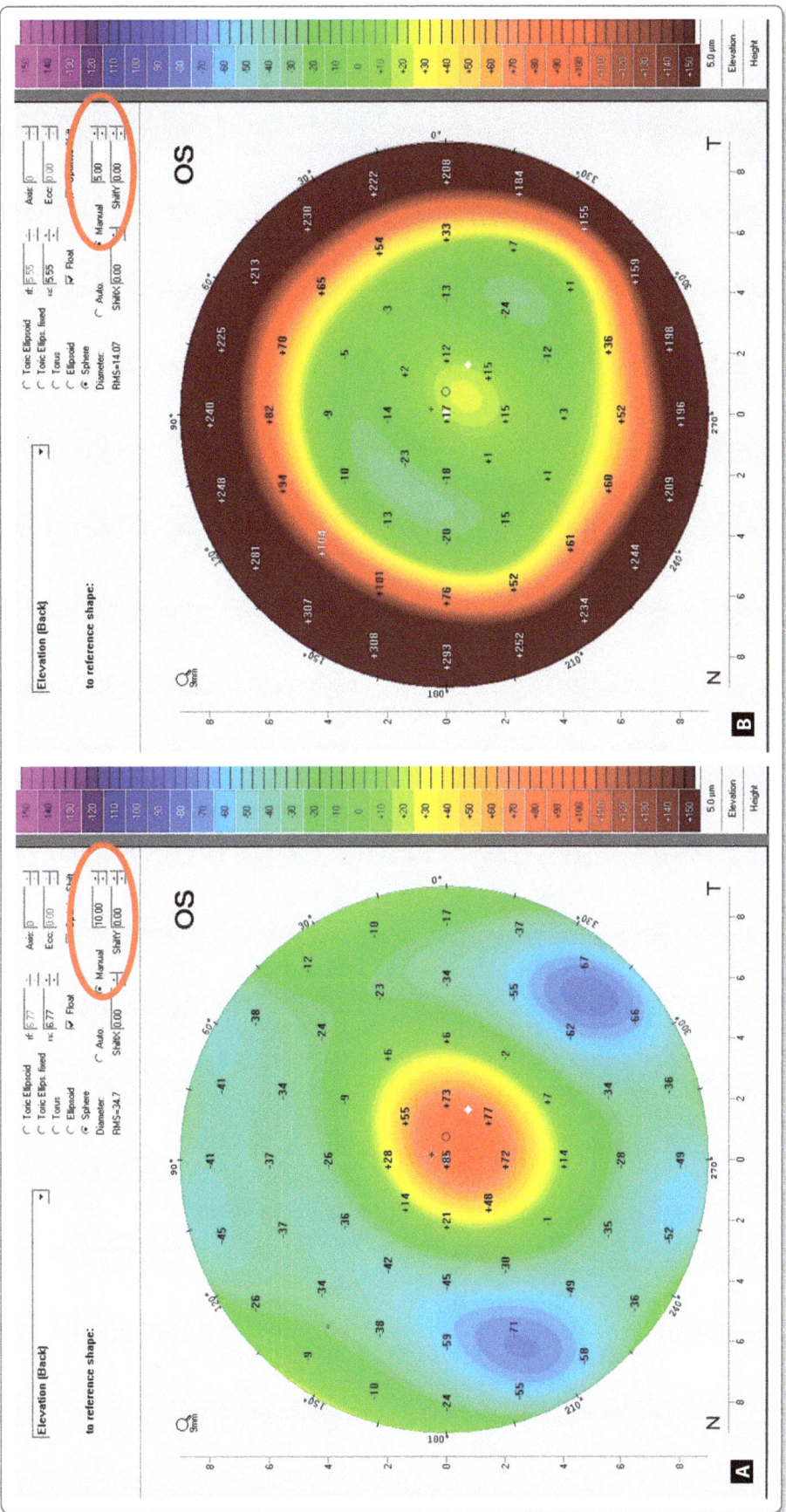

Figs. 6.11A and B: Effect of zonal diameter on the values and color display in the elevation map.

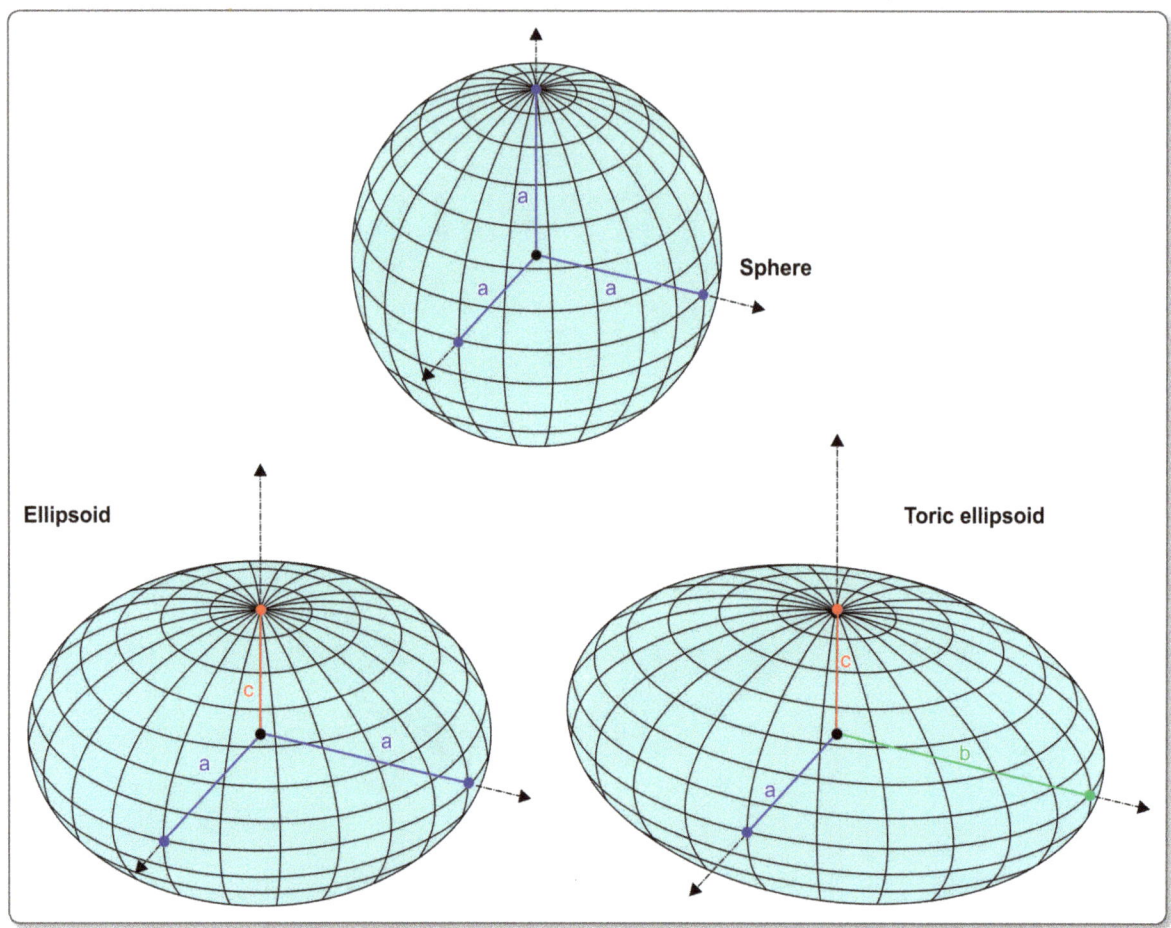

Fig. 6.12: Types of the reference surface.

evaluating the elevations. Since the shape of the cornea is conoid (aspherotoric), the BFS is able to describe and classify corneal patterns.

Based on the 8 mm BFS, Khachikian, Belin, and Ambrósio determined the cutoff values of elevations at the points corresponding to the thinnest location (Fig. 6.14). Tables 6.1 and 6.2 show the normative data for the Oculus Pentacam in myopic and hypermetropic populations, respectively, in one standard deviation (SD), two SD, and three SD matrix. The three SD parameters are used for quantification.

Moreover, the posterior elevation map with the BFS is the best map to localize and classify cone location (Figs. 6.15A to C). The cone is considered as central, paracentral, or peripheral when its apex is within the central 3 mm zone, between 3 mm and 5 mm central zones, and outside the 5 mm central zone, respectively.

2. *Best fit ellipsoid (BFE)*: This shape is rotationally symmetric according to two different axes, major and minor (see Figure 6.12). Therefore, it has two radii, but the steeper is fixed (Fig. 6.13B). This shape is usually not used.

3. *Best fit toric ellipsoid (BFTE)*: This shape is rotationally symmetric according to three different axes (see Figure 6.12). Therefore, it has three radii, but the steepest and the flattest ones are fixed (Fig. 6.13C). Because it is the closest RS to corneal shape, this RS fits well to a normal astigmatic cornea to display the remaining irregularities and the related higher-order aberrations (HOAs). This RS is used in Holladay report to detect early keratoconus (Chapter 23).

Elevation-based Patterns

Elevation-based patterns can best be studied by using the 8 mm BFS float mode. The patterns can be classified into two groups: (1) group A (symmetric patterns) and (2) group B (asymmetric patterns).

1. *Group A: Regular patterns (Figs. 6.16A and B)*: They are central island and symmetric hourglass. Contrary to the

Chapter 6: Elevation Maps

symmetric hourglass, a central island is found when the measured corneal surface has insignificant astigmatism (<1 D).

2. *Group B: Irregular patterns (Figs. 6.17A and B)*: They are tongue-like extension or skewed hourglass, and nonspecific irregular patterns. Tongue-like and skewed patterns can be encountered in cases with large angle kappa or misalignment.

Neither group A nor group B are considered as abnormal unless values are abnormal based on the cutoff values as mentioned earlier (see Tables 6.1 and 6.2).

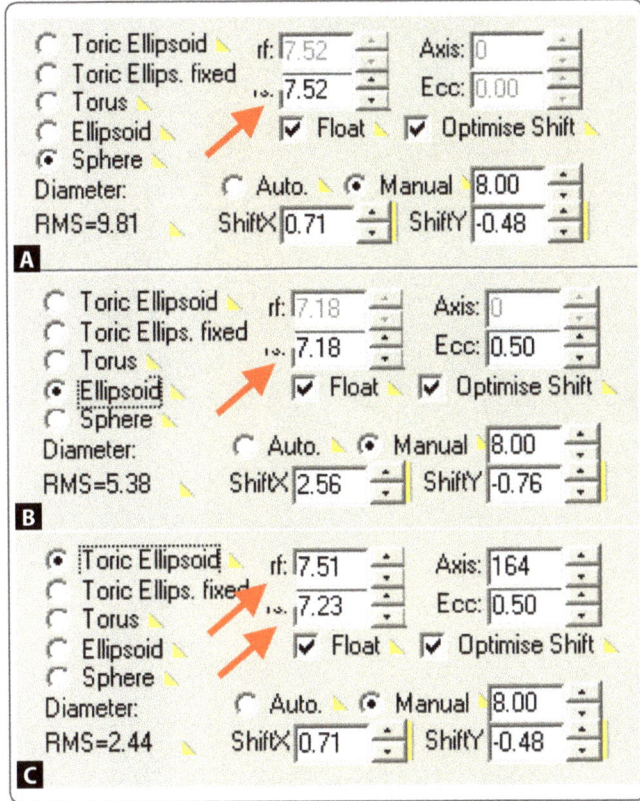

Figs. 6.13A to C: Radii adjusted by the computer for the (A) BFS; (B) BFE; and (C) BFTE. (BFE: best fit ellipsoid; BFS: best fit sphere; BFTE: best fit toric ellipsoid)

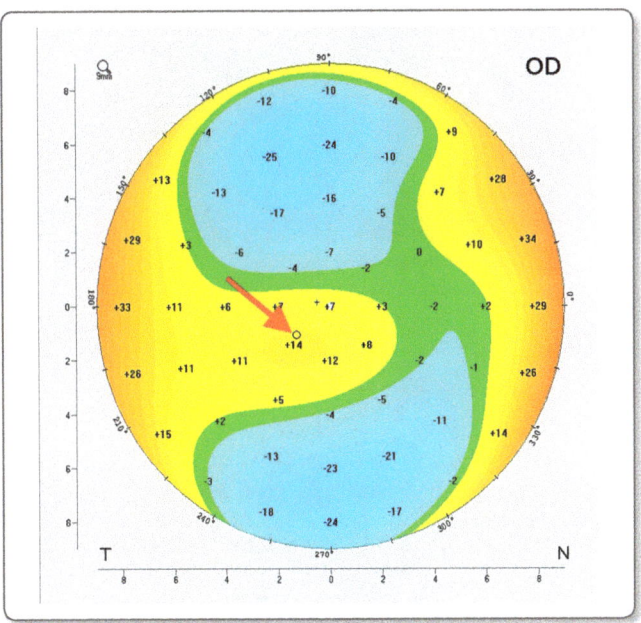

Fig. 6.14: When using the best fit sphere (BFS), the value that corresponds to the thinnest location is to be considered.

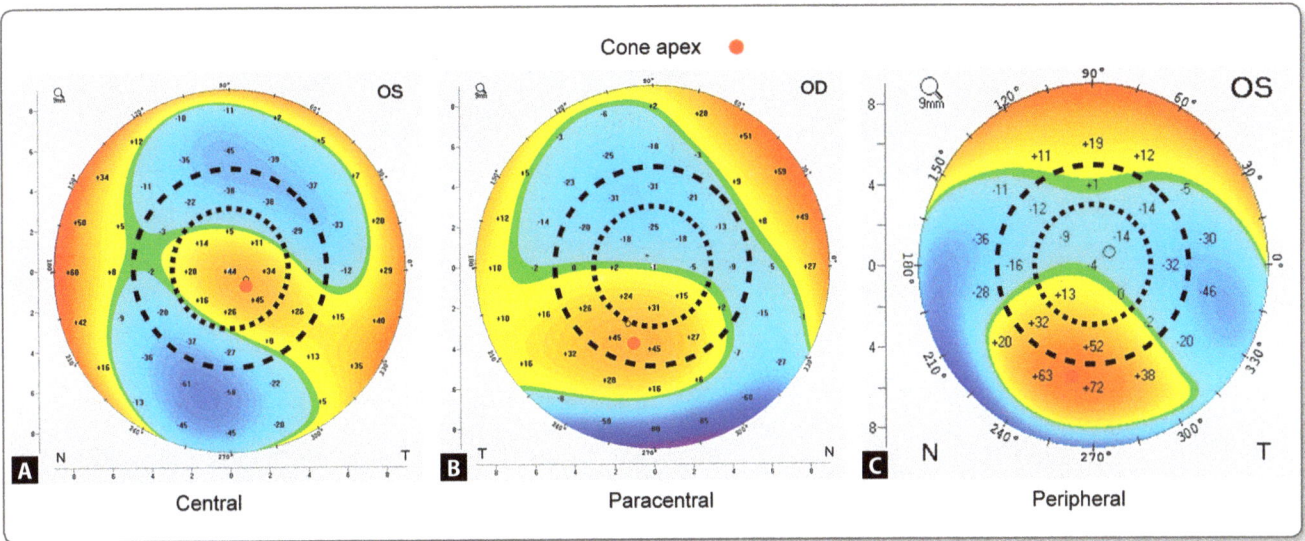

Figs. 6.15A to C: Classification of cone location by the posterior elevation map with 8 mm best fit sphere (BFS) float mode.

58 *Section 2: Corneal Maps and Profiles*

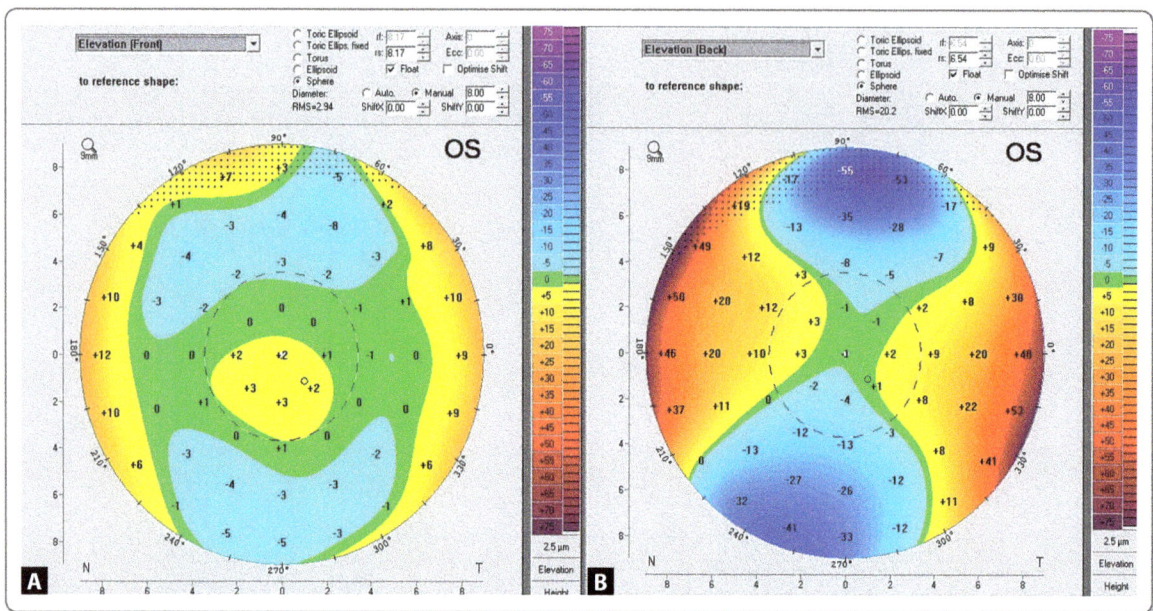

Figs. 6.16A and B: Regular patterns on the elevation maps. (A) Central island, indicating insignificant corneal astigmatism; and (B) Hourglass, indicating significant corneal astigmatism.

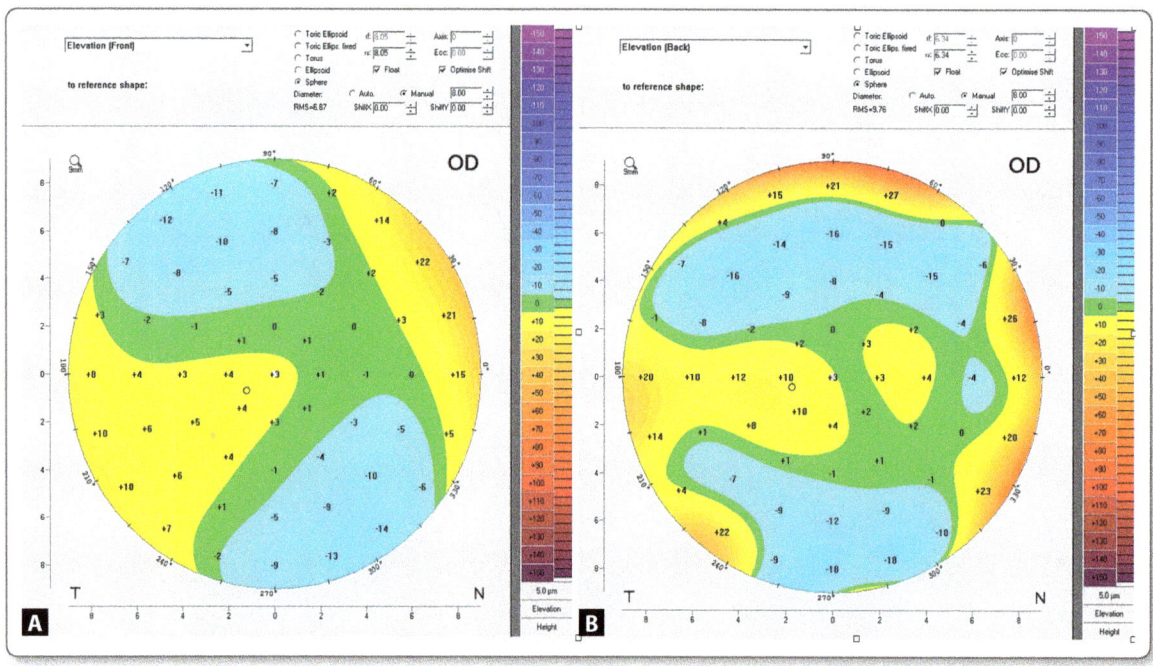

Figs. 6.17A and B: Irregular patterns on the elevation maps. (A) Tongue-like extension or skewed hourglass; and (B) Nonspecific irregular pattern.

Table 6.1: Cutoff elevation values for myopic population.

Location	1 SD	2 SD	3 SD
Anterior	3.7	5.7	7.7
Posterior	8.3	13	17.7

Table 6.2: Cutoff elevation values for hypermetropic population.

Location	1 SD	2 SD	3 SD
Anterior	2.1	4.3	6.5
Posterior	16.3	22.1	27.8

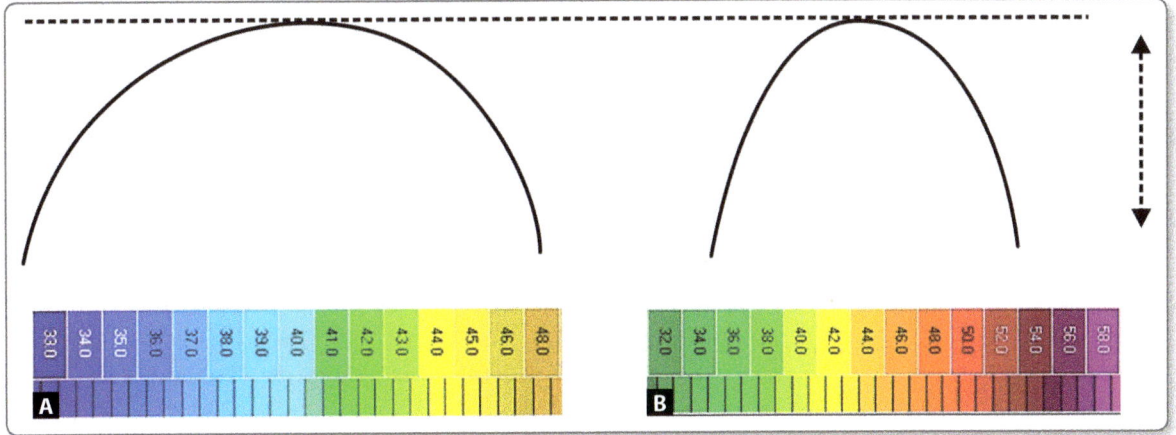

Figs. 6.18A and B: Difference between the curvature (slope) and the elevation (height) maps.

Elevation Maps versus Curvature Map

To understand the difference between the elevation maps and the curvature map, *see* Figures 6.18A and B. In this figure, both surfaces have the same height (elevation) but different slopes (curvature).

Belin/Ambrosio Enhanced Ectasia

INTRODUCTION

Belin/Ambrosio enhanced ectasia consists of the Belin/Ambrosio ectasia display (BAD), pachymetric data and numeric values (Fig. 7.1).

THE BELIN/AMBROSIO ECTASIA DISPLAY

The BAD is an elevation-based classification system developed by Belin, Ambrosia and Khachikian for early

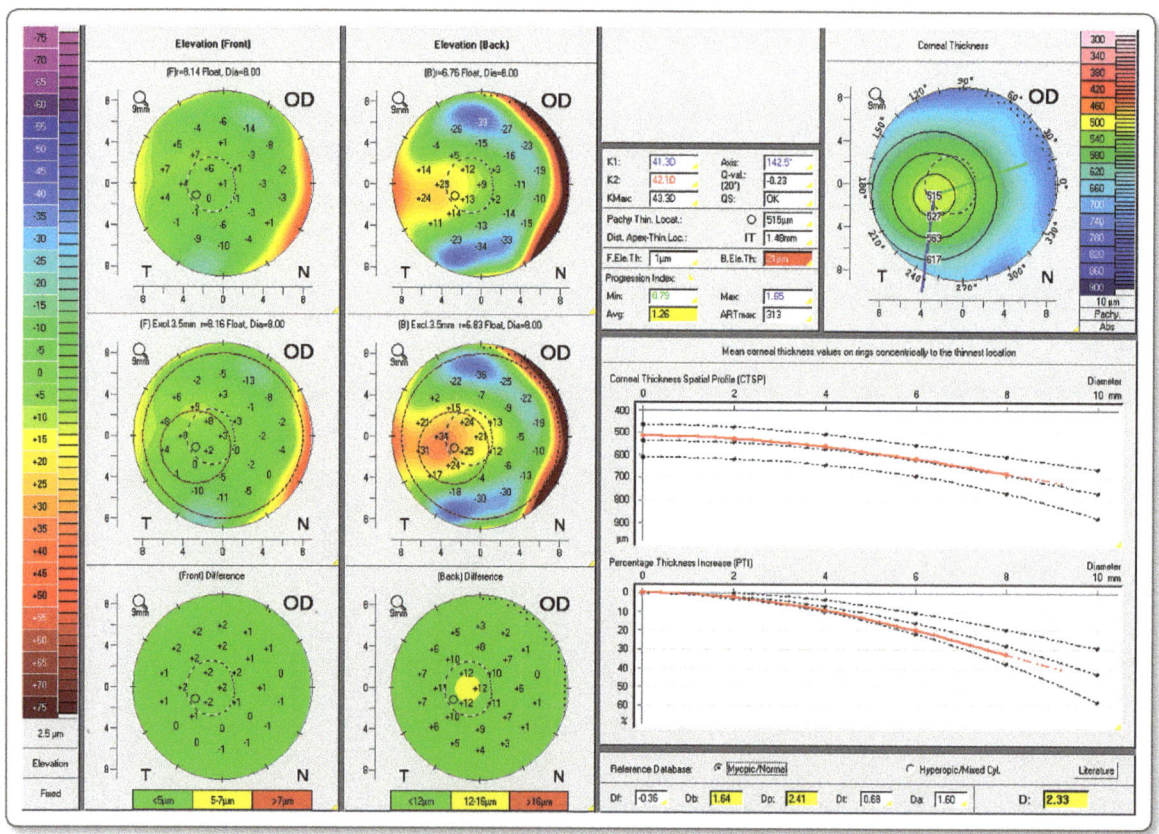

Fig. 7.1: Belin/Ambrosio enhanced ectasia.

detection of ectatic corneal diseases (ECDs). The BAD depends on the principle of "enhanced best-fit-sphere (BFS)."

The Enhanced Best-Fit-Sphere Reference Surface

Belin developed this concept to enhance the display of the cone in early or subclinical ECDs. Figure 7.2 is an illustration of an ECD. With the BFS float mode, the computer adjusts the best-fit reference surface (RS) (Fig. 7.2A: blue dotted curve) in a position that is based on the rule: a + b = c, as mentioned in Chapter 6. In the enhanced BFS, the computer excludes a variable area of 3.5–4 mm in diameter centered at the thinnest location. Therefore, the computer will choose another RS to achieve the same rule of a + b = c (Fig. 7.2B: red dotted curve). Then, the computer will use the new RS as an RS for the studied surface (Fig. 7.2C). In other words, the computer excludes a variable steep area in order to adjust a flatter RS to make the steep area more prominent. Figure 7.3 shows the elevation map before (A) and after (B) the application of the enhanced BFS. It is obvious that the cone became more prominent.

The display is based on elevation maps and does not take into consideration the curvature map and the pachymetry map.

The Display

Normal eyes and known keratoconic eyes were compared by using the baseline (standard) BFS and the enhanced BFS. The relative elevation changes were highly significant, which means that the difference in elevation between the standard and the enhanced BFS was minimal in normal eyes, while it was highly significant in the ectatic eyes. In Figure 7.4, the left column is for the anterior corneal surface and the right column is for the posterior corneal surface. Row (A) is the baseline elevation maps by using the standard BFS, row (B) is the enhanced elevation maps by using the enhanced BFS, and row (C) is the mathematical change in the elevation values between the baseline and the enhanced situations. At the bottom of the columns, the color bar shows

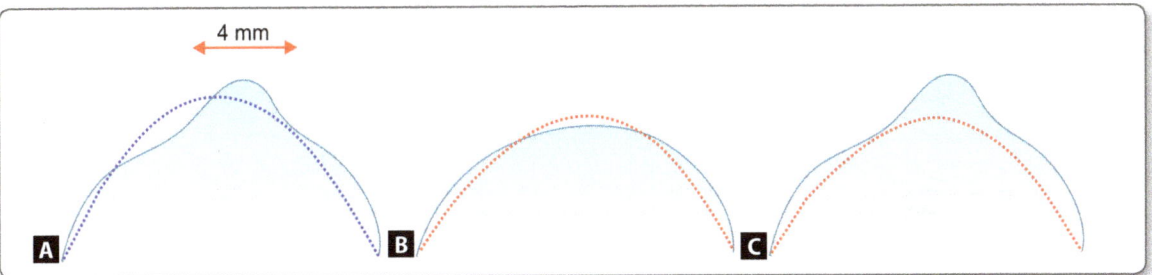

Figs. 7.2A to C: Principle of the Belin/Ambrosio ectasia display (BAD).

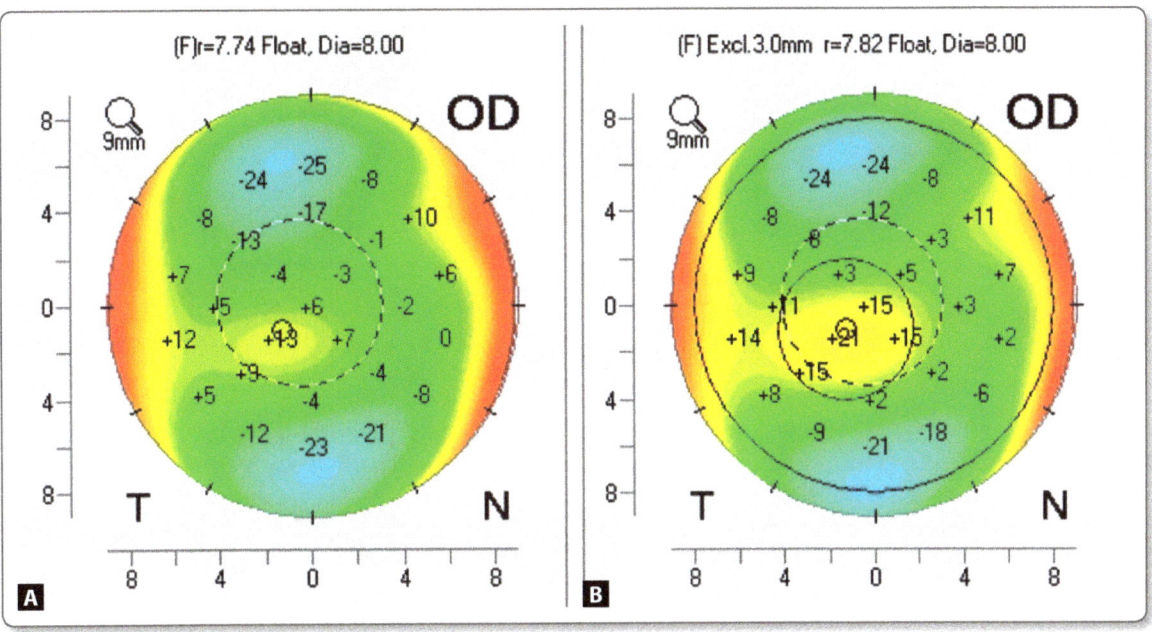

Figs. 7.3A and B: The elevation map (A) before and (B) after the application of the enhanced best-fit-sphere (BFS).

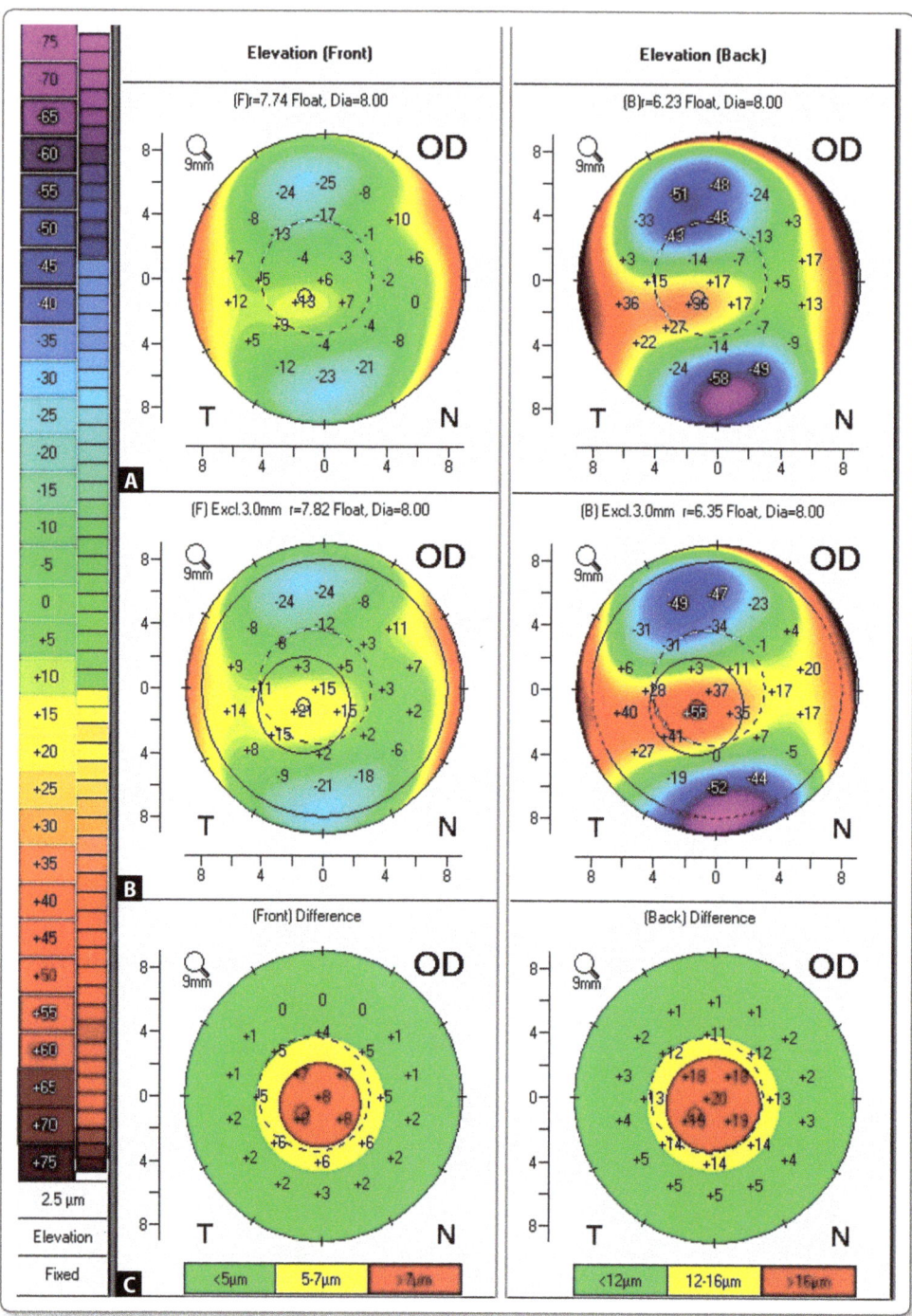

Figs. 7.4A to C: Belin/Ambrosio ectasia display (BAD).

the normal (in green), suspicious (in yellow) and abnormal (in red) range of changes. Therefore, green areas represent changes in values less than 5 μm for the anterior and less than 12 μm for the posterior, red areas represent changes more than 7 μm for the anterior and more than 16 μm for the posterior, and yellow areas represent the changes in between. In other words, if the display is totally green (Figs. 7.5A to C), the elevation maps are normal; if the display has a red flag (Figs. 7.6A to C), the elevation maps are abnormal; and if the display has a yellow flag (Figs. 7.7A to C: bottom right), the maps are suspicious.

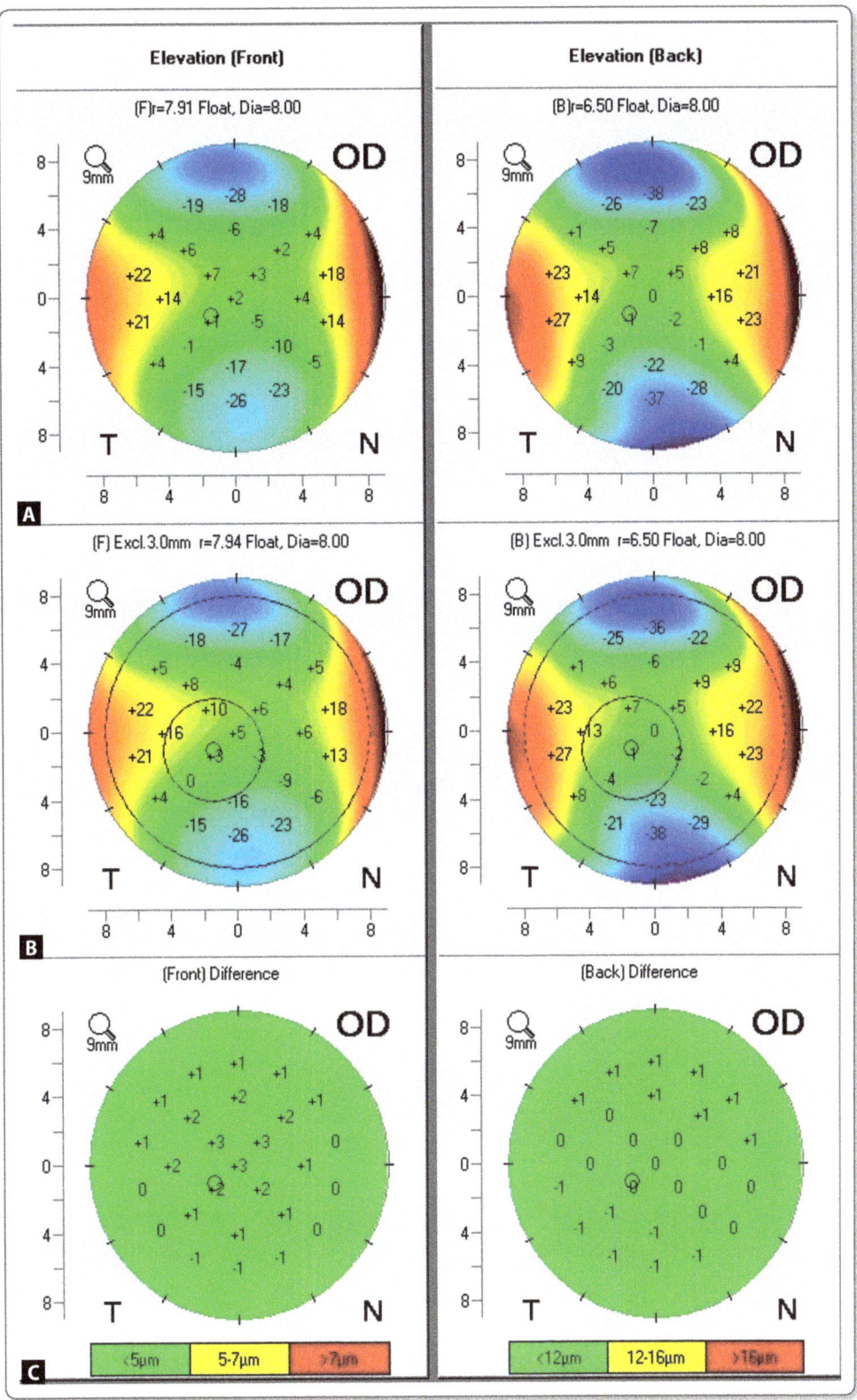

Figs. 7.5A to C: Belin/Ambrosio ectasia display in a cornea with normal elevation maps.

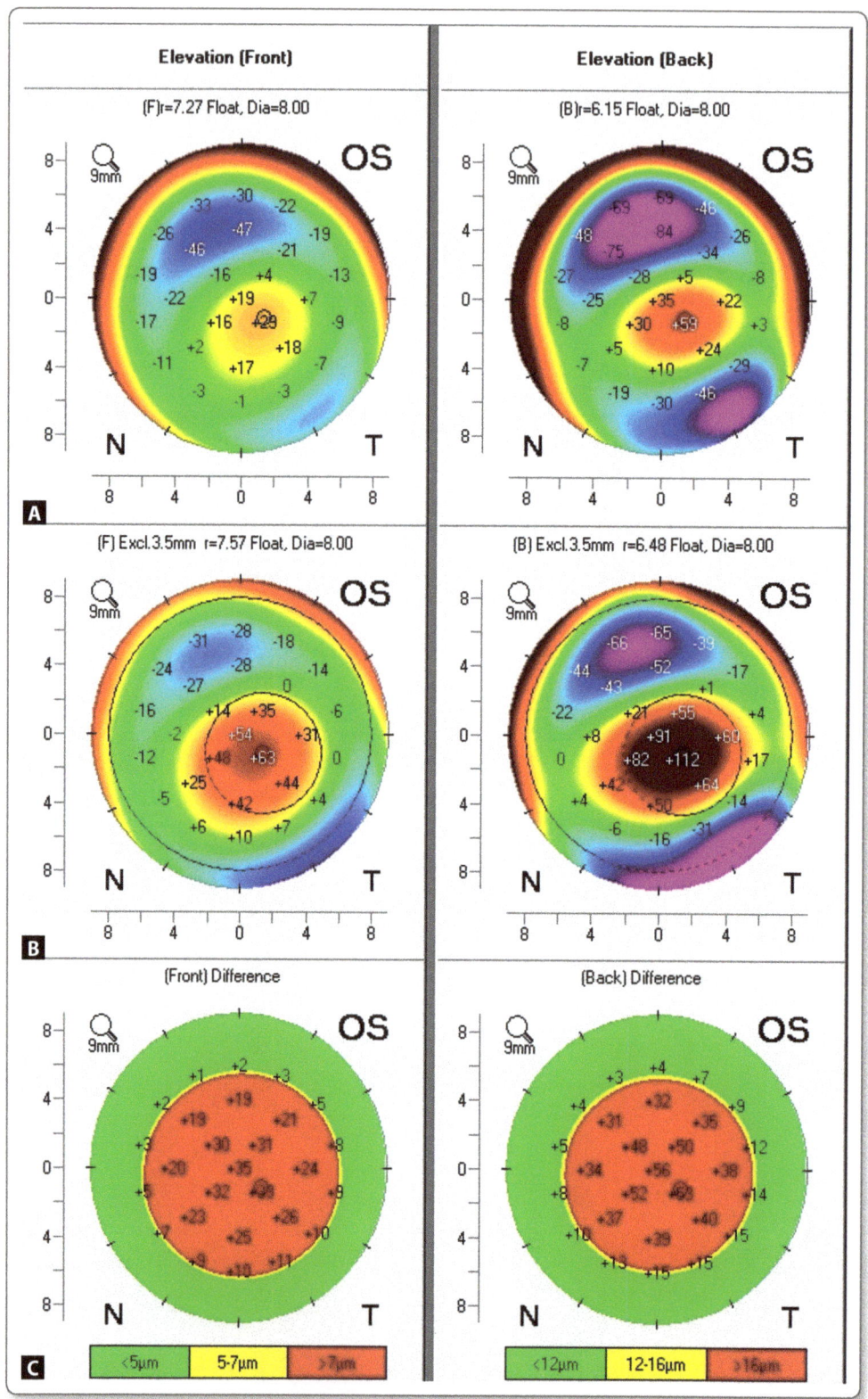

Figs. 7.6A to C: Belin/Ambrosio ectasia display in a cornea with abnormal elevation maps.

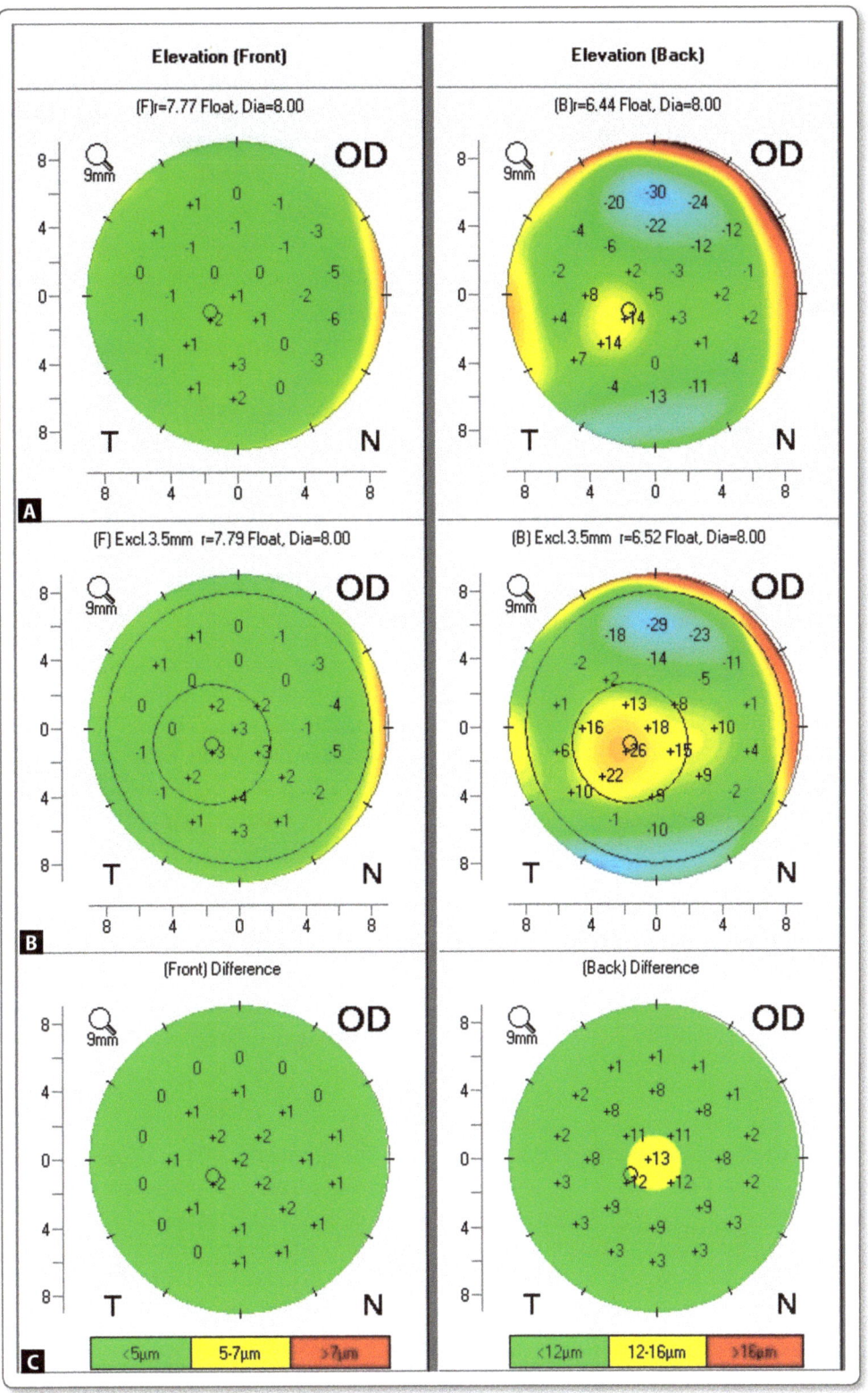

Figs. 7.7A to C: Belin/Ambrosio ectasia display in a cornea with a suspicious posterior elevation map.

PACHYMETRIC DATA

The pachymetric data consist of a full corneal thickness map, which identifies the value and location of the thinnest location, and thickness profiles. They are discussed in detail in Chapter 8.

NUMERIC VALUES

- *K_1 and K_2:* Flat and steep Sim-Ks.
- *Kmax:* Maximum K-reading on the anterior corneal surface.
- *Axis:* Axis of anterior corneal astigmatism related to the flat K (K_1).
- *Q-val (20°):* Q-value of the anterior corneal surface at 20°.
- *Qs:* Quality specification of the capture.
- *Pachy Thin. Locat.:* Corneal thickness at the thinnest location.
- *Dist. Apex-Thin. Loc:* The distance between the thinnest location and corneal apex. The orientation is given by a combination of two abbreviations: I = inferior, S = superior, N = nasal, T = temporal.
- *F.Ele.Th:* Front elevation at thinnest location.
- *B.Ele.Th:* Back elevation at thinnest location.
- *Progression index:*
  - *Min.:* The pachymetric progression index minimum: It defines the half meridian with the smallest progression index. It is displayed in green on the pachymetry map on the right.
  - *Max.:* The pachymetric progression index maximum: It defines the half meridian with the largest progression index. It is displayed in blue on the pachymetry map on the right.
  - *Avg.:* The pachymetric progression index average: It is the averaged ratio of individual progression to normative progression.
  - *ARTmax:* Ambrosio relational thickness. It is the ratio of the thinnest corneal thickness to the pachymetric progression index maximum.
- *Deviation parameters (Fig. 7.1 at the bottom right):* These parameters differ between myopic/emmetropic population and hypermetropic/mixed cylinder population. Therefore, they should be interpreted after refracting the patient. The parameters are color coded: white for normal, yellow for suspicious and red for abnormal. All D values are displayed as the standard deviation from the mean normal.
  - *Df:* Deviation of front elevation difference map.
  - *Db:* Deviation of back elevation difference map.
  - *Dp:* Deviation of average pachymetric progression.
  - *Dt:* Deviation of minimum thickness.
  - *Da:* Deviation of ARTmax.
  - *D:* It is the final D, which is the total deviation value. This final D value is based on Df, Db, Dp, Dt, Da, F.Ele. Th, B.Ele.Th, Pachy Thin. Locat, Dist. Apex-Thin. Loc, ART and Kmax. 100% sensitivity and 99% specificity is achieved with final D of 2.69.

APPLICATIONS OF BELIN/AMBROSIO ENHANCED ECTASIA

Since the BAD is elevation based, it reveals early abnormality on the elevation maps. However, early changes in the curvature map that are not associated with changes on the elevation maps cannot be detected by the BAD. Therefore, the BAD is not suitable to detect "para ectasia", such as forme fruste keratoconus and keratoconus suspect. This is discussed in detail in Chapter 19.

The BAD is important to detect ectasia and in post-laser vision correction (LVC) study.

Ectasia

The definition of the ECDs and the role of the BAD in the diagnosis are discussed in Chapter 19.

Post-Laser Vision Correction Study

A thorough history taking is essential in the workup for refractive surgery. In some cases, and for some reasons, patients may not mention a previous surgery to the cornea. The BAD can be used to detect post-LVC corneas. This is discussed in detail in Chapter 22.

CHAPTER 8

Corneal Thickness Maps and Profiles

INTRODUCTION

Corneal thickness map, relative thickness map (relative pachymetry), corneal thickness spatial profile (CTSP) and percentage thickness increase (PTI) are used for:
- Diagnosing ectatic corneal diseases (ECDs).
- Confirming the diagnosis of Fuchs' endothelial dystrophy and cornea guttata.
- Observing the progression of the previous diseases.
- Making the right decision for laser vision correction (LVC), intracorneal rings (ICRs) implantation and corneal cross-linking (CXL).
- Deciding the exact amount of correction in LVC by applying the rules of residual stromal bed and percent of tissue altered (PTA).
- Planning for ICRs in the management of ECDs in terms of location of the ring and depth of the tunnel as discussed below in patterns.

CORNEAL THICKNESS MAP (PACHYMETRY MAP)

Principle

The computer measures the thickness of the cornea at all points depending on the elevation maps; the difference between the front and back surface elevations is corneal thickness.

Patterns

The shape of the normal cornea is a negative meniscus lens (back surface radius of curvature is steeper than the front) which is thin at its optical center and thickens by the square of the distance from the center. The positive total power is a result of air in front and aqueous behind. The normal pattern is usually circular. Figure 8.1 represents the circular pattern, in which the pachymetry zones are almost central, circular, concentric and symmetric. However, this pattern can be encountered in keratoconus (KC) as well.

Abnormal pachymetry patterns are:
- *Horizontal displacement pattern (Fig. 8.2)*: This pattern may occur due to misalignment, large angle kappa and rarely due to ECDs.
- *Vertical displacement pattern (Fig. 8.3)*: It is also known as "dome shape." It is usually encountered in ECDs.

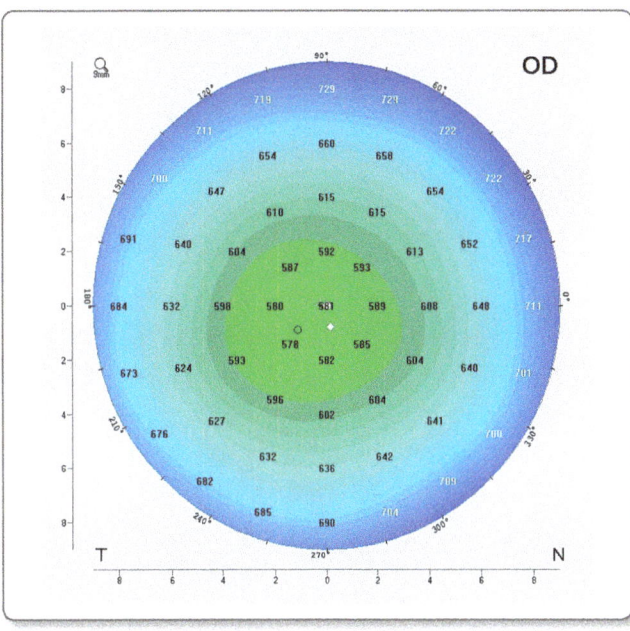

Fig. 8.1: The circular pattern.

Section 2: Corneal Maps and Profiles

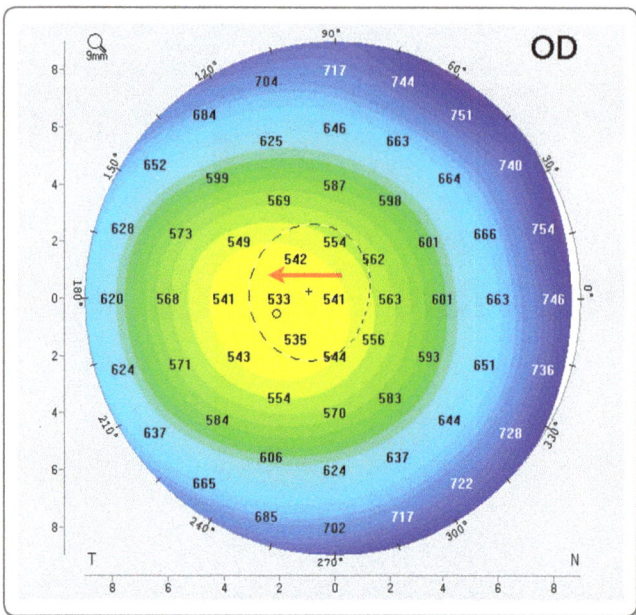

Fig. 8.2: Horizontal displacement pattern.

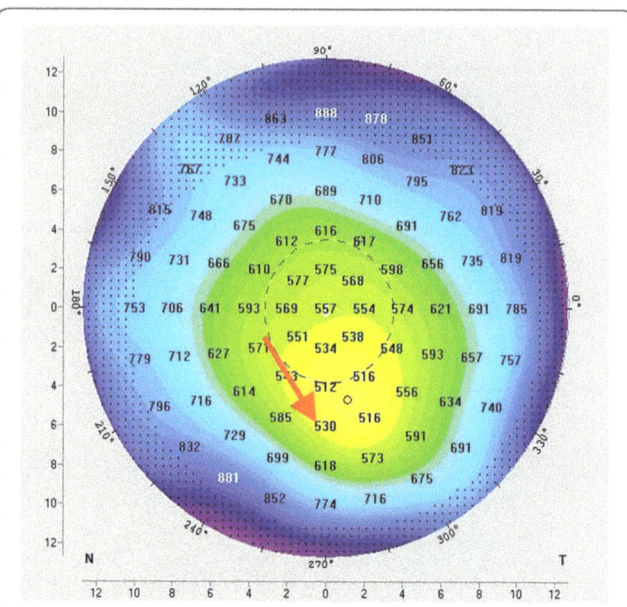

Fig. 8.3: Vertical displacement pattern.

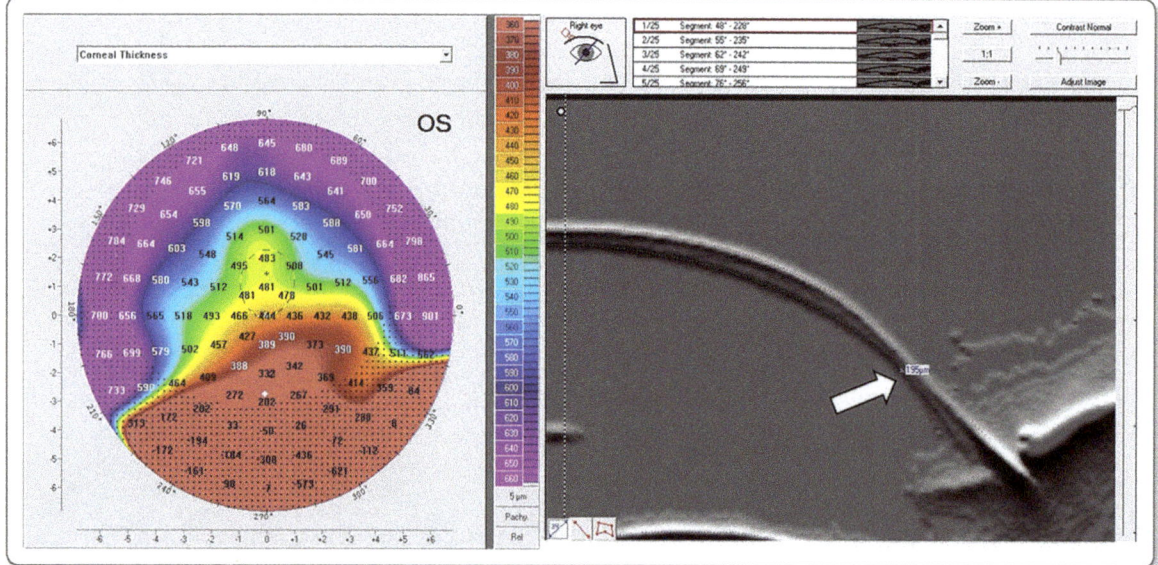

Fig. 8.4: Bell pattern.

However, it can be seen in patients with constant rubbing, in whom the dome will be inferior-temporal due to the direction of band rubbing. When ICRs implantation is planned in this pattern, a special precaution to the depth of the tunnel is essential because the thinnest location (TL) will be very close to the tunnel, bearing the risk of introducing the ICR into the anterior chamber during insertion. When calculating the depth of the tunnel in this pattern, it is recommended to consider the thickness at the TL rather than the thinnest point along the tunnel.

- *Bell pattern (Fig. 8.4):* This pattern is a hallmark of pellucid marginal degeneration (PMD). It is characteristic for inferior band thinning. In this pattern, the risk of corneal perforation during ICR implantation is very high due to two reasons: (1) the inferior area is usually very thin, and the proper place to insert the ICR is usually inferior; and (2) due to highly distorted cornea in PMD, the inferior part is usually extrapolated as shown in the Figure (black dots), making the tomographic thickness map unreliable at that area; in this case, anterior segment optical coherence tomography (AS-OCT) is strongly recommended.

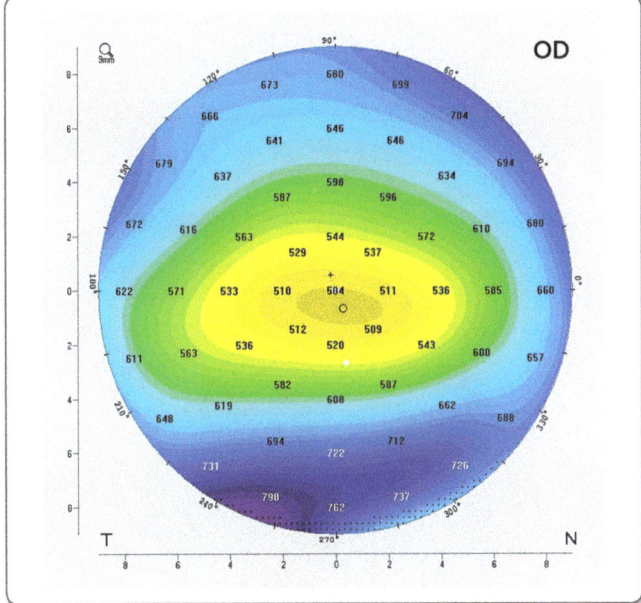

Fig. 8.5: Droplet pattern.

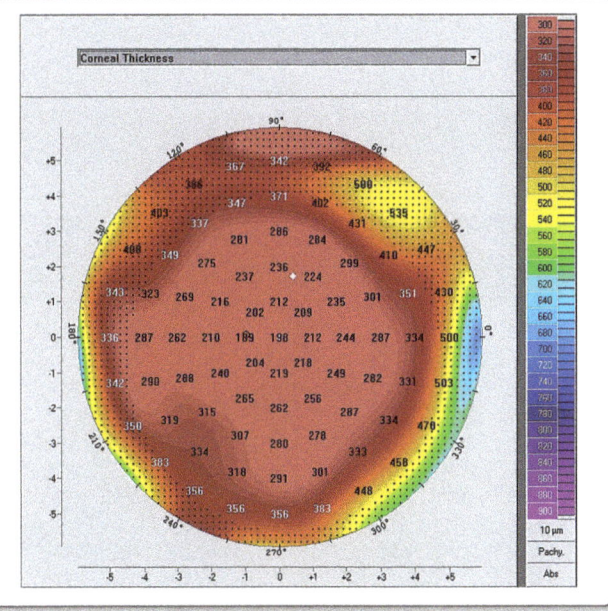

Fig. 8.6: Globus pattern.

- *Droplet pattern (Fig. 8.5):* It takes a triangular shape. It is usually encountered in KC, but might be an early sign of PMD.
- *Globus pattern (Fig. 8.6):* It is characterized by generalized thinning extending to the limbus. It is a hallmark of keratoglobus (KG). In this pattern, ICR implantation and traditional corneal transplantation are contraindicated.

Limitations

One limitation of corneal thickness map is corneal opacities. The beam light suffers from scattering in the areas of scars, leading to artifacts, extrapolated data and misinterpretation. The area of the scar is usually displayed as flat area which is true but exaggerated. In addition, scarred areas are interpreted as thin, which is not always true. The anterior OCT is more reliable in such cases. Figures 8.7 to 8.10 are for a typical corneal scar.

Figure 8.7 is the slit lamp view—the scar is oval and partially interferes with the pupillary zone, and hence affecting vision.

Figure 8.8 is the four-composite refractive map—a flat area on the anterior curvature map and anterior elevation map, a steep corresponding area on the posterior elevation map, and a corresponding thin area on the corneal thickness map. Many surgeons may misinterpret this case as ectasia or KC. The important sign that differentiate this case from ectasia and KC is the flat corresponding area on the anterior curvature map rather than the hot spot (steep area) that should be found in ectasia and KC.

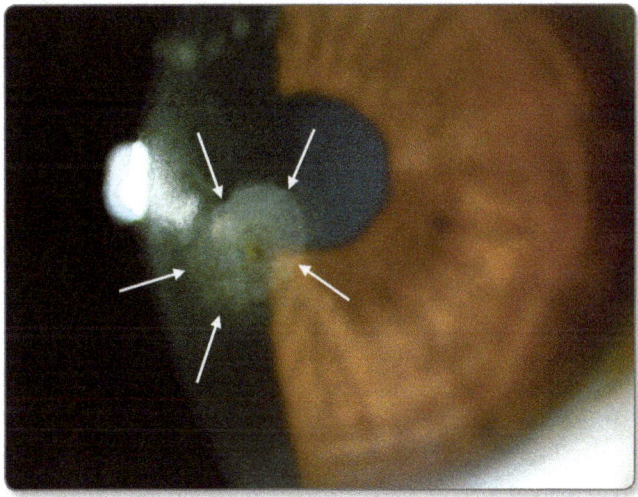

Fig. 8.7: Corneal scar: the slit lamp view.

Figure 8.9 is the four-composite selective map—the flat area is more prominent on the anterior tangential map and the relative pachymetry.

Figure 8.10 is the AS-OCT view—a horizontal linear cross-section along the scar shows the real thinning of the cornea over and under the scar. Since the epithelium has a filling effect (remodeling), it thickens over the scar to smoothen the anterior surface, and therefore masks the real flattening caused by the scar (Fig. 8.11). Look at the bulging on the posterior surface which explains the very high elevation values on the posterior elevation map.

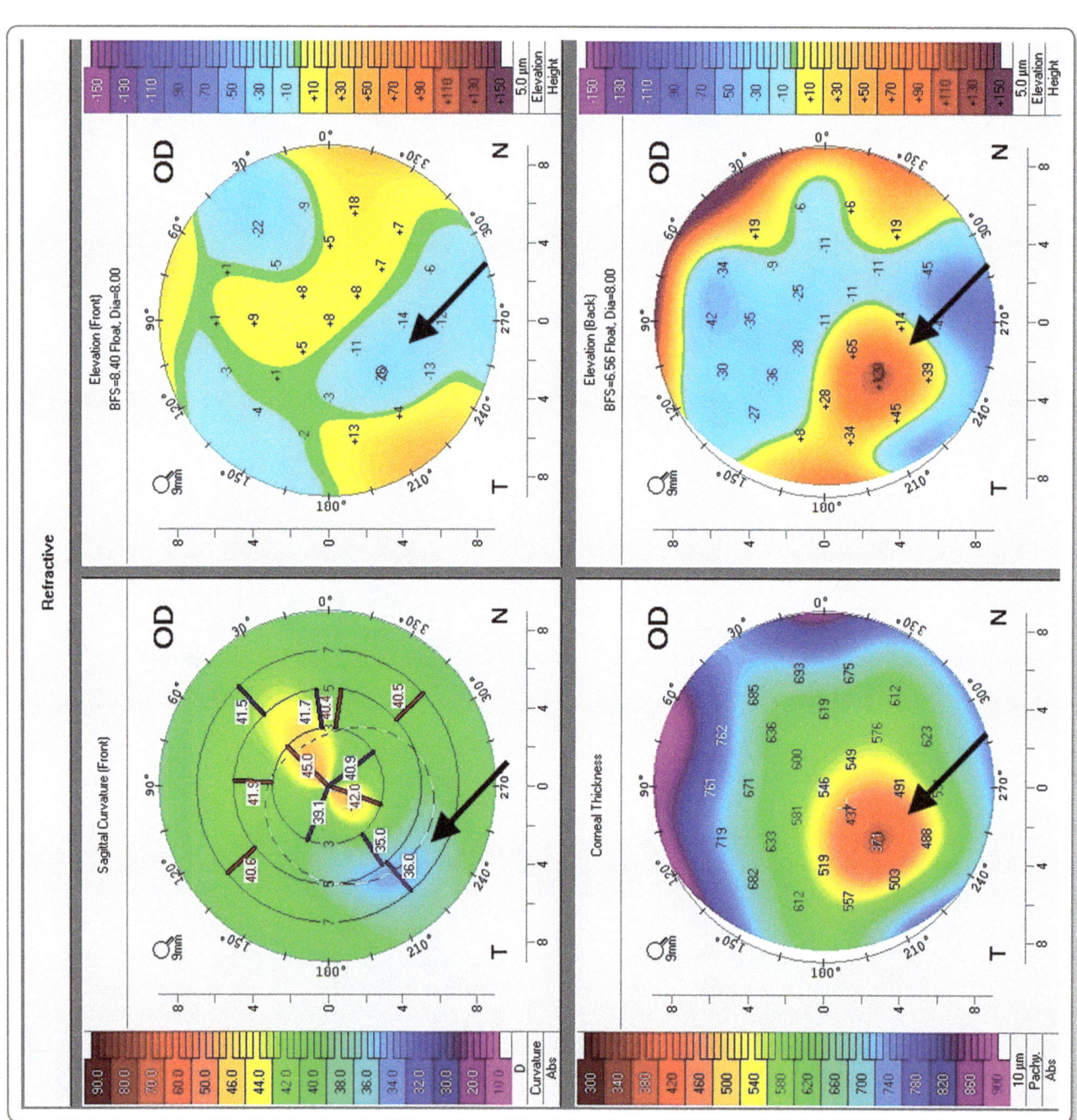

Fig. 8.8: Corneal scar: the four-composite refractive map.

Chapter 8: Corneal Thickness Maps and Profiles

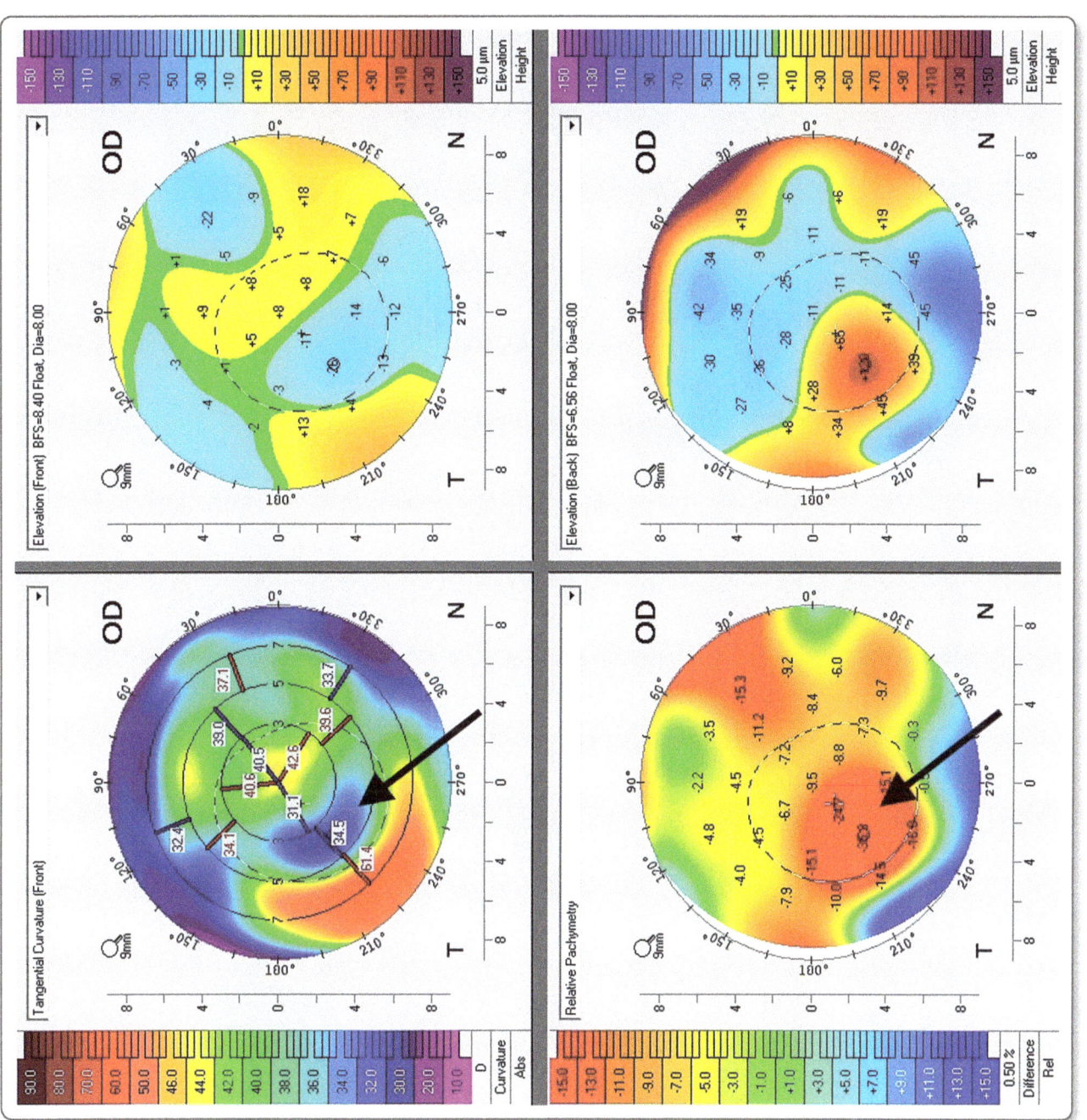

Fig. 8.9: Corneal scar: the four-composite selective map.

Section 2: Corneal Maps and Profiles

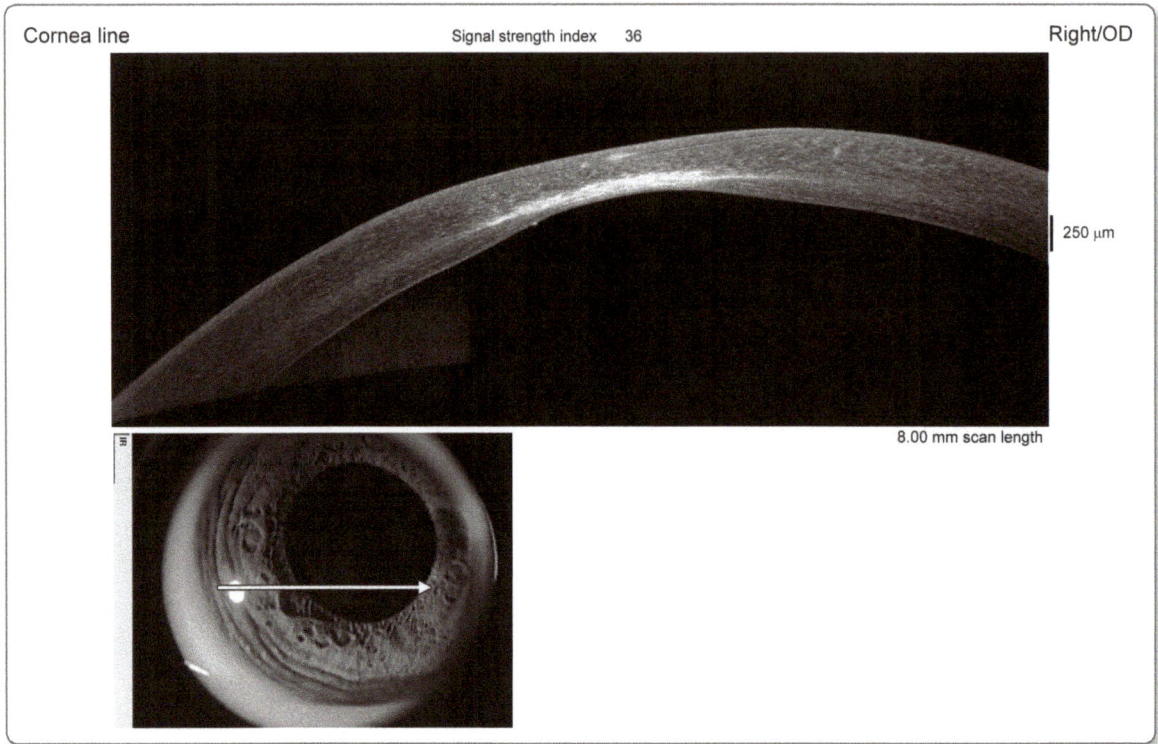

Fig. 8.10: Corneal scar: the anterior segment optical coherence tomography (AS-OCT) cross-section view.

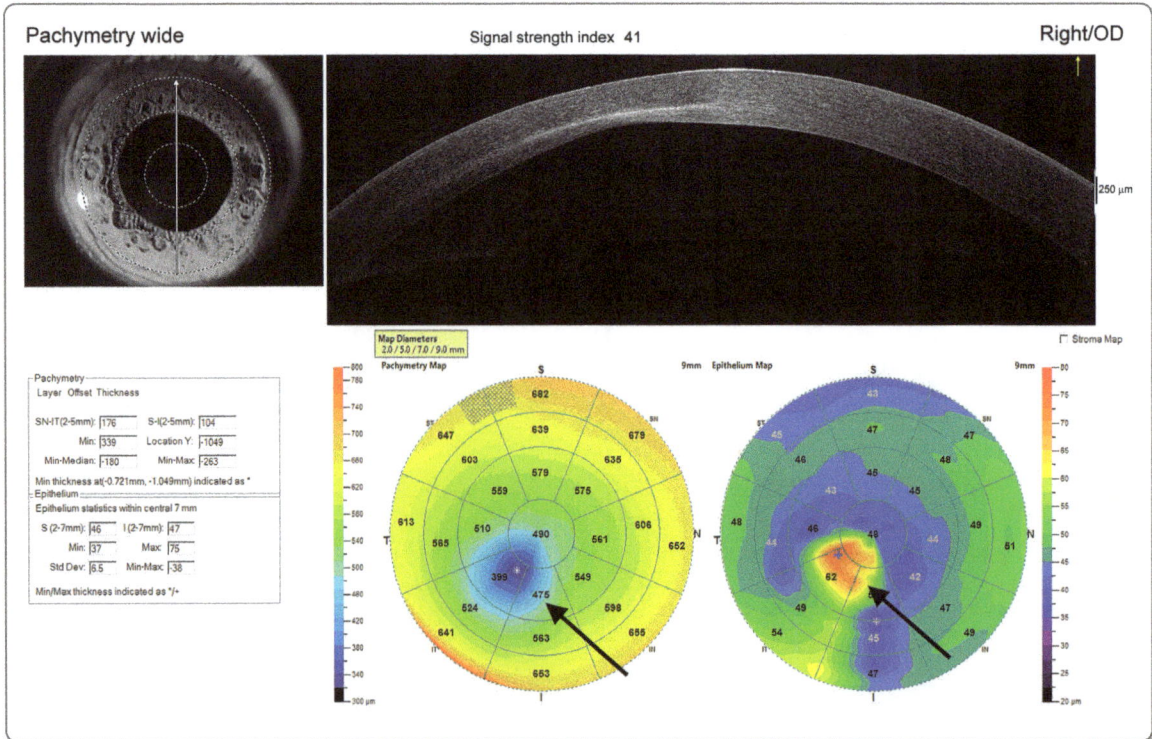

Fig. 8.11: Corneal scar: the pachymetry map and the epithelial map by the anterior segment optical coherence tomography (AS-OCT).

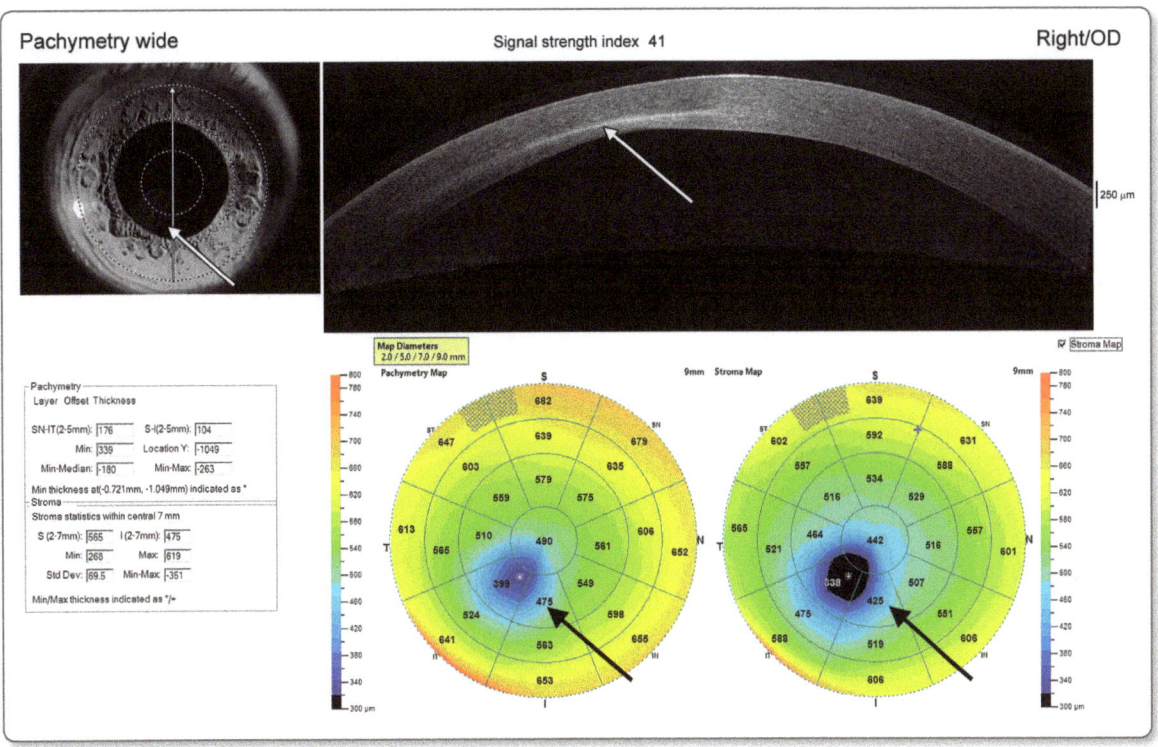

Fig. 8.12: Corneal scar: the pachymetry map and the stromal map by the anterior segment optical coherence tomography (AS-OCT).

Figure 8.11 is the AS-OCT pachymetry map with epithelial thickness map—look at the thinning in the pachymetry map on the left side and the corresponding thickening of the overlying epithelium in the epithelium map on the right.

Figure 8.12 is the AS-OCT pachymetry with stromal map on the right. It shows a larger zone of thinning in the stroma in comparison with the thinning seen on the pachymetry map on the left. That is because the pachymetry map is the algebraic sum of epithelium remodeling effect and stromal changes.

CORNEAL THICKNESS SPATIAL PROFILE AND PERCENTAGE THICKNESS INCREASE

Principle

The CTSP describes the progression of corneal thickness in relation with corneal zones, while the PTI describes the percentage of this progression (Fig. 8.13). The horizontal axis represents 2 mm, 4 mm, 6 mm, 8 mm and 10 mm corneal rings concentric to the TL. The vertical axis represents corneal thickness in the CTSP and the percentage of thickness increment in the PTI. The red curve represents the captured cornea. The black-dotted curves are the average normative data in general normal population for two standard deviation [Confidence interval (CI):95%].

Patterns

The normal pattern of both CTSP and PTI is a curved line plotted in red, following (but not necessarily within) the course of the normative black-dotted curves, with an average less than 1.20. In other words, the shape of the curve should show a gradual increment. The reference in this regard is the 6 mm zone. If the curve deviates before this zone, it is considered as abnormal.

Abnormal patterns are:

- *Quick slope (Fig. 8.14)*: The red curve deviates before the 6-mm zone. It is encountered in ECDs and corneas with high potential (Chapter 19).
- *S-shape*: The red curve slopes down then up. This might be before the 6-mm zone (Fig. 8.15), or after it (Fig. 8.16). It can be seen in ECDs and corneas with high potential (Chapter 19).
- *Flat slope (Fig. 8.17)*: It is seen in diseased thickened corneas, such as Fuchs' endothelial dystrophy and cornea guttata.
- *Inverted slope (Fig. 8.18)*: It is a hallmark of PMD. However, not every PMD has this pattern.

Section 2: Corneal Maps and Profiles

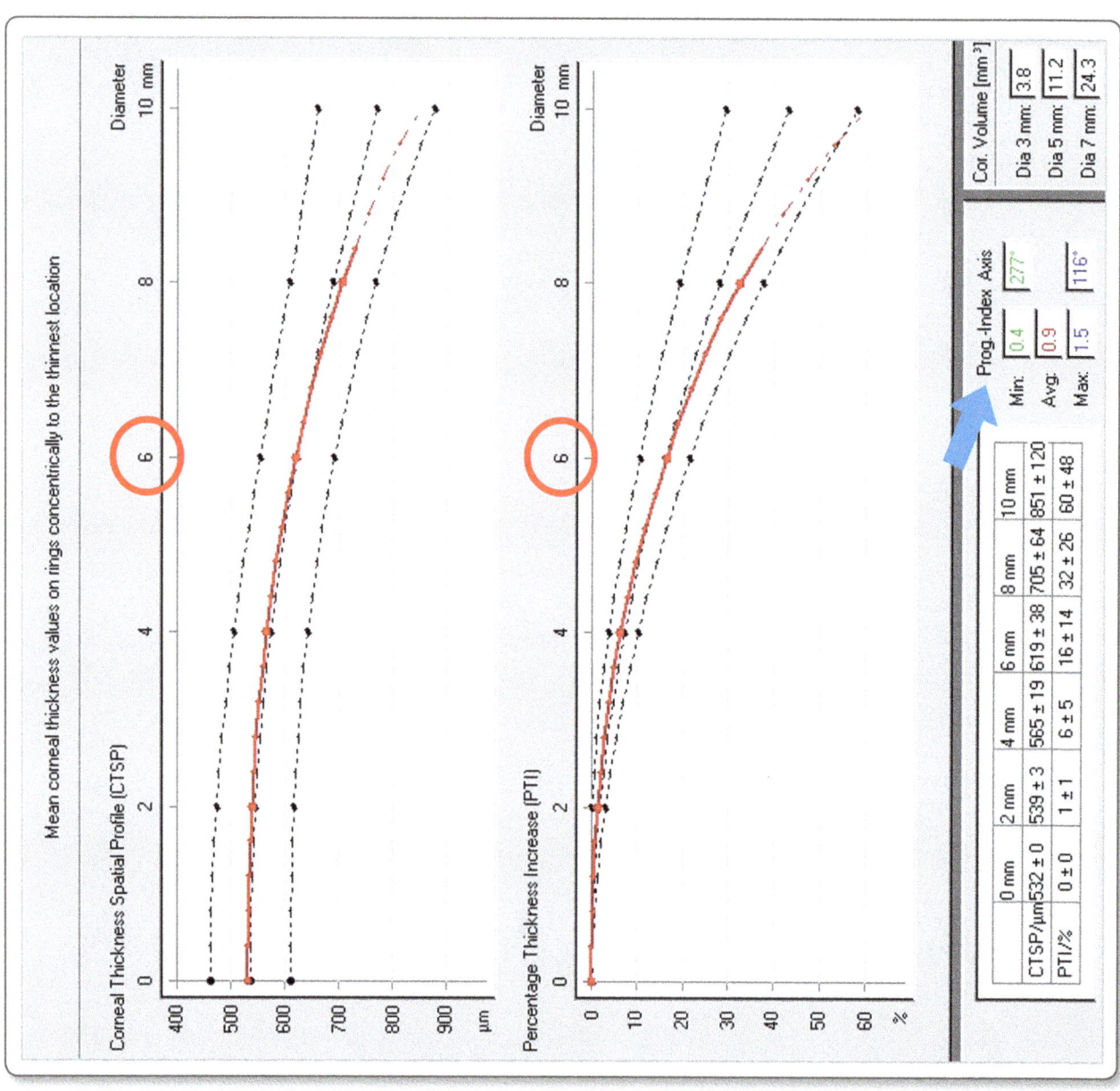

Fig. 8.13: Corneal thickness spatial profile, percentage thickness increase and pachymetric progression index.

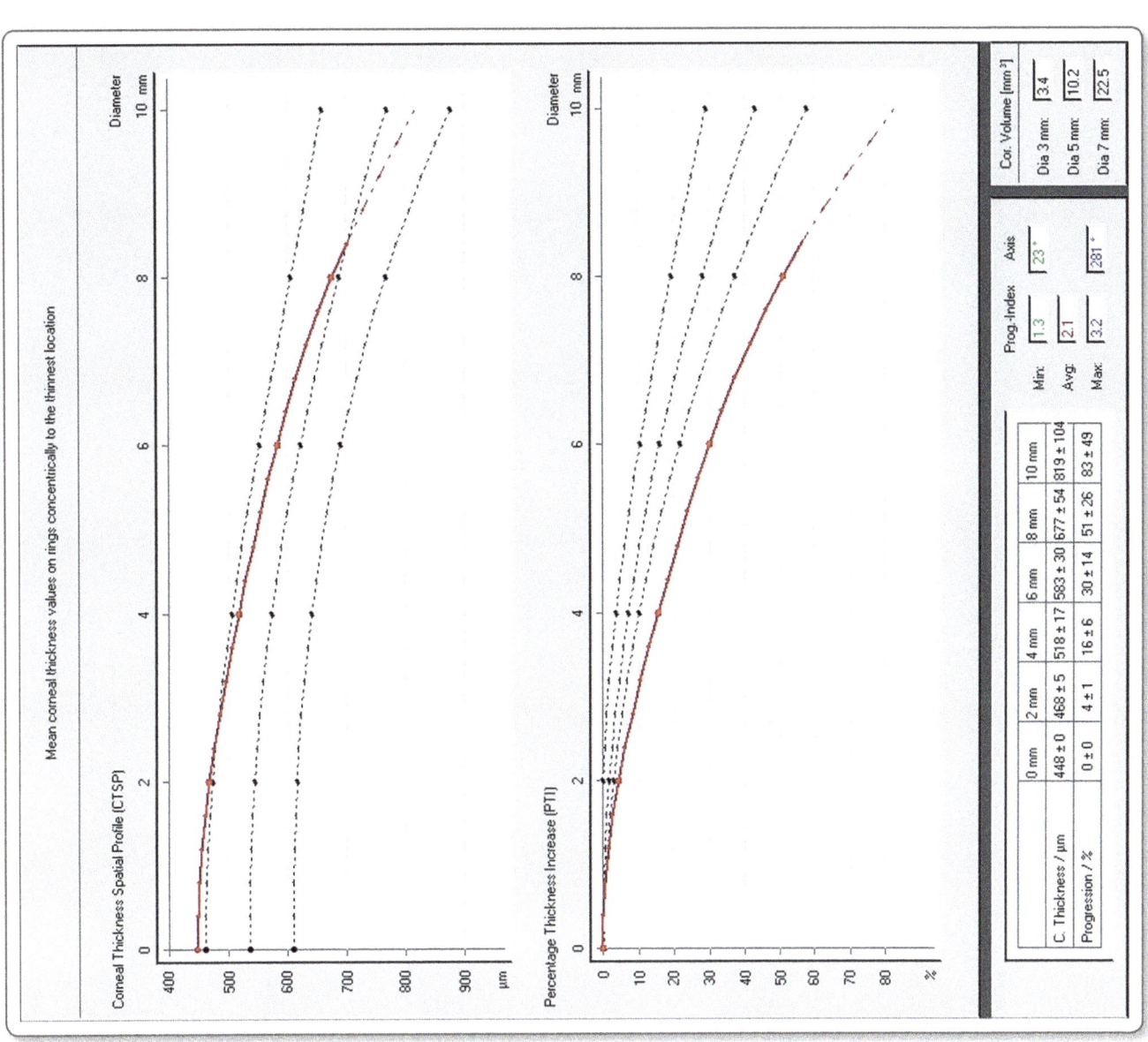

Fig. 8.14: Quick slope.

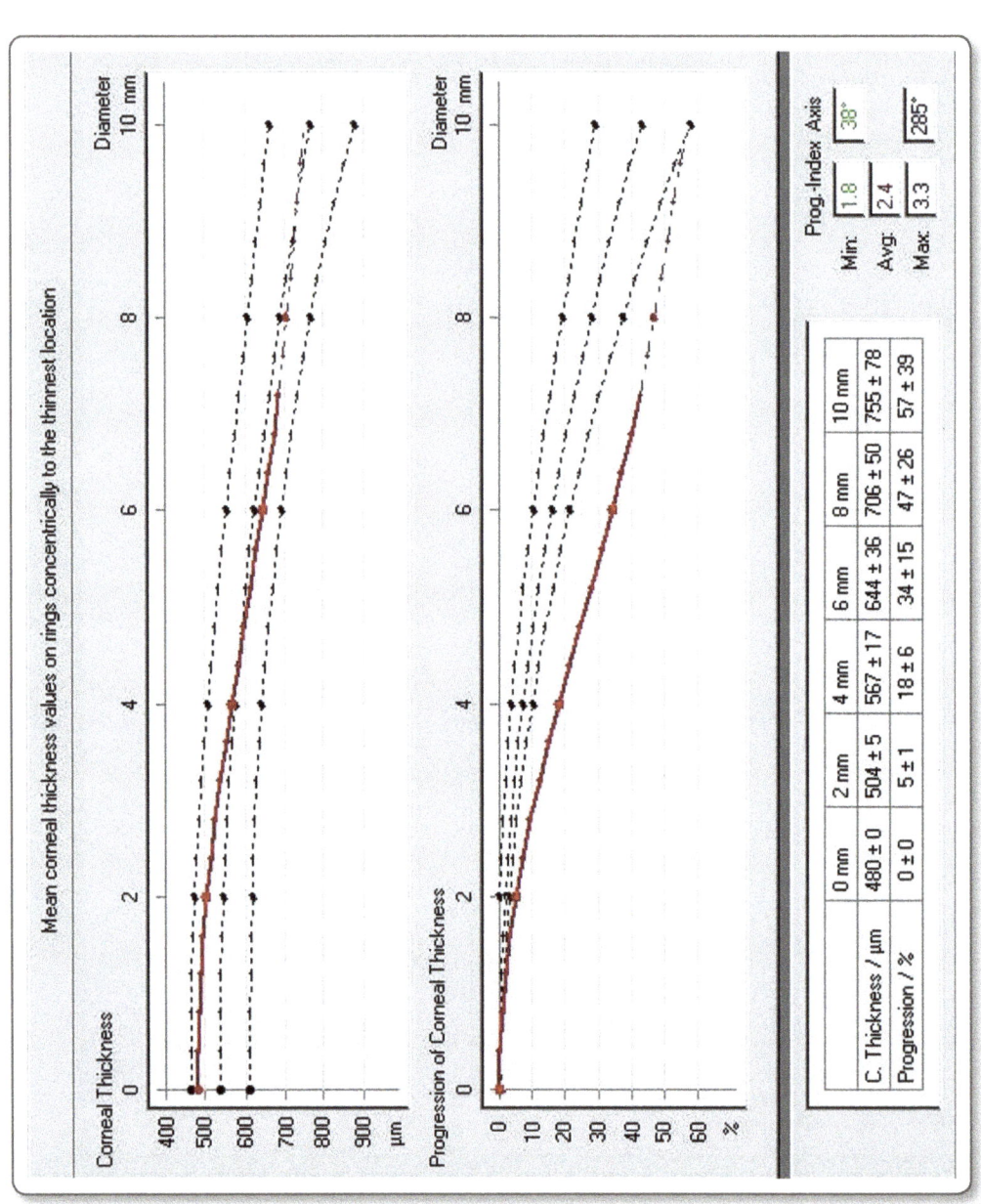

Fig. 8.15: S-shape before the 6 mm.

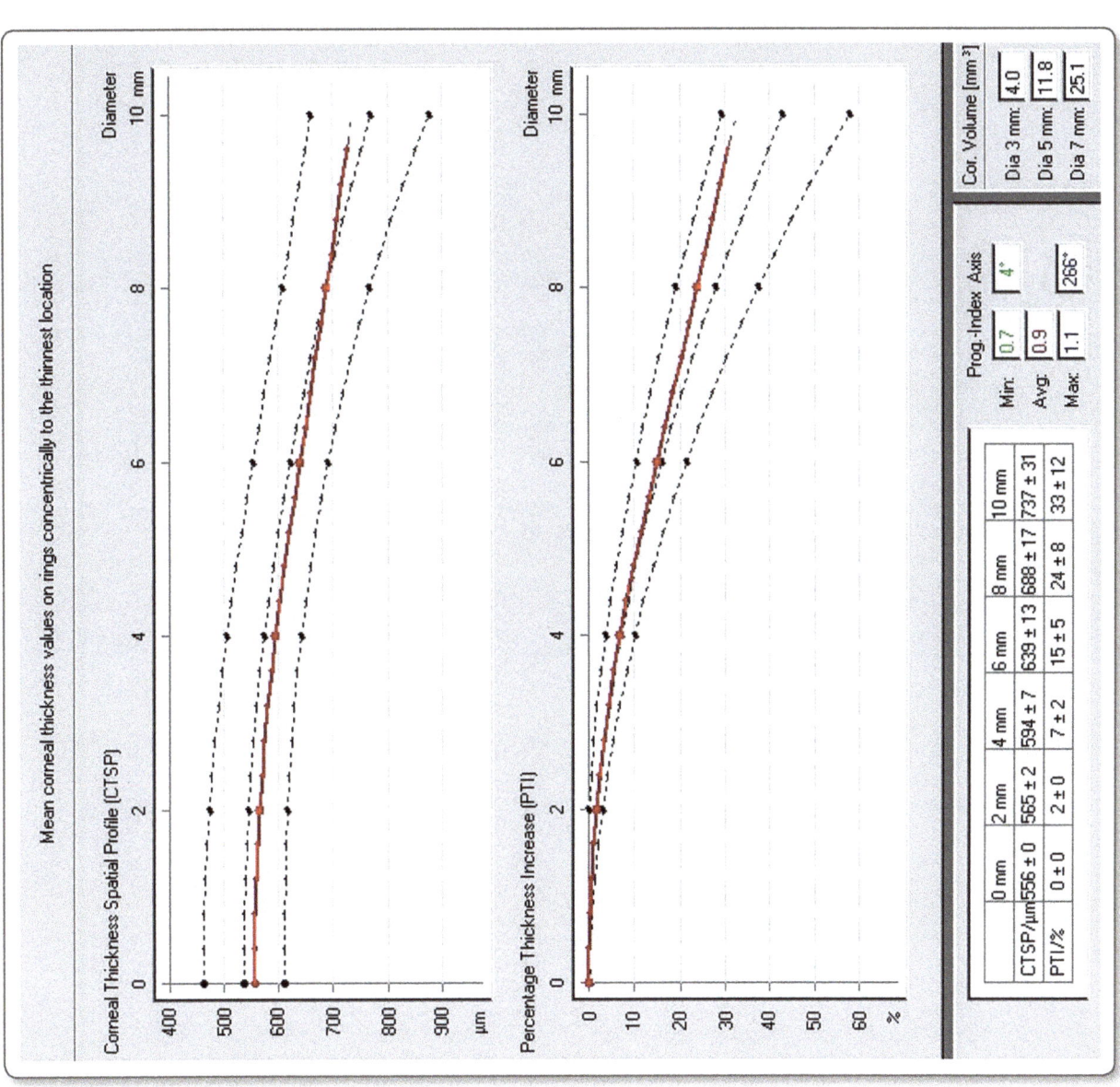

Fig. 8.16: S-shape after the 6 mm.

Section 2: *Corneal Maps and Profiles*

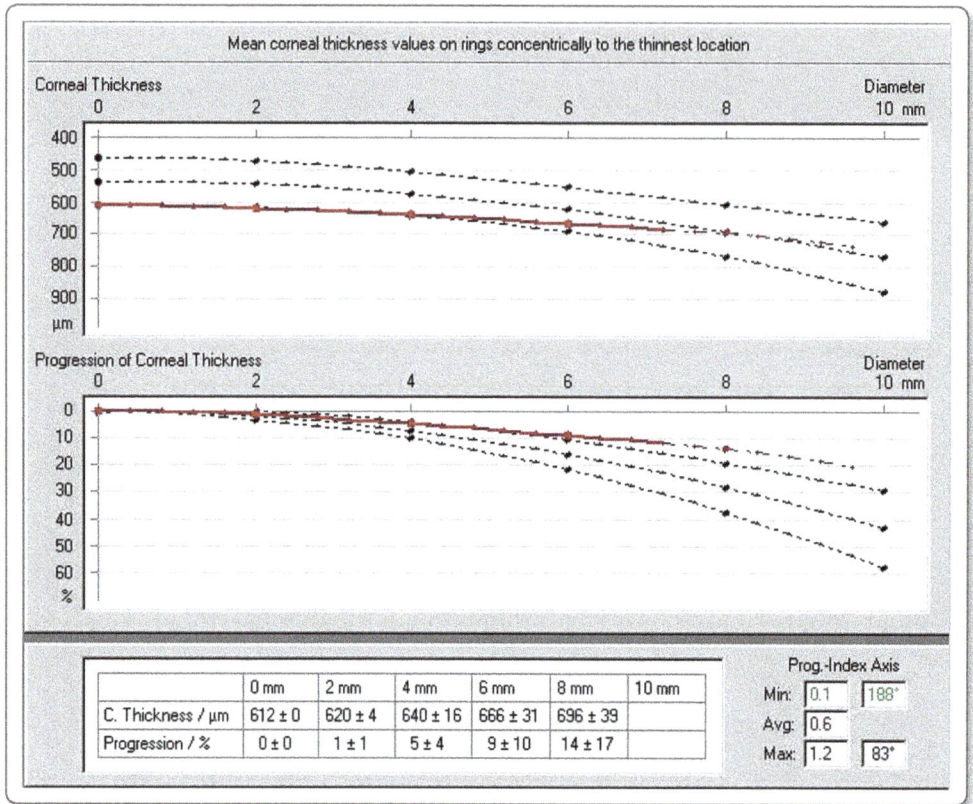

Fig. 8.17: Flat slope.

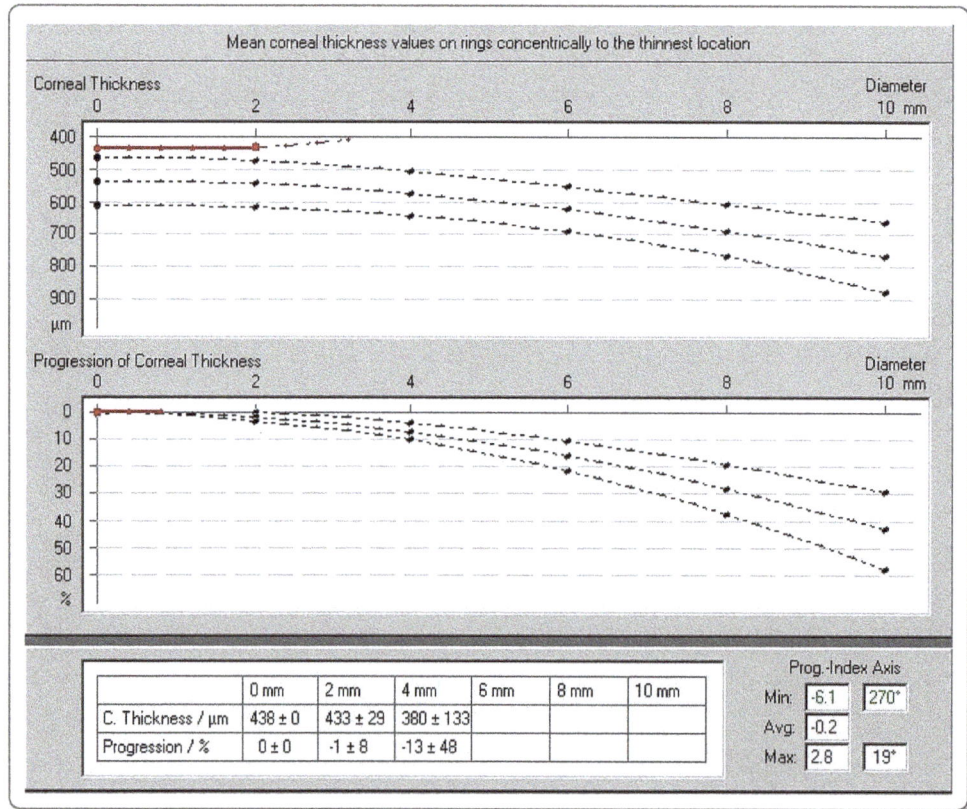

Fig. 8.18: Inverted slope.

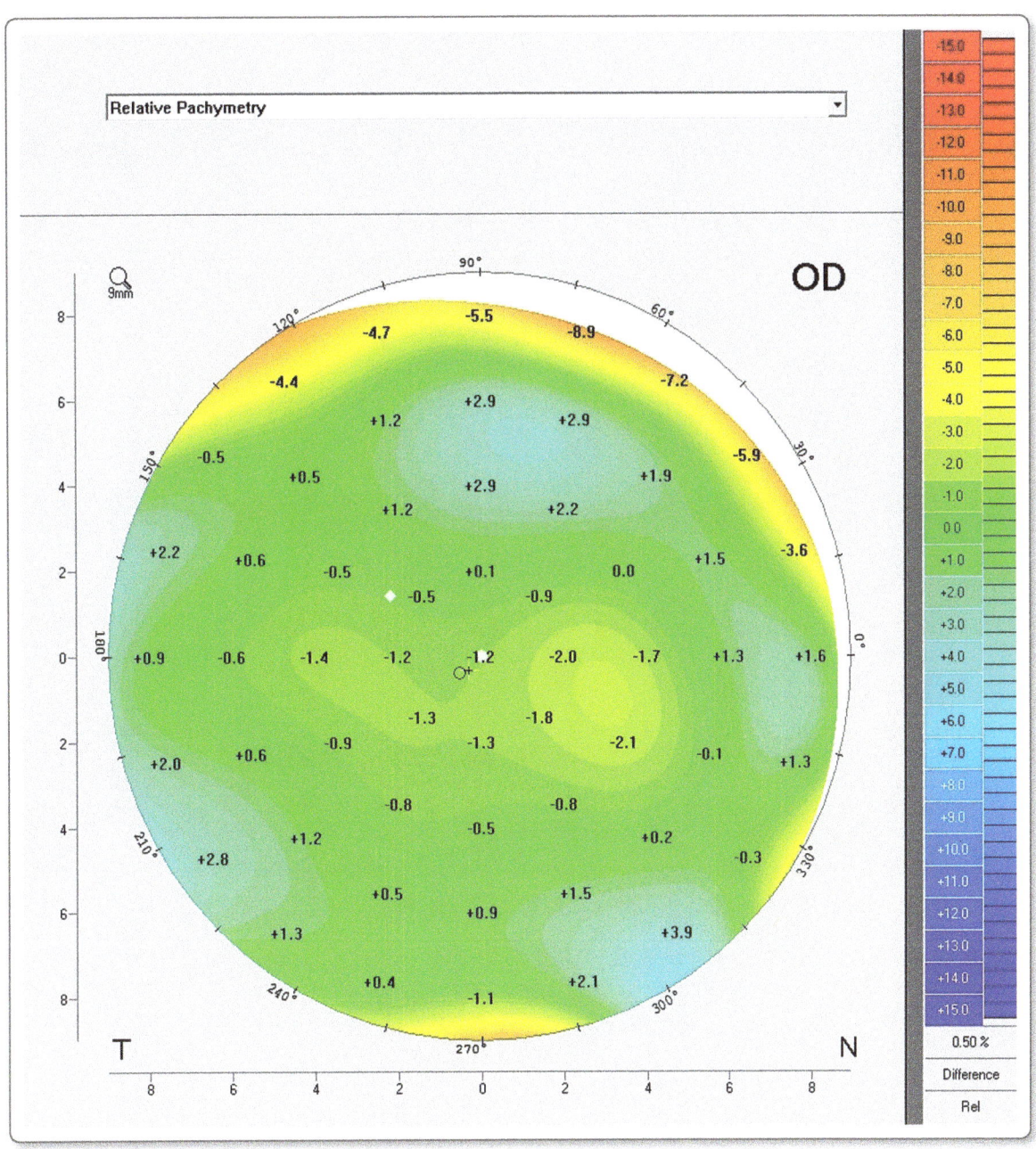

Fig. 8.19: The relative thickness map.

PACHYMETRIC PROGRESSION INDEX

Thickness/location relationship can be introduced as an index known as the pachymetric progression index (PPI) (bottom of Figs. 8.13 to 8.18). This index represents the maximum, minimum and average progression of the captured cornea in comparison with the normative data. The normal average value of the PPI is 0.8–1.1 (Fig. 8.13). When the average is <0.8, the cornea is diseased and thickened as in corneal edema, cornea guttata and Fuchs' endothelial dystrophy (Fig. 8.17). When the average is ≥1.2, the cornea is most probably abnormal and may be ectatic (Figs. 8.14 and 8.15). In S-shape pattern, the average is usually normal when the S is after the 6-mm zone (Fig. 8.16).

There are three important values of the progression index, namely min, max and average (Chapter 7).

THE RELATIVE PACHYMETRY

The principle of this map is very similar to the principle of the elevation map. In the elevation map, the captured

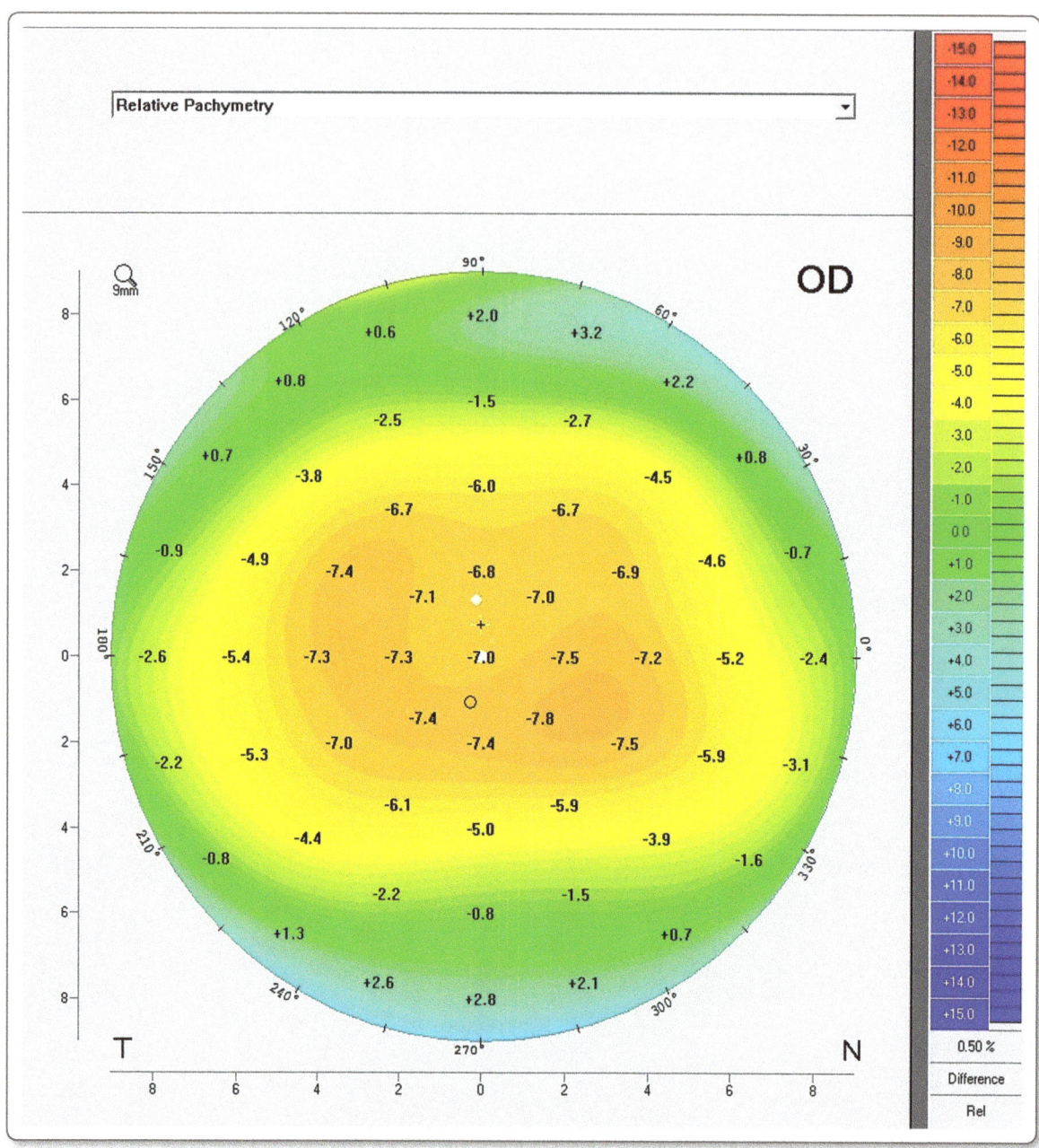

Fig. 8.20: Suspicious relative thickness map.

cornea is measured in relation to a reference surface. In the relative pachymetry, the thickness map of the captured cornea is compared with a standard normative thickness map in normal population.

The relative pachymetry is displayed as percentage values (Fig. 8.19). Areas thicker than the similar areas in the standard map will be displayed in positive values and vice versa. For example: +7 and +9 values are thicker than the standard map by 7% and 9%, respectively, and vice versa when the values are negative. In general, areas with −5 to −8 are suspicious (Fig. 8.20), while areas with less than −8 (e.g. −10) are abnormal and are usually encountered with ECDs (Fig. 8.21).

This map has three main applications:
1. In the workup for refractive surgery (Chapter 18).
2. In differentiating ECDs from entities mimicking ECDs (Chapter 22)
3. In Holladay Report (Chapter 23).

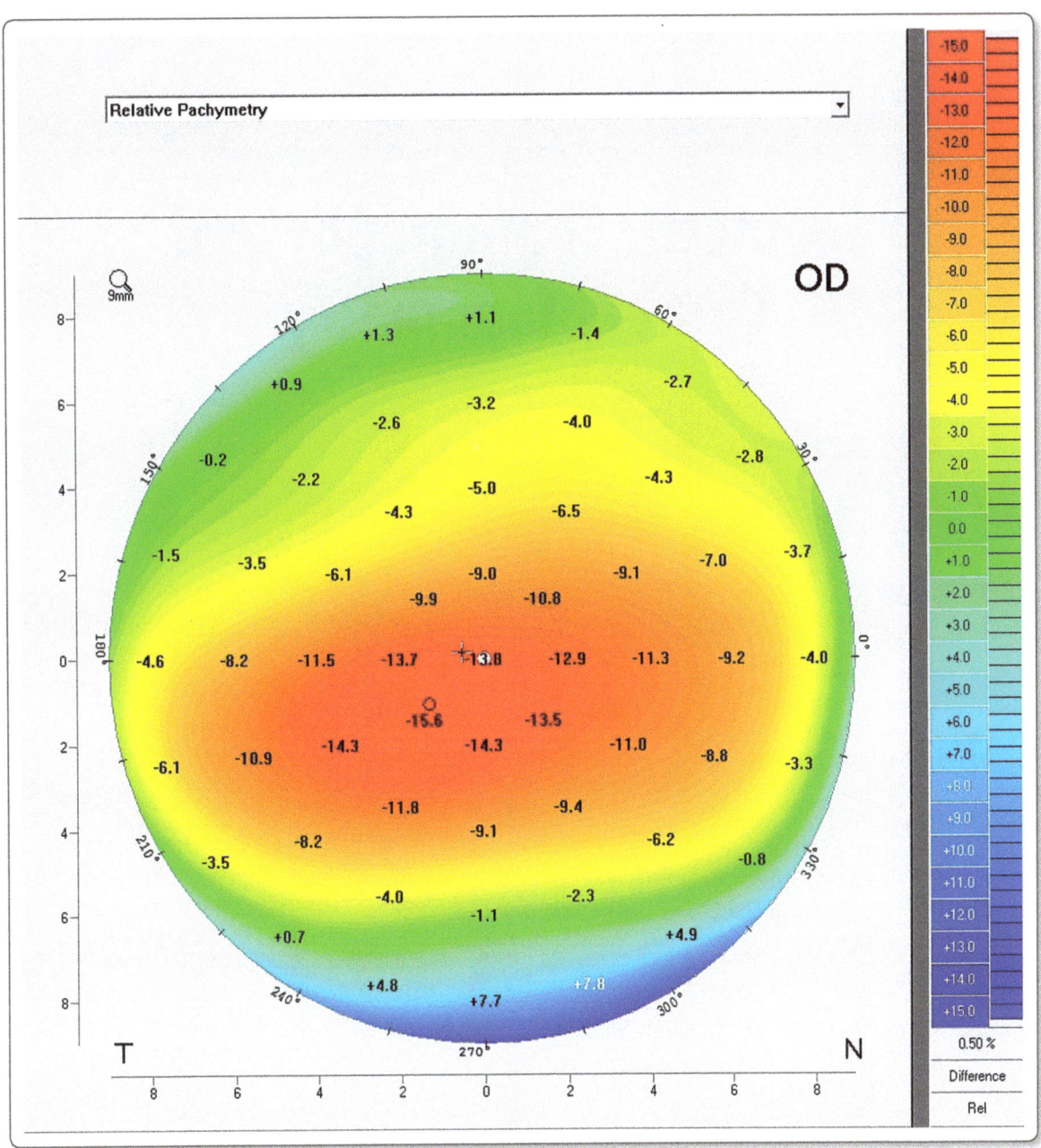

Fig. 8.21: Abnormal relative thickness map.

CHAPTER 9

Geometric Tomography and Corneal Topometry

INTRODUCTION

As mentioned in Chapter 1, corneal shape is "conoidal" (refer Fig. 1.3). It is a composition of toricity, asphericity and asymmetry. From a meridional viewpoint, the cornea is "toric", which is the source of corneal astigmatism. From the zonal viewpoint, the cornea is "aspheric" because the radius of curvature differs between the center and the periphery. From a sectorial viewpoint, the cornea is asymmetric because the nasal sector is usually flatter than the temporal sector. In this chapter, toricity, asphericity and asymmetry will be discussed from curvature and elevation viewpoints.

CORNEAL TORICITY

The cornea is toric because its base is an ellipse. In children and adults, the vertical diameter of the base is larger than the horizontal diameter. In adults, the vertical diameter is 10.6 mm, while the horizontal diameter is 11.7 mm in average. As the eye becomes older in age, the diameters flip so that the vertical becomes larger than the horizontal. This toricity has its effect on both the curvature and the elevation maps.

Corneal Toricity on the Curvature Maps

Corneal toricity is the source of corneal astigmatism. In children and adults, the astigmatism is with-the-rule (WTR) because the vertical meridian is steeper than the horizontal meridian. In older population, the astigmatism is usually against-the-rule (ATR) because the vertical meridian becomes flatter than the horizontal meridian. When WTR or ATR astigmatism is significant (≥1D), the curvature map will show the bowtie pattern. In WTR astigmatism, the bowtie is vertical, while in ATR astigmatism, it is horizontal. In some cases, the astigmatism is oblique and the bowtie is oblique (refer Figs. 5.17 to 5.20).

Corneal Toricity on the Elevation Maps

Corneal toricity is seen on elevation maps when the best-fit-sphere (BFS) is used as a reference surface (RS). In case of significant corneal astigmatism (≥1D), the hourglass pattern is encountered. This pattern results from the difference in radius of curvature between the steep and the flat corneal meridians. The flat meridian is located above the RS, while the steep is located below (refer Fig. 6.4). This is why the steep meridian is plotted in negative values and coded in cold colors. The hourglass is oriented vertically, horizontally or obliquely in WTR, ATR or oblique astigmatism, respectively (refer Figs. 6.6 to 6.8).

CORNEAL ASPHERICITY

The cornea is not a piece of a sphere; it has an aspherical shape. Corneal asphericity results from the difference in radius of curvature among corneal zones (Fig. 9.1).

Corneal asphericity is measured by a number of values, such as numeric eccentricity (e), corneal shape factor, p-value and Q-value. The mathematical relationship between these values is beyond the scope of this book. However, the most commonly used value to describe corneal asphericity is Q-value.

Chapter 9: Geometric Tomography and Corneal Topometry

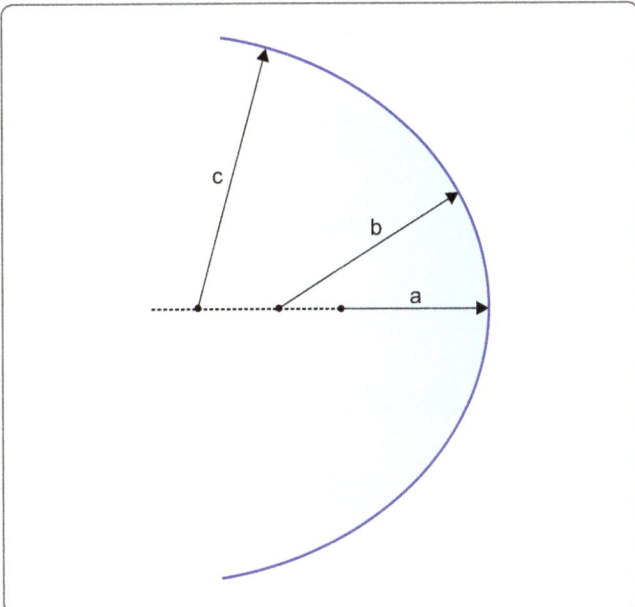

Fig. 9.1: Corneal asphericity.

Patterns of Asphericity

There are three main aspheric shapes: oblate, prolate and hyperprolate.

In the *spherical surface*, the radii of curvature are equal at all points. As a result, all curvature readings are also equal. The peripheral incident light rays on a sphere are refracted more than the axial and paraxial rays because the angle of incidence (and consequently the angle of refraction) at the periphery is larger than that around the center. Consequently, the refracted rays are unfocused leading to what is known as spherical aberration (SA) (refer Fig. 5.1). In this shape, Q-value = 0.00.

1. In the *oblate surface*, the radii of curvature become smaller toward the periphery, and consequently the refractive power increases toward the periphery. In other words, the center is flatter than the periphery. This increases the problem of large angle of incidence at the periphery, inducing more SA (refer Fig. 5.2). This shape is encountered after myopic keratorefractive procedures. In this shape, Q-value is >0.00.
2. In the *prolate surface*, the radii of curvature increase toward the periphery, therefore the refractive power at the periphery is smaller than that at the center. In this shape, the cornea is steeper at the center than at periphery. This compensates for the larger angle of incidence at the periphery, leading the rays to be focused with the least amount of defocus; i.e. minimum tolerable SA. The normal cornea has a prolate shape. In this shape, Q-value is between 0 and –1 (see Fig. 5.3).
3. The *hyperprolate surface* is an exaggeration of the prolate surface. The incident rays are defocused due to the big difference in radii between the center and the periphery, inducing SA (refer Fig. 5.4). This shape is encountered in ectatic corneal diseases (ECDs) and after hypermetropic keratorefractive procedures. In this shape, Q-value is ≤–1 (e.g. –1.2, etc.).

Spherical Aberration

Spherical aberration results from abnormal Q-value. It usually affects peripheral vision, affects measurements of sphere, and results in halos around oncoming lights. The Q-value at which all rays are focused in one point (no SA) is –0.53 (refer Fig. 5.5). When Q-value is > –0.53 (more positive), positive SA is encountered. When Q-value is < –0.53 (more negative), negative SA is found. In normal population, Q-value ranges between -0.10 and -0.30, and is almost –0.27 on average. This means that in normal population, the cornea has positive SA. SA is discussed in detail in Chapter 14.

The Effect of Corneal Asphericity on Refraction

Corneal asphericity affects cycloplegic refraction when refracting the patient by retinoscopy. Due to the difference in power between central and peripheral cornea, the light reflex through the dilated pupil shows a paradoxical movement, e.g. central segment with while peripheral segments against. Therefore, it is recommended to focus on and consider the movement of only the central segment.

The Effect of Corneal Asphericity on Vision

The effect of corneal asphericity on vision differs according to the status of refraction:
- Corneal asphericity in emmetropia:
  - If Q >–0.53 (more positive), positive SA is present. When the eye is refracted in dim light (larger pupil size), it shows an amount of hypermetropia.
  - If Q = –0.53, no SA is present. The eye is emmetropic in both scotopic and photopic light conditions.
  - If Q <–0.53 (more negative), negative SA is present. When the eye is refracted in dim light (larger pupil size), it shows an amount of myopia. This explains why some people suffer from myopia at night.

- Corneal asphericity in myopia:
  - If Q > –0.53 (more positive), positive SA is present. When the eye is refracted in dim light (larger pupil size), it shows less myopia (hypermetropic shift).
  - If Q = –0.53, no SA is present. The eye has the same amount of myopia in both scotopic and photopic light conditions.
  - If Q < –0.53 (more negative), negative SA is present. When the eye is refracted in dim light (larger pupil size), it shows larger amount of myopia (myopic shift). This explains why the symptoms of some myopic people exaggerate at night.
- Corneal asphericity in hypermetropia:
  - If Q > –0.53 (more positive), positive SA is present. When the eye is refracted in dim light (larger pupil size), it shows larger amount of hypermetropia (hypermetropic shift).
  - If Q = –0.53, no SA is present. The eye has the same amount of hypermetropia in both scotopic and photopic light conditions.
  - If Q < –0.53 (more negative), negative SA is present. When the eye is refracted in dim light (larger pupil size), it shows less amount of hypermetropia (myopic shift).

Corneal Asphericity on the Curvature Maps

- In *spherical* corneas, the curvature maps show similar K-readings at every point. In other words, the difference between K-readings all over the cornea is less than 1D, and the difference between Sim-Ks and Kmax is less than 1D as well (Fig. 9.2).
- In *prolate* and *hyperprolate* corneas, the center is steeper than the periphery. Therefore, the concentric color zones show progressive cooling toward the periphery (Fig. 9.3).
- In *oblate* corneas, the center is flatter than the periphery, and the concentric color zones show progressive warming of colors toward the periphery (Fig. 9.4).

In all cases, the gradient of color is proportional to Q-value.

Corneal Asphericity on the Elevation Maps

When the BFS RS in the *float* mode and a 5-μm color scale are used:
- The *spherical* cornea shows an almost homogeneous green color because it is consistent with the RS, especially

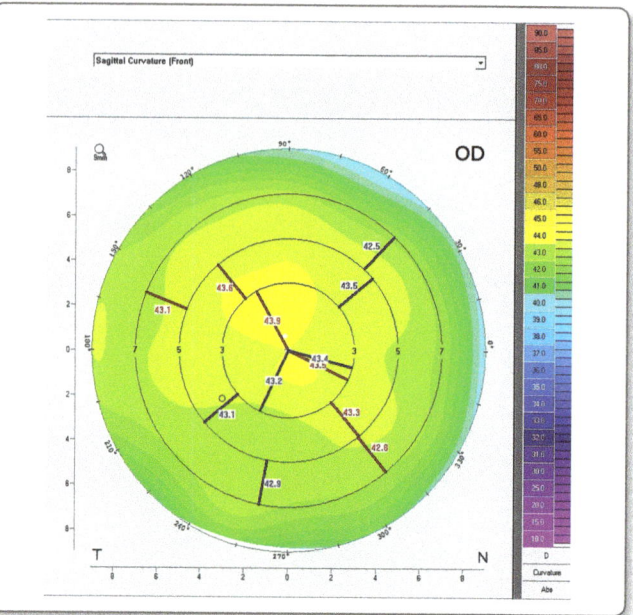

Fig. 9.2: Curvature pattern in spherical cornea.

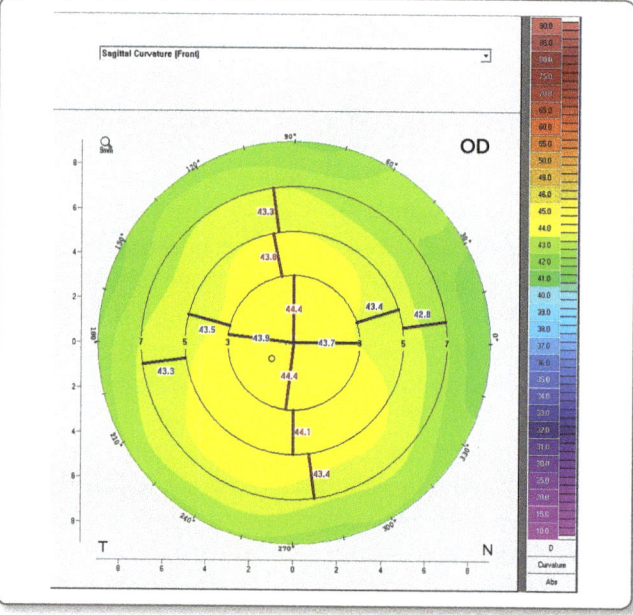

Fig. 9.3: Curvature pattern in prolate cornea.

in the center and mid-periphery (Fig. 9.5). The periphery may show different colors due to the difference between corneal diameter and the diameter of the used zone of the BFS (standard 8 mm).
- The *prolate* and *hyperprolate* corneas show central yellow protrusion, which is the central portion of the cornea that is above the RS (Fig. 9.6). The more negative the Q-value, the larger the protrusion and the larger the plus numbers within it.

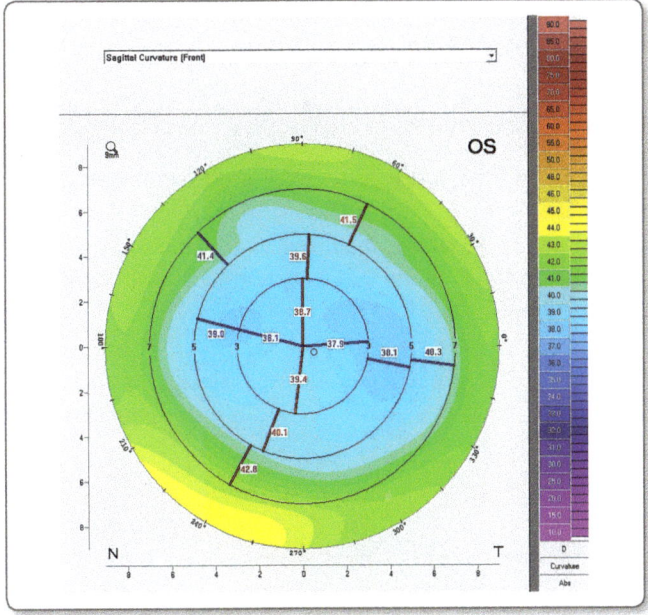

Fig. 9.4: Curvature pattern in oblate cornea.

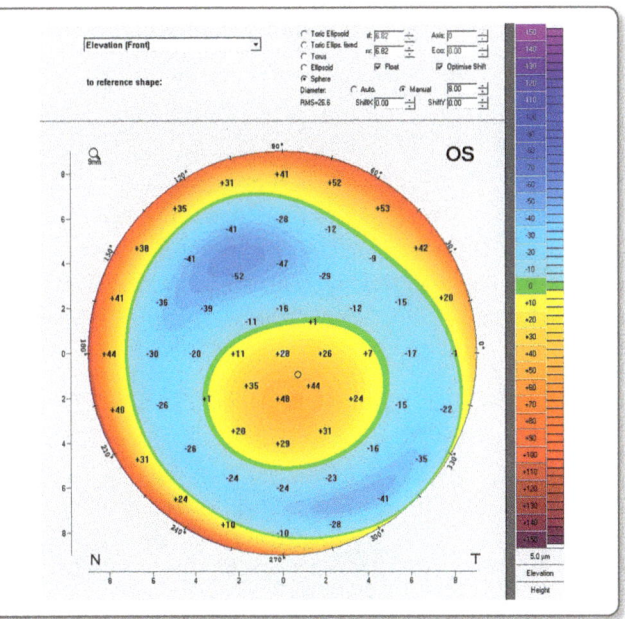

Fig. 9.6: Elevation pattern in prolate and hyperprolate cornea.

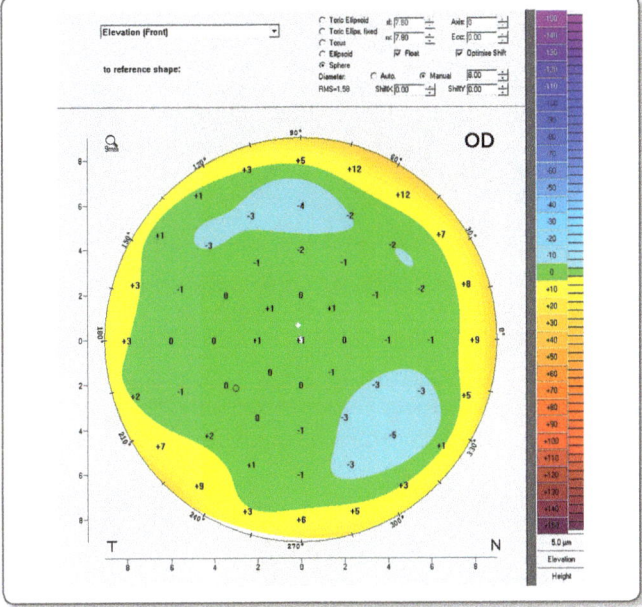

Fig. 9.5: Elevation pattern in spherical cornea.

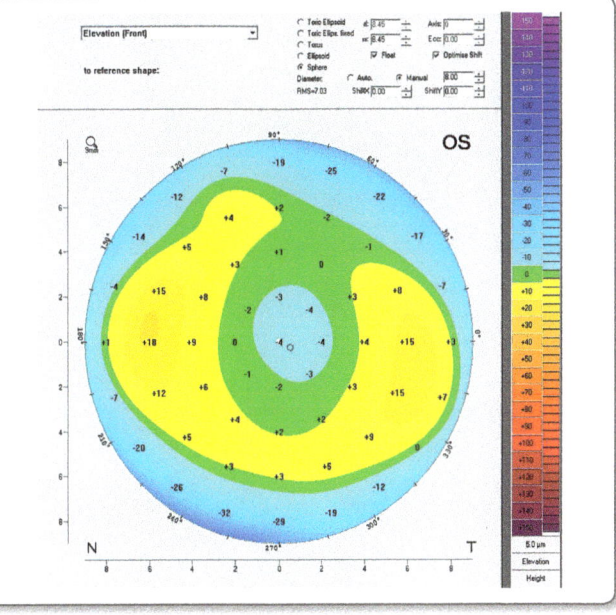

Fig. 9.7: Elevation pattern in oblate cornea.

- The *oblate* cornea shows a flat blue central island with minus values because corneal center is flat and below the RS (Fig. 9.7). The central blue zone is surrounded by a green paraxial ring which represents the intersection between the cornea and the RS. That is surrounded by yellow or red colors with plus values representing corneal periphery that is above the RS because the periphery is steeper than the center in the oblate cornea.

CORNEAL ASYMMETRY

The normal cornea is horizontally asymmetric. It flattens progressively from center to periphery, with the nasal portion being flattening slightly more than the temporal portion.

Corneal Asymmetry on Curvature Maps

- In the normal cornea, corneal asymmetry appears as colder colors in the nasal versus the temporal sectors of the cornea (refer Fig. 1.4).
- In ECDs, the asymmetry is higher than normal and is usually vertical or oblique rather than horizontal (Fig. 9.8). As the ECDs progress, the asymmetry combines with the hyperprolate asphericity, inducing the off-center conic pattern, characteristic of ECDs (Fig. 9.9).

Corneal asymmetry is one of the most important indices to detect early ECDs.

Corneal Asymmetry on Elevation Maps

When the BFS RS in the *float* mode and a 5-μm color scale are used:

- In the normal cornea, the horizontal corneal asymmetry is responsible for the slight temporal skewing or temporal decentration (Fig. 9.10).

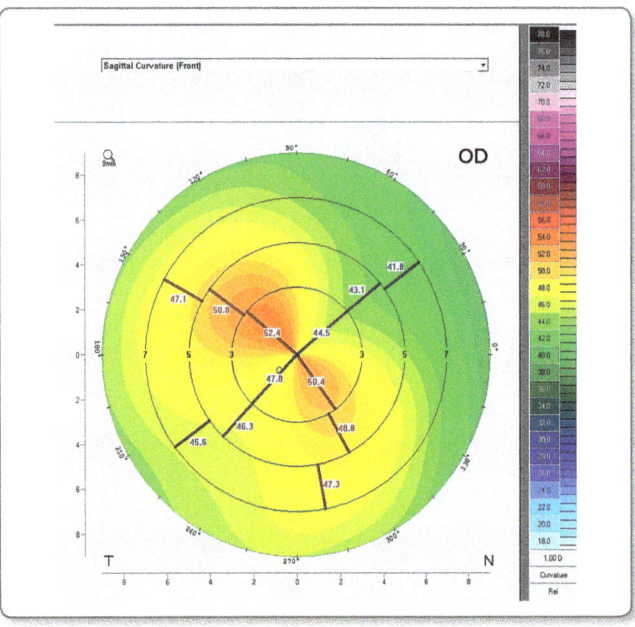

Fig. 9.8: Curvature asymmetry in ectatic corneal diseases.

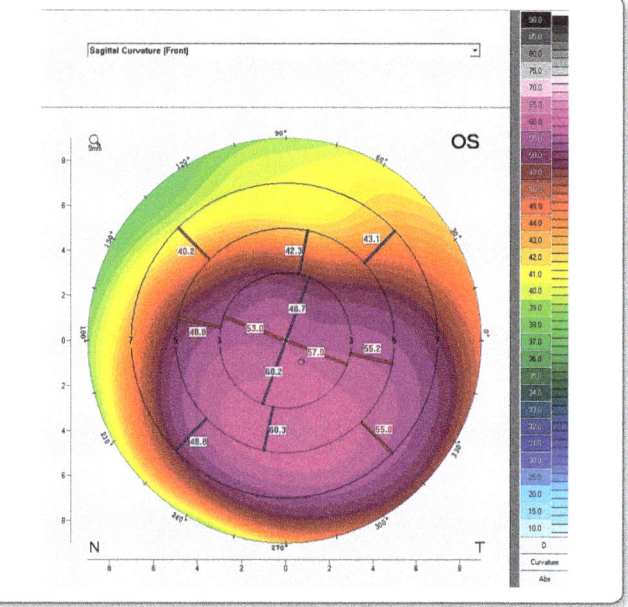

Fig. 9.9: Off-center conic pattern in ectatic corneal diseases.

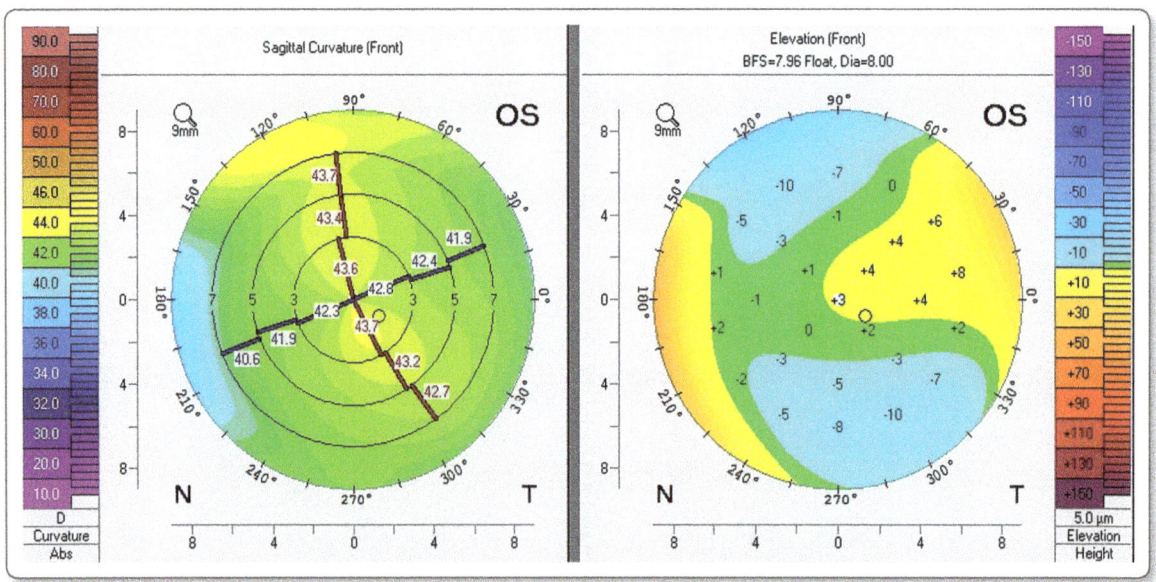

Fig. 9.10: Horizontal corneal asymmetry in normal cornea.

Chapter 9: Geometric Tomography and Corneal Topometry

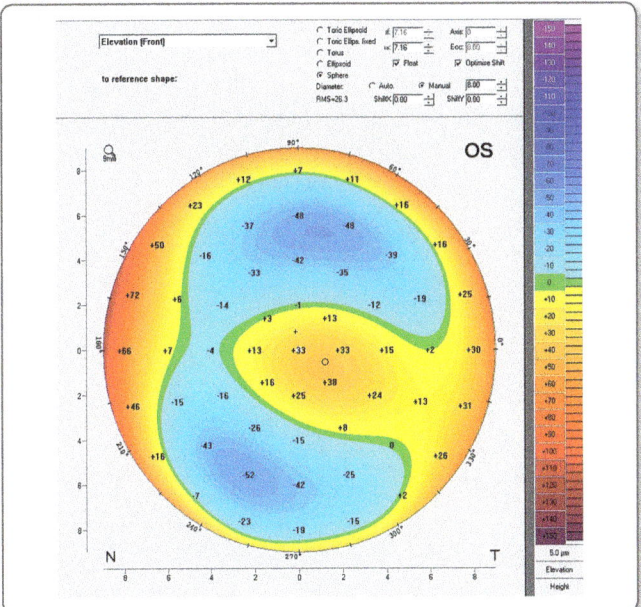

Fig. 9.11: Corneal asymmetry in ectatic corneal diseases—tongue-like extension.

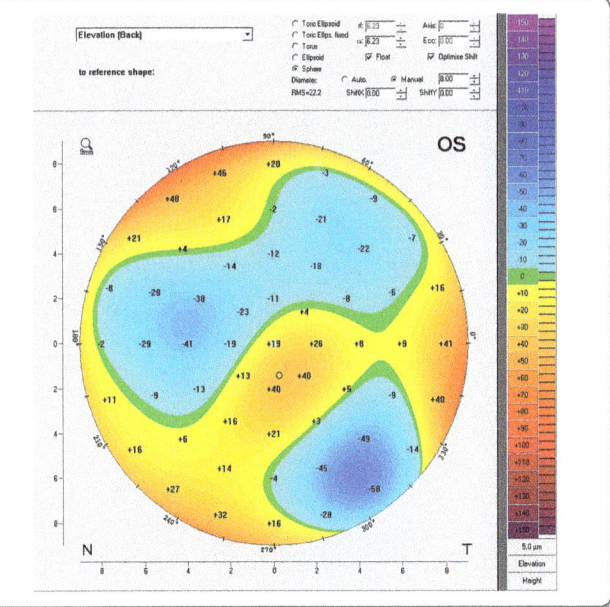

Fig. 9.12: Corneal asymmetry in ectatic corneal diseases—segmental asymmetry.

- In the ECDs, corneal asymmetry is usually vertical or oblique. In all cases, the asymmetry appears as overskewed hourglass, tongue-like extension or segmental asymmetry as shown in Figures 9.11 and 9.12.

To differentiate these patterns from misalignment or large angle kappa, values corresponding to the thinnest location should be considered. In ECDs, the values are abnormal.

SECTION 3

Understanding Corneal Refraction

SECTION OUTLINE

10. Corneal Astigmatism
11. Objective Corneal Dioptric Power
12. Astigmatic Dissociation

Corneal Astigmatism

DEFINITIONS AND CLASSIFICATIONS OF ASTIGMATISM

Astigmatism is a term that was first introduced by Thomas Young in the early 1800s. It refers to the refractive error in which there is a difference in the power of refraction between different meridians. It occurs whenever any one of the refracting surfaces in the optical system assumes a toric shape. Therefore, it can be of corneal origin, intraocular origin, or both.

There are two types of astigmatism, regular and irregular.

Regular Astigmatism

In regular astigmatism, there are two principle meridians, one is of minimum power (minimum curvature or flattest) and the other is of maximum power (maximum curvature or steepest). The steepest and flattest meridians are perpendicular to each other. As mentioned in Chapter 5, the tomographic presentation of regular astigmatism is symmetric bowtie on the curvature maps and symmetric hourglass on the elevation maps.

Regular astigmatism is described by five criteria (Fig. 10.1):

1. There is only one flattest meridian and one steepest meridian.
2. The two meridians are at right angles.
3. The gradient of power between the two meridians is similar in all sectors.
4. It induces astigmatic lower-order aberration (LOA).
5. It is corrected by a spherocylindric lens.

If the optical system has regular astigmatism, the image of a point source at infinity is not focused at one point, it is distributed between two principal linear images, one is generated by, and parallel to, the principal meridian of maximum power of refraction, and the other one is generated by, and parallel to, the principal meridian of minimum power of refraction. The interval that is bracketed by these two linear images is referred to as the interval of Sturm. Within this interval, the circle of least confusion is located at the plane where the vertical and horizontal meridians are equally defocused. Images generated by other meridians are distributed along the interval of Sturm (Fig. 10.2).

Based on the relationship between the formed images and the retina (location-based), or on the position of the refracting meridians (meridian-based), regular astigmatism can further be subclassified into:

- *Location-based:*
  - *Simple astigmatism*: When one of the two principal linear images falls on the retina.
    - If the other image falls in front of the retina, it is described by "simple myopic astigmatism". It induces astigmatic LOA (Chapter 14) and is corrected by a minus cylindric lens.
    - If the other image virtually falls behind the retina, it is described by "simple hypermetropic astigmatism". It induces astigmatic LOA (Chapter 14) and is corrected by a positive cylindric lens.
  - *Compound astigmatism*: When both principal linear images fall on same side in relation with the retina.
    - If they fall in front of the retina, it is described by "compound myopic astigmatism". It is a combination of myopia and simple myopic astigmatism. Therefore, it induces defocus because of myopia and astigmatic LOA because of the astigmatism component (Chapter 14). This type is corrected by a minus spherocylindric lens.

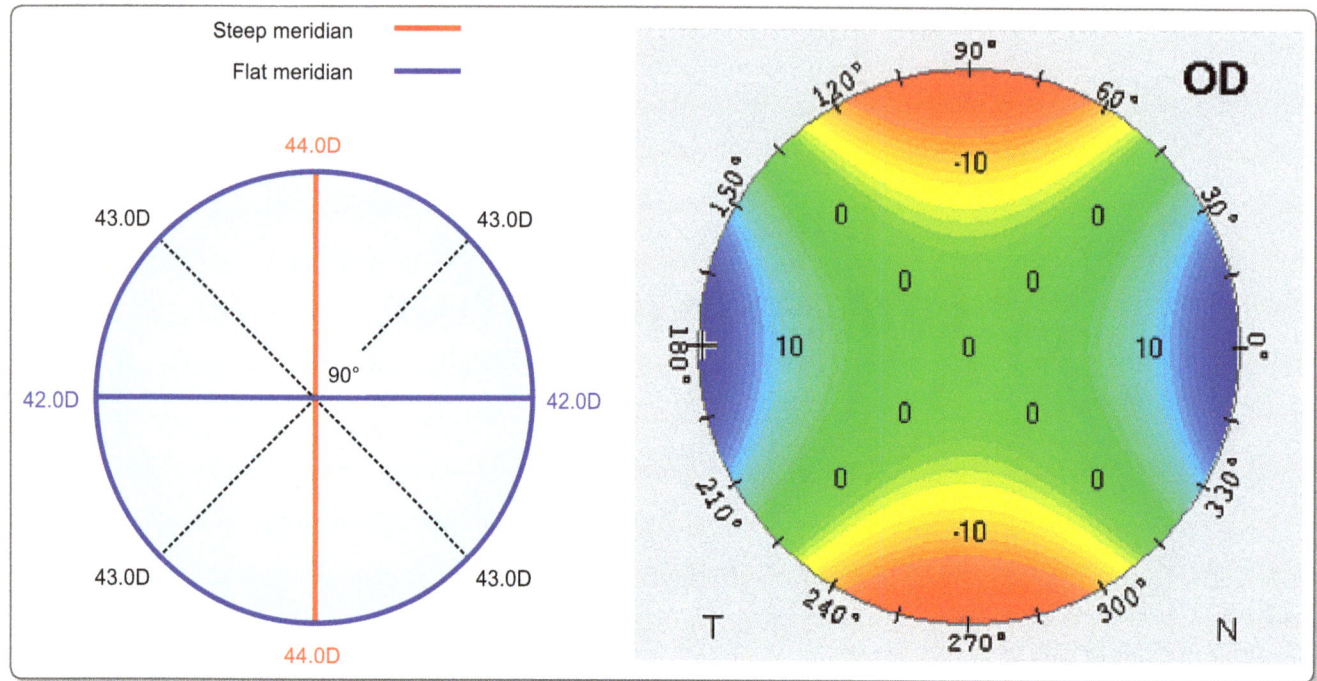

Fig. 10.1: Regular astigmatism.

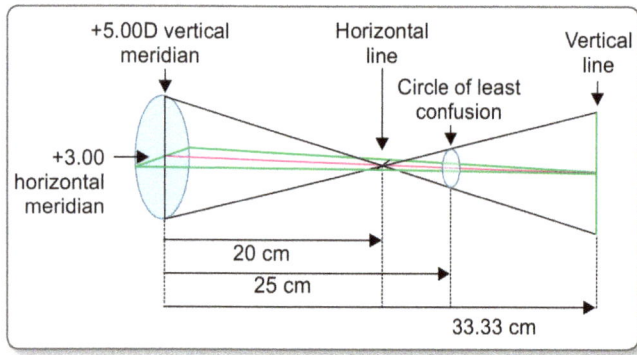

Fig. 10.2: The interval of Sturm.

- If they virtually fall behind the retina, it is described by "compound hypermetropic astigmatism". It is a combination of hypermetropia and simple hypermetropic astigmatism. Therefore, it induces defocus because of hypermetropia and astigmatic LOA because of the astigmatic component (Chapter 14). This type is corrected by a positive spherocylindric lens.
- *Mixed astigmatism*: It occurs when one of the principal linear images falls in front of, and the other one virtually falls behind, the retina. Depending on the sign of the equation used, it can be considered either as a combination of hypermetropia and simple myopic astigmatism, or as a combination of myopia and simple hypermetropic astigmatism. It induces defocus and astigmatic LOA (Chapter 14), and can either be corrected by a minus spherical lens combined with a plus cylindric lens, or by a plus spherical lens combined with a minus cylindric lens.
- *Meridian-based*:
  - *With-the-rule astigmatism (WTR)*: When the meridian of maximum power of refraction is within 90° ± 30° (refer Figs. 5.17 and 5.20). In this type, the vertical image formed by this meridian is frontal to the horizontal one.
  - *Against-the-rule astigmatism (ATR)*: When the meridian of maximum power of refraction is within 180° ± 30° (refer Figs. 5.18 and 5.20). In this type, the horizontal image formed by this meridian is frontal to the vertical one.
  - *Oblique astigmatism*: When the two principle meridians are neither vertical nor horizontal (refer Figs. 5.19 and 5.20).

Irregular Astigmatism

Irregular astigmatism occurs when the orientation of the principal meridians changes from one point to another across the pupil, or when the amount of astigmatism changes from one meridian to another. Based on that, irregular astigmatism is described by five criteria:

1. There might be more than one steep meridians or semimeridians, and are not at right angles.
2. There might be more than one flat meridians or semimeridians, and are not at right angles.
3. The gradient of power between and along the meridians may or may not be similar in all sectors.
4. It induces higher-order aberrations (HOAs).
5. It cannot be corrected by a spherocylindric lens.

Based on the relationship among the meridians or semimeridians, irregular astigmatism can further be subclassified into regularly irregular astigmatism (periodic), irregularly irregular astigmatism (nonperiodic), and a combination of both (mixed irregular astigmatism).

Periodic Irregular Astigmatism

It is characterized by (Fig. 10.3):
- Two or more similar flat meridians and two or more similar steep meridians.
- The angle between meridians is periodic and of same angular frequency.
- The gradient of power between the meridians is regular in a periodic angular frequency.
- It cannot be corrected by a spherocylindric lens.
- This type of astigmatism induces peripheral HOAs that usually affect night vision.
- Based on the change in the gradient of refractive power along every meridian, this type is subclassified into *simple periodic* and *mixed periodic*.

- Based on the number of the similar meridians, there are six subtypes of the *simple periodic*, inducing six types of HOAs; they are—(1) trefoil, (2) tetrafoil, (3) pentafoil, (4) hexafoil, (5) heptafoil, and (6) octafoil. These HOAs affect peripheral (night) vision, causing starbursts images.
- Based on the number of the similar meridians, there are nine subtypes of the *mixed periodic*, inducing nine types of HOAs; they are—(1) secondary astigmatism, (2) tertiary astigmatism, (3) quaternary astigmatism, (4) secondary trefoil, (5) tertiary trefoil, (6) secondary tetrafoil, (7) tertiary tetrafoil, (8) secondary pentafoil, and (9) secondary hexafoil. These HOAs affect central and peripheral vision, causing starbursts images with ghost images.

All the above expressions and their criteria are explained in detail in Chapter 14.

Nonperiodic Irregular Astigmatism

It is characterized by (Fig. 10.4):
- Two meridians at right angles.
- The gradient of power between the two meridians is irregular.
- The gradient of power along one of the two meridians is regular, while it is irregular along the other one.
- This type of astigmatism induces central HOA that affects central vision, inducing ghost images.
- It cannot be corrected by a spherocylindric lens.

Based on the severity of irregularity along the irregular meridian, there are three subtypes, inducing three types of HOAs; they are—(1) coma, (2) secondary coma, and (3) tertiary coma.

All the above expressions and their criteria are explained in detail in Chapter 14.

Mixed Irregular Astigmatism (Fig. 10.5)

This is the most common type of irregular astigmatism. This type is a combination of the previous two types. It represents a variety of mixed unclassified irregular irregularities, inducing a mixture of HOAs.

All the above expressions and criteria are explained in detail in Chapter 14.

ETIOLOGY OF IRREGULAR ASTIGMATISM

Irregular astigmatism can be of intraocular origin or corneal origin.

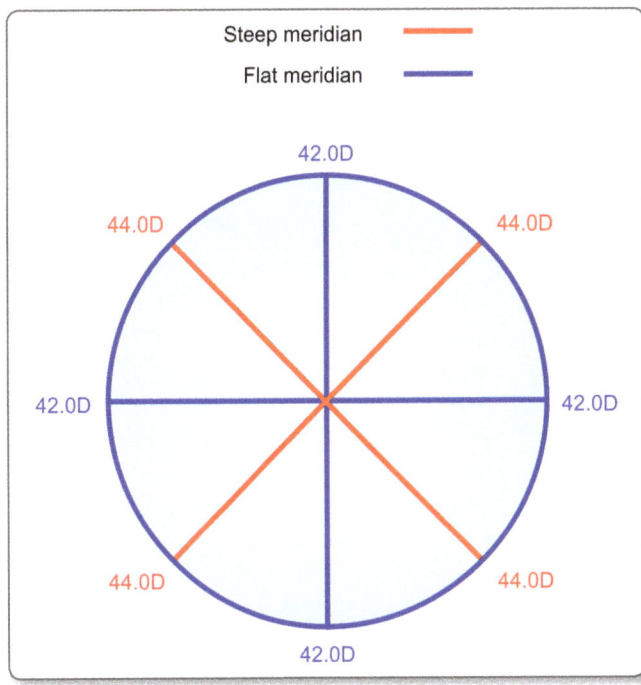

Fig. 10.3: Periodic irregular astigmatism.

Section 3: *Understanding Corneal Refraction*

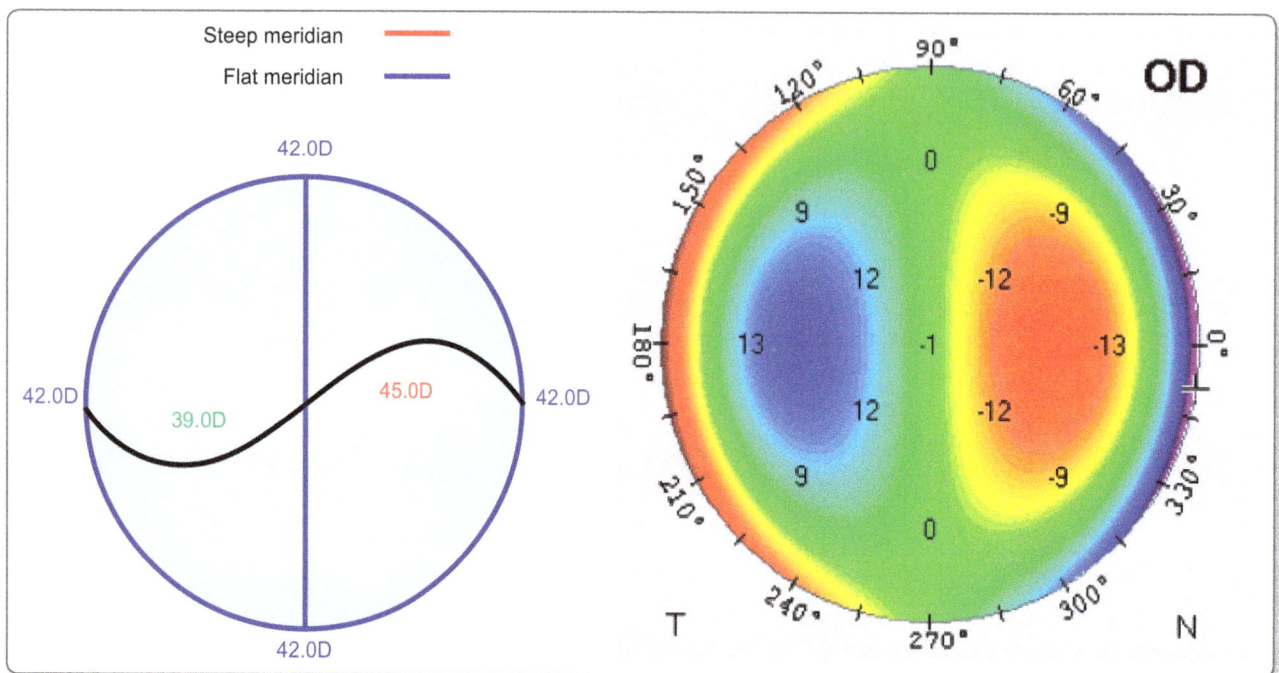

Fig. 10.4: Nonperiodic irregular astigmatism.

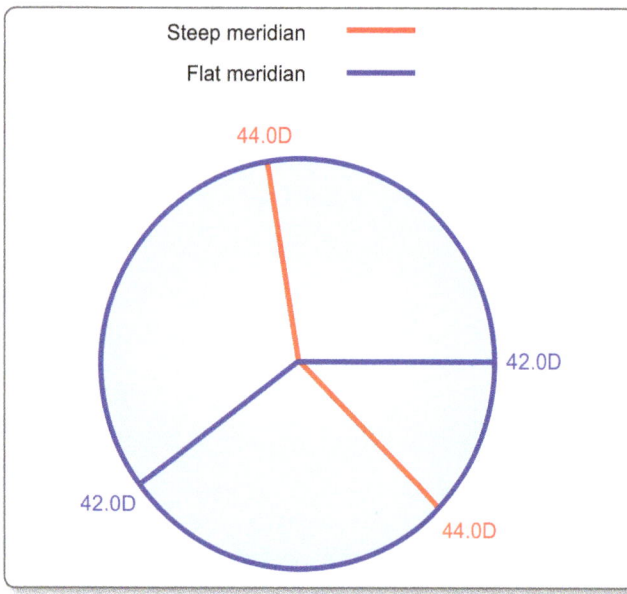

Fig. 10.5: Mixed irregular astigmatism.

Intraocular-induced Irregular Astigmatism

This type can either be induced by the crystalline lens, phakic intraocular lens (PIOL), or pseudophakic IOL.
- *Crystalline lens:* Irregular astigmatism is induced by crystalline lens subluxation.
- *Phakic intraocular lens and pseudophakic IOL:* Irregular astigmatism is induced by IOL decentration, tilting, or subluxation.

Corneal-induced Irregular Astigmatism

This is the most common source of irregular astigmatism. It can be classified into ectatic and nonectatic.

Ectatic Corneal Irregular Astigmatism

Ectatic corneal diseases are discussed in detail in Chapter 19.

Nonectatic Corneal Irregular Astigmatism

Irregular astigmatism may be induced by surgical interventions or trauma, or related to corneal pathologies.
- *Surgically induced*: Irregular astigmatism can be induced by keratorefractive procedures and keratoplasty.
  - *Keratorefractive procedures:* They include radial keratotomy (RK) and laser vision correction (LVC).
    ♦ *Radial keratotomy*: Healing of the incisions is usually very slow and unpredictable. Due to irregular fibrous tissue formation and epithelial inclusions, central asymmetric flattening occurs. Vision disturbance and glare are more pronounced when the incisions are eight and more, the incisions extend within the central 3 mm zone, or when there is hypertrophic scarring.

- *Laser vision correction*: LVC consists of—(1) surface ablation (PRK: photo refractive keratectomy, Trans-PRK: trans epithelial photo refractive keratectomy, LASEK: laser subepithelial keratomileusis, and Epi-LASIK: epipolis laser *in situ* keratomileusis), (2) lamellar ablation (LASIK: Laser *in Situ* keratomileusis, Femto-LASIK: femtosecond laser *in situ* keratomileusis, SBK: sub-Bowman keratomileusis), and (3) small incision lenticule extraction (SMILE).

Corneal irregularities can generally result from LVC due pre-, intra-, or post-operative factors.

- *Preoperative factors*: Irregular corneal tomography; bad calibration; and bad laser suite conditions, such as improper room humidity and poor quality of room air.
- *Intraoperative factors*:
  - *Surface ablation:* Stromal incursions during mechanical epithelial removal, improper laser dynamics, central blockage of the laser treatment by the laser plume, poor or decentered alignment during laser ablation, poor laser calibration leading to steep islands or decentered zones, poor cyclotorsion compensation in astigmatic treatment, and liquid accumulation on the corneal bed.
  - *Lamellar ablation*: Complications during the flap creation such as an incomplete flap, irregular flap, free flap, and button-hole flap; and ablating the inner surface of the flap hinge and out-of-bed ablation. This commonly occurs in hypermetropic treatments and can be avoided by proper pupil offset technique and proper centralization of the flap with the 1st Purkinje image.
- *Postoperative factors:*
  - *Surface ablation*: Poor wound healing response, delayed epithelialization, haze, scarring, and dry eye.
  - *Lamellar ablation*: Complications such as interface debris, epithelial ingrowth, diffuse lamellar keratitis (DLK), central toxic keratopathy (CTK), distorted and dislocated flap, macrostriae, dry eye, and corneal melting or scarring.

In addition, corneal irregularities resulting from LVC can be classified into Macro-Irregular and Micro-Irregular Patterns. The former is usually due to decentration and the latter is usually due to flap complications. However, a mixture of both is very common.

Macroirregular pattern: The main source for visual disability is an area larger than 2 mm steeper or flatter than the surrounding area. There are two types—(1) decentration and (2) a central island.

1. *Decentered ablated zone (Fig. 10.6)*: It is defined as an unintentional asymmetric alteration in the optical system of the eye. The main reasons are misalignment, uneven uptake, or uneven emission of laser energy, or asymmetric or abnormal wound healing. It is best evaluated by the elevation maps and the tangential curvature map rather than the sagittal curvature map due to the difference between the reference axis of the sagittal map, line of sight, and corneal apex. Decentration induces HOAs, particularly coma.
2. *Central island*: It is a central area that measures more than 1 mm in size and has a relatively different steepness from the surrounding by more than 1D in power and does not extend to the periphery. It may be flatter (Fig. 10.7) or steeper (Fig. 10.8) than the periphery. In both cases, it results in night glare if it is smaller than the mesopic pupil. The etiology is multifactorial, including wound healing process, pupil size, amount of correction, ablation diameter and profile, quality of the ablation, and quality of the flap. Central island induces positive spherical aberrations if it is flat and negative spherical aberrations, if it is steep.

Microirregular pattern: It is defined as discrete irregularities, not specifically creating a well-defined steeper or flatter area of the cornea. This pattern may resemble para ectasia pattern (Chapter 22); therefore, history taking is a very important key factor.

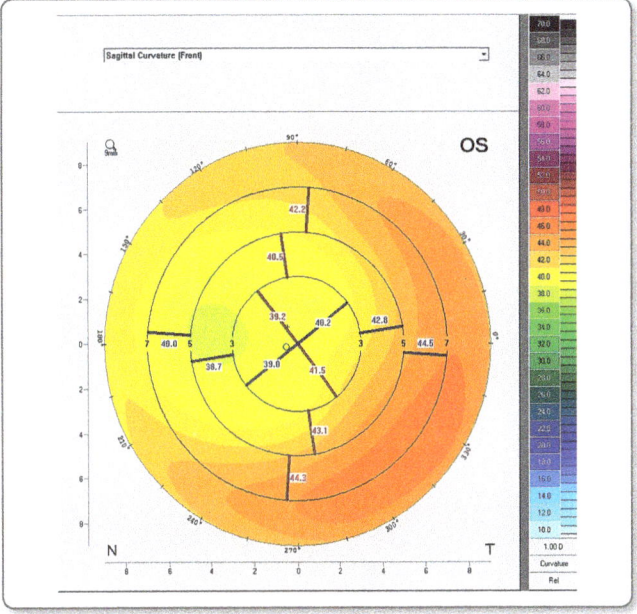

Fig. 10.6: Decentered ablated zone.

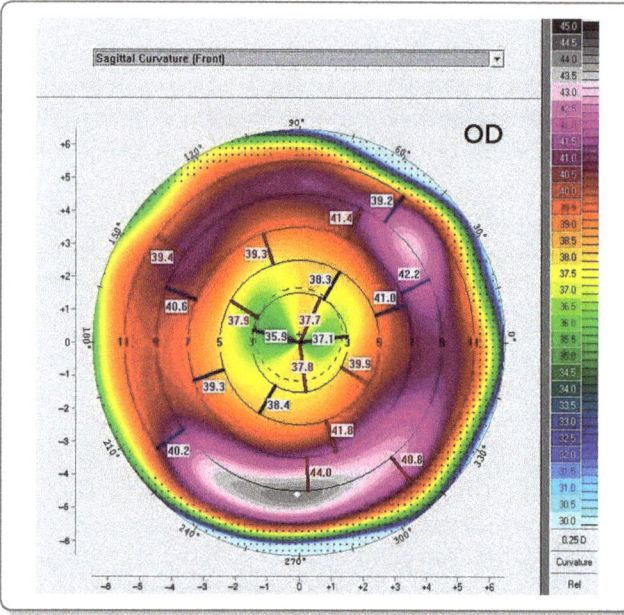

Fig. 10.7: Central flat island.

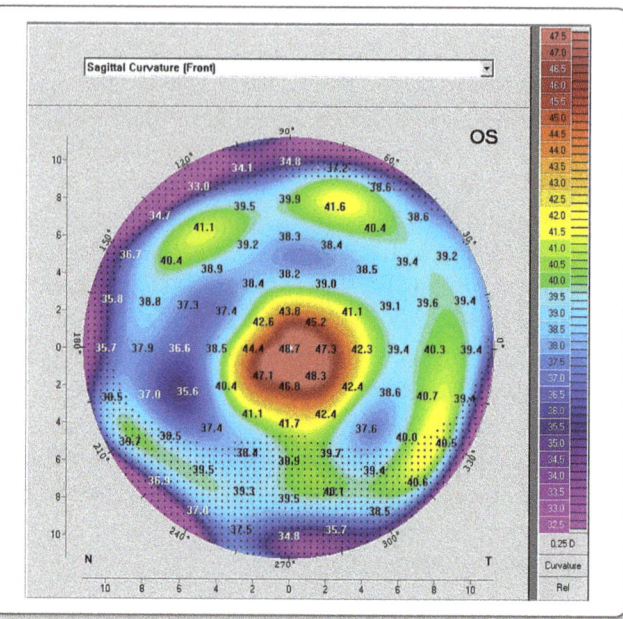

Fig. 10.8: Central steep island.

Moreover, corneal irregularities induced by LVC can be graded into four grades based on their clinical impact. Table 10.1 represents the clinical grading of post-LVC corneal irregularities.

- *Keratoplasty:*
  - *Penetrating keratoplasty (PKP):* PKP induces irregular astigmatism due to the following determinants:
    ◆ *Preoperative determinants:* Donor age, size of recipient's cornea, and pathologic properties of the recipient's cornea such as peripheral thinning or ectasia, focal edema or scar, defects of Bowman's layer, degree of vascularization, and previous PKP or other corneal surgery.
    ◆ *Intraoperative determinants:* Decentration of donor and/or recipient trephination; "vertical tilt" due to discrepancies of wound configuration, application of different trephination techniques in donor and recipient, tilt of the trephine away from the optical axis, limbal plane not horizontal, creation of steps due to change of trephination direction, high or low intraocular or intracameral pressure, and overlap of dehiscence due to vertical cut incongruence; "horizontal torsion" due to asymmetric placement of second cardinal suture and unfavorable alignment of the graft due to horizontal shape incongruence; excessive over or under sizing of the donor; distortion and squeezing of the cornea (for example, dull trephine); traumatizing of the cornea by surgical instruments; suture-related factors such as suture material, suture technique (single, running, double running, and combined),

Table 10.1: Grading of post-LVC corneal irregularities

Grade	Signs and symptoms
1	- Mild symptoms at night or daylight conditions - Loss of 1–2 lines of BCVA useful vision for reading, driving and walking - No disability for normal life, but with discomfort - No monocular diplopia - Ray tracing abnormal. Distortion = 2–8 μm - Aberrometry: RMS = 2–3 μm
2	- Moderate disability - Loss of 3–4 lines of BCVA - Reading and driving partially affected, especially in dim-light conditions - Some patients prefer not to use the eye - Moderate monocular diplopia - Ray tracing affected. Distortion = 8–14 μm - Aberrometry: RMS = 3–6 μm
3	- Severe disability - Eye not useful for visual performance - Loss of >5 lines of BCVA patients prefer not to use the eye - Reading and driving affected at light conditions - Severe monocular diplopia or polyopia - Ray-tracing disaster. Distortion > 14 μm - Aberrometry: RMS > 6 μm
4	- Eye not useful, legally blind - BCVA = 20/200 or less - Aberrometry, ray tracing, and topography not possible to capture due to the severity of irregularities

(BCVA: best corrected visual acuity; RMS: root mean square; LVC: laser vision correction)

suture length, suture angle relative to graft-host-junction, suture tension, and "depth disparity"; simultaneous intraocular interventions (triple procedures, IOL exchange, etc.); fixation rings and lid specula; and surgeon's experience.

- *Postoperative determinants*: Suture-related factors such as "cheese wiring" of sutures, suture loosening, suture adjustment or selective suture removal, timing of suture removal, and sequential or all-at-a-time suture removal; wound healing processes including wound dehiscence, retrocorneal membrane, incarceration of overlapping cut edges, and focal vascularization; medication (for example, corticosteroids); and postoperative trauma.

In addition, trephination can either be mechanical or non-mechanical (Femtosecond Laser). The latter is superior to the former in avoidance of trauma to intraocular tissues, avoidance of radial and tangential forces effecting tissue "squeezing", reduction of horizontal torsion (Erlangen orientation teeth), reduction of vertical tilt ("perfect" congruent cut surfaces of donor and recipient), and reduction of recipient and donor decentration.

- *Lamellar keratoplasty (LKP)*: What has been mentioned in PKP can be applied on LKP. However, some of the intraoperative determinants may have less impact in LKP in comparison with PKP.

Both PKP and LKP induce corneal irregularities. This can be due to sutures, especially if they were asymmetric, or even after suture removal, if it was uncontrolled by tomography. Figure 10.9 shows the orientation of corneal astigmatism on a corneal graft before suture removal. It shows a steep 120° meridian with high astigmatism. Figure 10.10 shows the new orientation of astigmatism after removal of the 120° sutures.

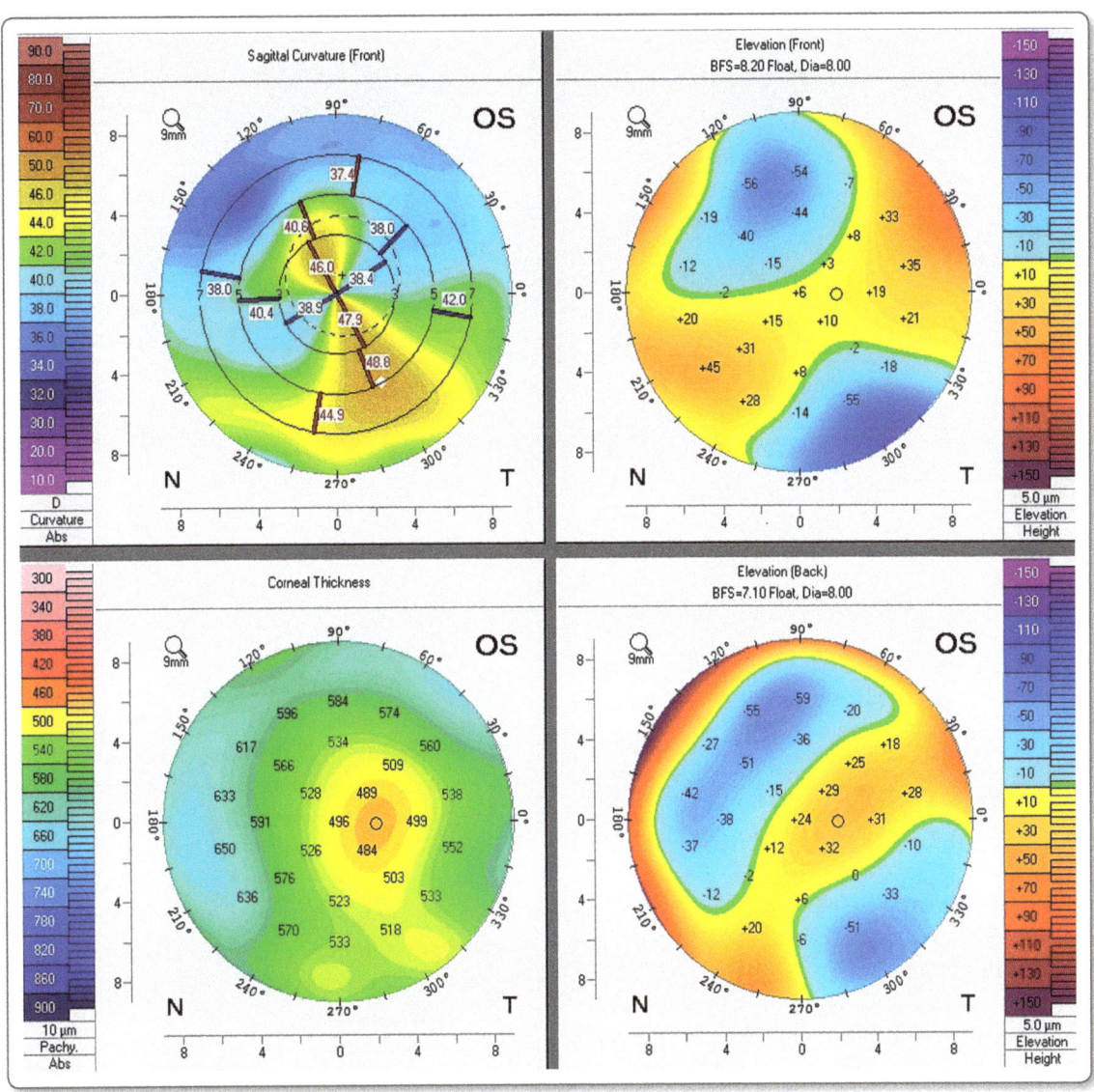

Fig. 10.9: Corneal graft before suture removal.

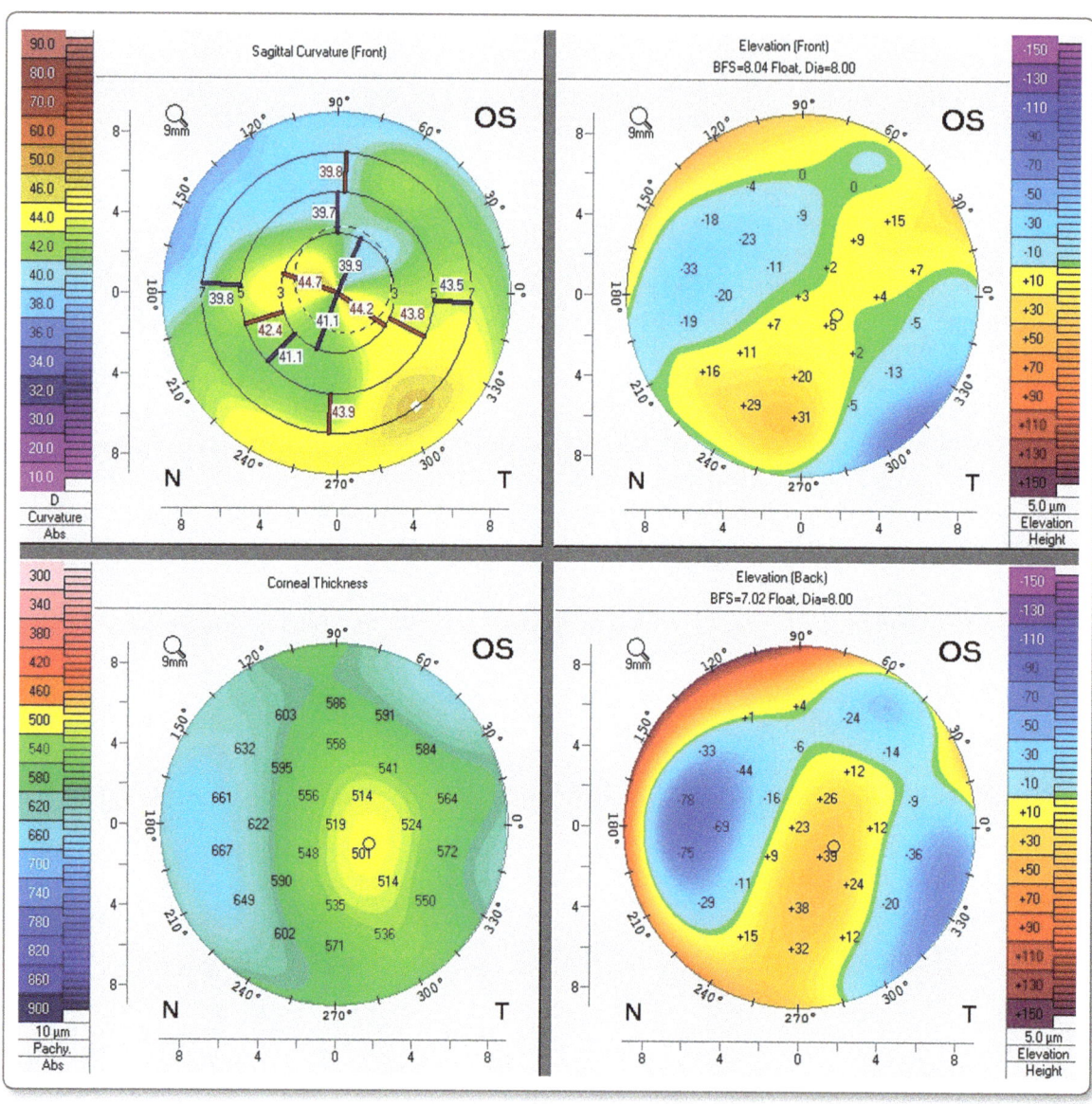

Fig. 10.10: Corneal graft after removal of the 120° sutures.

Traumatic

Corneal trauma may result in irregular astigmatism relative to the type of trauma and to the surgical technique used in the initial approach. Corneal wounds affect vision by two mechanisms—(1) scars across the visual axis and/or (2) scars inducing irregular astigmatism. The location, size, texture, and depth of the scar are all critical to the patient's visual potential.

Tomographic features of corneal scars differ according to their size, location, and density. In general, small scars cannot be detected by the quality specification (QS) of the tomographer because the area of the scar may be extrapolated (Figs. 10.11 and 10.12). However, corneal scars are characterized by the following tomographic features:

1. True flattening over the area of the scar.
2. *A corresponding false over estimated thinning:* There might be some thinning due to stromal contracture, but due to light scattering, the tomographer cannot give a real measurement of thickness through the scar as mentioned in Chapter 8 (refer Figs. 8.7 to 8.12).
3. *A corresponding false over estimated bulging in the posterior elevation map:* There might be some posterior elevation due to stromal contracture, but due to light scattering, the tomographer cannot give a real measurement of posterior elevation through the scar.

The above three criteria differentiate the tomography of the scar from the tomography of an ectatic corneal disease (ECD), as the latter is described by a steepening of the anterior curvature map rather than flattening in addition to abnormal posterior elevation. This is described in detail in Chapters 19 and 22.

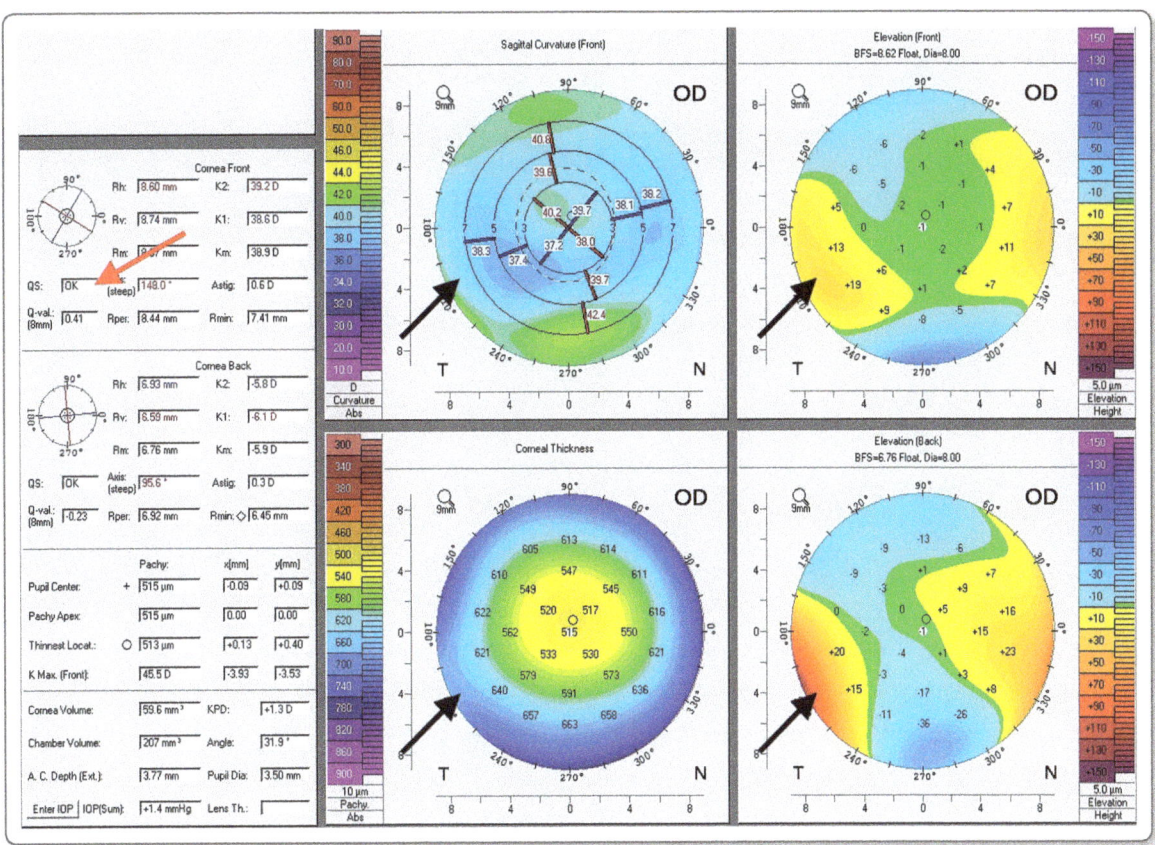

Fig. 10.11: Peripheral corneal scar. The four-composite map. Data were extrapolated and overlooked by the computer (QS=OK). The black arrows point at the location of the scar (see next figure).

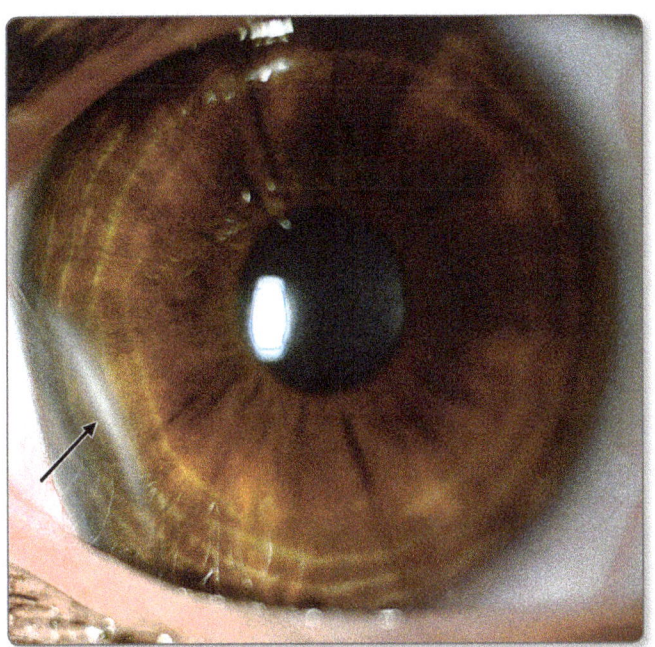

Fig. 10.12: Peripheral scar. Slit lamb view of same previous figure.

Pathologic

Any corneal disease, inflammation, infection, dystrophy, or degeneration that alters corneal structure can potentially cause irregular astigmatism. Ocular surface disease is a significant source of irregular astigmatism. In general, dry eye, contact lens warpage, pterygium, and herpetic disease are the most common causes for induced astigmatism in nonectatic corneas.

- Dry eye affects the accuracy of K-readings and induces focal irregularities, most commonly central or inferior steepening, which may mimic an early ECD (Fig. 10.13).
- Extended wear of contact lenses usually induces corneal steepening and corneal thinning in both epithelium and stroma. In some cases, constant rubbing of the contact lens against the epithelium causes hypertrophy as shown in Figure 10.14. The average time required for these changes to resolve after discontinuing the contact lenses is 8 weeks.

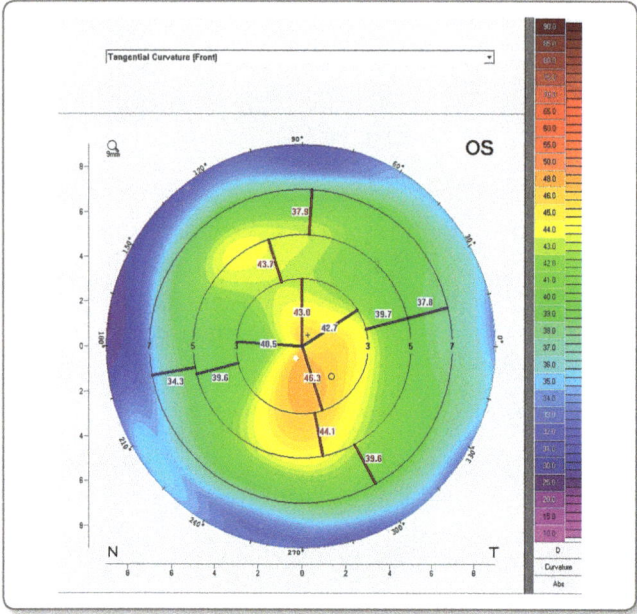

Fig. 10.13: Hot spot caused by dry eye.

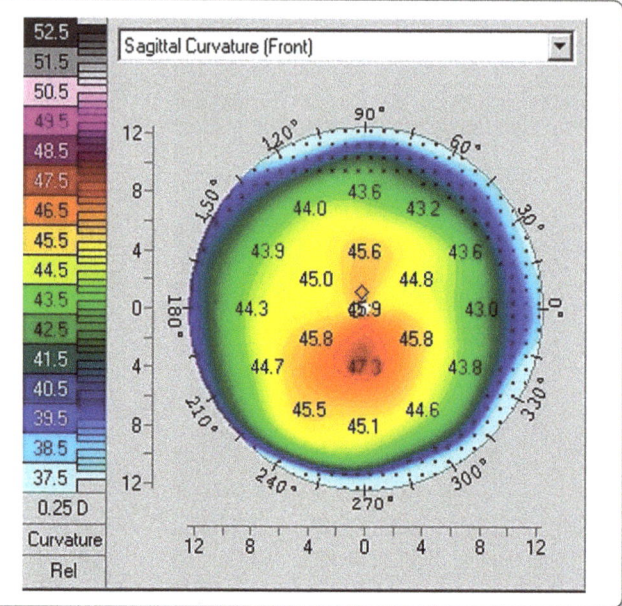

Fig. 10.14: Hot spot caused by soft contact lens.

- Pterygium usually causes irregular WTR astigmatism (Figs. 10.15 and 10.16). Several mechanisms were suggested—obscuration of the underlying corneal tissue, leading to extrapolated data; pooling of tear at the apex of the pterygium; compression of the underlying stroma; and asymmetric contraction along the semimeridian of the pterygium. The magnitude of the induced astigmatism is related to the size of the pterygium.
- Herpetic disease may be complicated by linear dendritic and/or spot scars. Tomographic features of the traumatic scars apply here. Scars induced by other infections are usually more severe and diffuse, giving the tomographic pattern of unspecific microirregular astigmatism.

EVALUATION OF IRREGULAR ASTIGMATISM

Both qualification and quantification of irregular astigmatism are important. Qualification is performed objectively, while quantification is performed subjectively and objectively.

Subjective Evaluation of Irregular Astigmatism

Subjective evaluation starts with suspicion followed by examination.

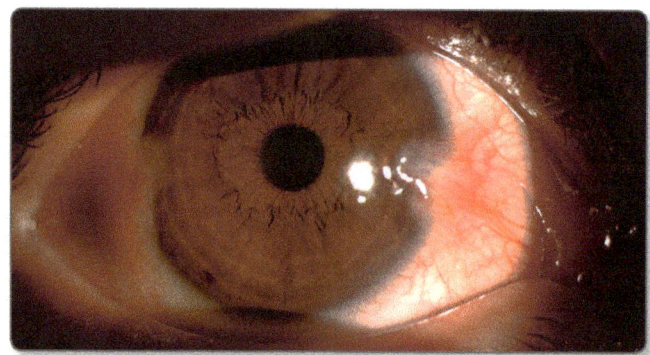

Fig. 10.15: Bilateral pterygium. Slit lamp view.

Suspicion of Irregular Astigmatism

Irregular astigmatism is suspected in the following cases:
- *Symptoms*: Patients complain of bad quality of vision due to shadows, glare, starbursts, ghost images, distortion of images, and monocular diplopia.
- A positive family history of an ECD.
- *Unusual manifest astigmatism*: Manifest astigmatism is considered by some physicians to be unusual when it is WTR more than 3D, ATR more than 1.5D, and oblique more than 2D.
- *Irregular reflex on retinoscopy*: Retinoscopy is a part of the subjective refraction. Irregular reflex is known as a scissoring reflex, which is the earliest sign of a subclinical

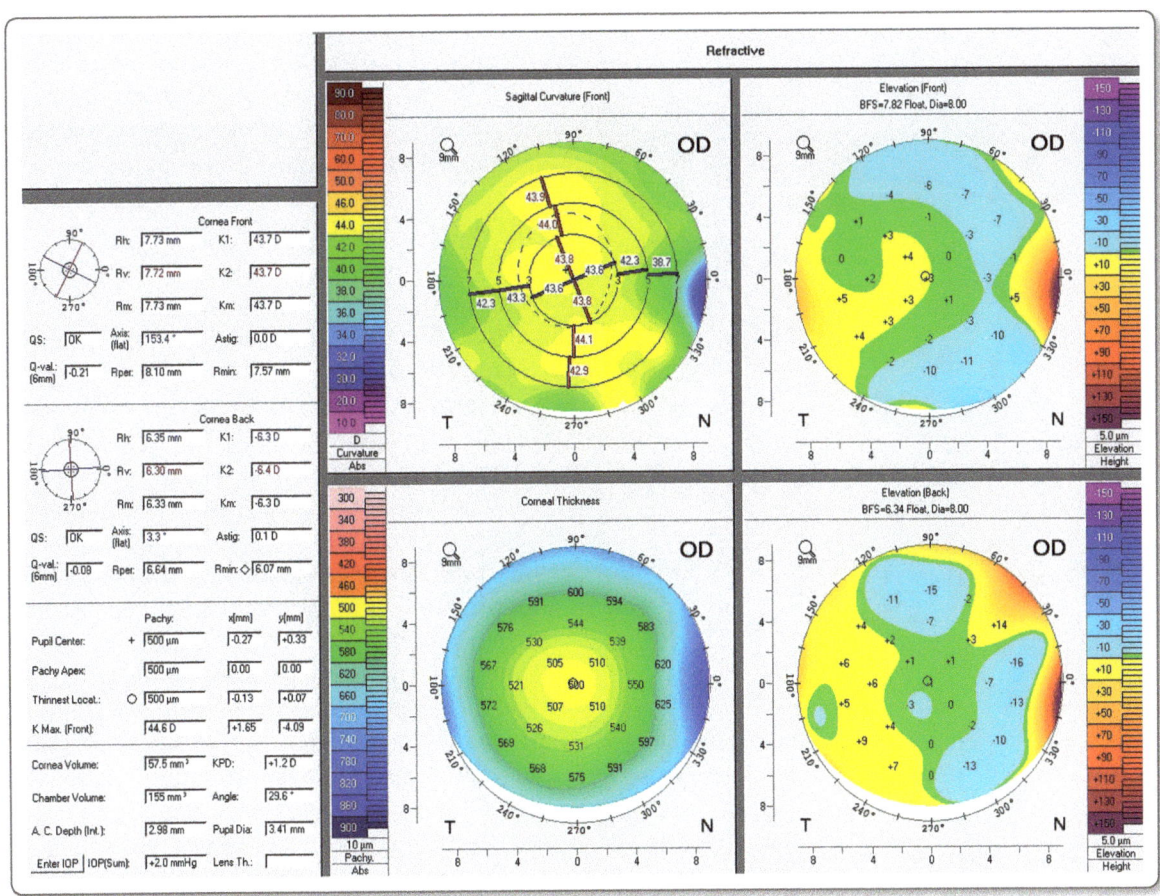

Fig. 10.16: Bilateral pterygium. The four-composite refractive map for the same previous figure.

ECD, but can be seen in cases with other causes of irregular astigmatism or media opacities.

- Nonoptimum spectacle corrected distance visual acuity (CDVA), but with optimum potential visual acuity (PVA), where PVA is vision measured with spectacles and pinhole test (PHT) or with rigid gas permeable (RGP) contact lenses. This can be explained by corneal irregularities that can be overcome by reducing the area of irregularity (by PHT) or creating an artificial perfect surface over the cornea (by an RGP lens).
- *Difficulty in determining the axis of manifest astigmatism*: When the patient hesitates, and gives different answers for different axes, or when they cannot give a final answer when using the astigmatic fan and the astigmatic dial.
- *Inconsistency between CDVA and different amounts and axes of manifest refraction (MR)*: When the objective refraction shows a significant amount of astigmatism, but it is not accepted by the patient who is achieving the same visual acuity despite correction of the cylinder at a different axis.
- *Anisometropia*: It is defined by a significant difference in refractive error between the two eyes of more than 1D in any meridian. Figure 10.17 is an example of anisometropia on the horizontal meridian. In case of oblique astigmatism (Fig. 10.18), the refraction on the vertical and horizontal meridians is calculated by the following formula:

$$F_\theta = (F_{cyl}) \sin^2 \theta$$

where "F_θ" is the power in the vertical meridian, "F_{cyl}" is the power in the oblique meridian, and "θ" is the angle between the vertical meridian and the correcting cylinder axis.

Subjective Refraction

Subjective refraction consists of MR, cycloplegic refraction (CR), and postmydriatic test (PMT). In mild cases of irregular astigmatism, determination of the MR is straight forward, while in moderate cases, it becomes a challenge, and becomes impossible in severe cases. However, all subjective measures should be tried to obtain an accurate MR, such as the astigmatic dial, astigmatism fan, cross-

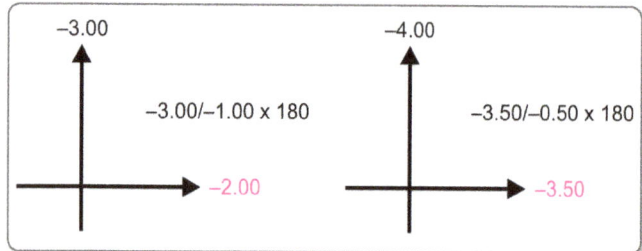

Fig. 10.17: Anisometropia on the horizontal meridian.

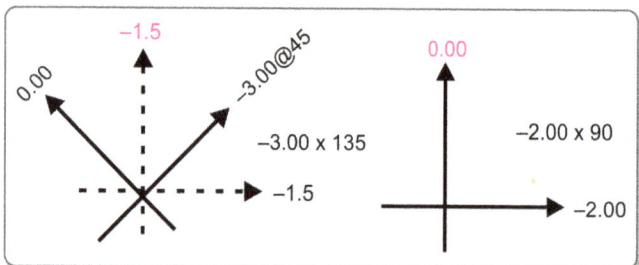

Fig. 10.18: Anisometropia on an oblique meridian.

cylinder, and over-refraction techniques. Although there are manipulations to be used in binocular balance, they are important only for the prescription of glasses, but not for customized LVC. CR is indicated in the above points 5–8

and when there is a difference between the "corrected" MR and corneal refraction. This is discussed in detail in the next Chapter 12. PMT is important to refine the results after CR. This is performed after the effect of cycloplegia has resolved, usually after 3 days.

Objective Evaluation

Irregular astigmatism is qualified (diagnosed, graded, and classified) by the objective evaluation, which also quantifies the astigmatism by measuring the induced HOAs and calculating corneal refraction. The objective evaluation is performed by corneal tomography or topography and wavefront analysis.

- *Corneal tomography and topography*: Normal and abnormal tomographic patterns are discussed in Chapters 5 to 8.
- *Wavefront aberrometry*: There are two types of wavefront aberrometry—(1) corneal and (2) ocular (total). The former measures, the HOAs induced by the irregular astigmatism in the cornea, while the latter measures the HOAs generated by the irregular astigmatism in the whole refractive system of the eye, mainly cornea and the crystalline lens. Wavefront aberrometry qualifies (classifies) and quantifies the HOAs. Chapters 13, 14, and 15 are devoted to address this topic.

CHAPTER 11

Objective Corneal Dioptric Power

INTRODUCTION

Objective corneal refraction is a term given to the calculated spherocylindric dioptric power of the cornea. Corneal power is usually measured and expressed in keratometric dioptric power (K-readings) rather than a spherocylindric dioptric power. Measuring the objective spherocylindric dioptric power (ODP) of the cornea is of clinical importance. It can assist with evaluating the refraction in the situations wherein manifest refraction (MR) is not applicable such as in young children and toddlers, patients with neurological deficits whose subjective responses are not reliable, and ocular media obstructions such as cataracts, vitreous hemorrhage, and hyphema. Moreover, measuring ODP is very helpful in ectatic corneal diseases (ECDs) and irregular corneas wherein determination of MR may be difficult or even misleading especially in moderate and severe cases. In such cases, ODP can be compared with the MR to check the reliability of the latter, especially in terms of axis and amount of astigmatism. Nevertheless, ODP can explain how the topography-guided software calculates the spherocylindric power (sphere, cylinder, and axis) in irregular and ectatic corneas.

To understand how ODP is calculated, maps measuring keratometric corneal power should first be reviewed in Chapter 5.

CALCULATING OBJECTIVE CORNEAL DIOPTRIC POWER

Since the total corneal refractive power (TCRP) uses ray tracing to calculate keratometric corneal power, K-readings obtained by this method are most reliable. Therefore, ODP is calculated by using the K-readings (K_1 and K_2) obtained from the TCRP map, and referring them to the normal mean K-reading that is considered as a reference K-reading (K_{ref}). The K_{ref} differs depending on the method used to measure it and the studied population. In this regard, I will use K_{ref} = 43D because the average normal corneal power is 43.05D. However, any other value can be used.

Having said that, ODP can be calculated by the following systematic steps:

- *Step 1*: Mesopic pupil should be determined. It is best measured by the pupillometer.
- *Step 2:* K-readings (K_1 and K_2) are obtained from the TCRP map. Readings of the zone corresponding to the mesopic pupil are considered. For example, if the mesopic pupil size is 4 mm, readings from the 4 mm zone cantered on the pupil center are considered. In case the mesopic pupil size is not available, readings from the 5 mm zone are considered. The $K_2 - K_1$ difference represents the magnitude of corneal astigmatism.
- *Step 3:* To simplify the matter, ODP is calculated by using the plus cylinder equation and following the following steps:
  - K_1 is pushed toward K_2 by a plus cylinder, which equals $K_2 - K_1$.
  - The axis of the plus cylinder is the axis of K_2.
  - K_2 is pushed to K_{ref} by a sphere, which equals $K_{ref} - K_2$.
  - The resultant sphere, cylinder and axis represent the ODP.
- *Step 4:* MR is corrected at corneal plane by the following equation:

$$MRc = MR/[1 - (d \times MR)]$$

where "MRc" is the manifest refraction corrected at corneal plane, "d" is back vertex distance (BVD) in meters (usually 0.012 m or 0.015 m).

This formula should be applied on meridional power in the following steps:
- Correct flat meridian power.
- Correct steep meridian power.
- Corrected astigmatism = corrected steep–corrected flat meridians' power.
- MRc = sphere (corrected steep meridian)/corrected astigmatism X axis of steep meridian.

- *Step 5:* The MRc is expressed in plus cylinder equation and checked against ODP.

N.B: The ODP sphere is related to the chosen K_{ref}. ODP astigmatism is not affected by the chosen K_{ref}. In other words, if K_{ref} is chosen to be other than 43.0D, the sphere of ODP will change, while the astigmatism will not because it is the difference between K_1 and K_2 regardless of the chosen K_{ref}.

CLINICAL EXAMPLES

Example 1

A patient with right eye MR = +4D Sph/ + 3D Cyl × 90° for BVD = 15 mm.

Figure 11.1 shows the cornea with its two meridians (K_1 and K_2), and shows the position of the K_{ref} value.
- *Step 1:* The mesopic pupil size is 4 mm. TCRP K_1 = 37.5D × 180°, K_2 = 40D × 90° at the 4 mm zone.
- *Step 2:* Corneal astigmatism = $K_2 - K_1$ = 40 – 37.5 = +2.5D
- *Step 3:* The ODP is calculated by using the plus cylinder equation and following the following steps:
  - K_1 is pushed toward K_2 by: $K_2 - K_1$ = 40 – 37.5 = +2.5D Cyl.
  - The axis of the +2.5D Cyl is 90° (K_2 axis).
  - K_2 is pushed to K_{ref} by: $K_{ref} - K_2$ = 43 – 40 = +3D Sph.

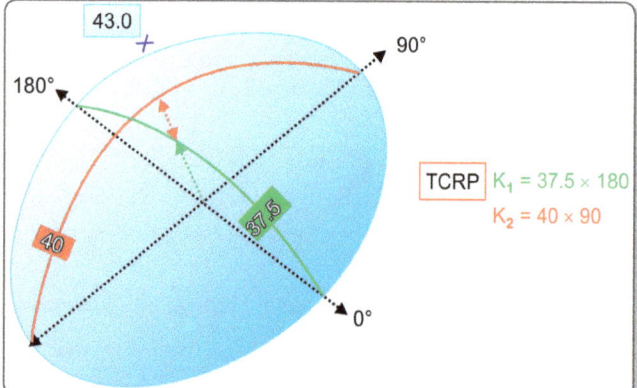

Fig. 11.1: Example 1—meridional power of the cornea.

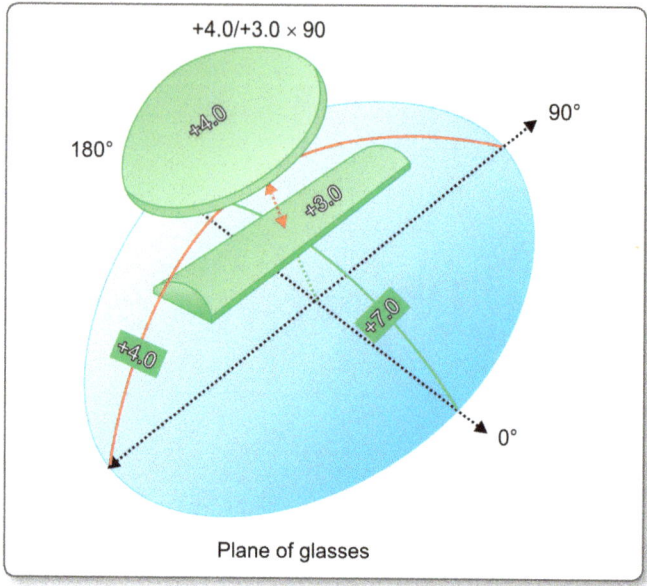

Fig. 11.2: Example 1—meridional power of the manifest refraction at spectacle plane.

- ODP = +3D Sph/+2.5D Cyl × 90° in reference to K_{ref} = 43D.
- *Step 4:* The MR is +4D Sph/+3D Cyl × 90°. It is corrected at the corneal plane by meridional correction. Figure 11.2 illustrates the meridional power of MR at the spectacle plane. This MR has a steep meridian = +4D (sphere) at the 90° meridian, and a flat meridian = +4D (sphere) + 3D (cylinder) = +7D at the 180° meridian. The MRc is calculated as follows:
  - Corrected flat meridian power = +7/(1 – 0.015 × +7) = +7.82D on 180° meridian.
  - Corrected steep meridian power = +4/(1 – 0.015 × +4) = +4.26D on 90° meridian.
  - Corrected astigmatism: corrected flat – corrected steep = +7.82 – 4.26 = +3.56D.
  - MRc= sphere (corrected steep meridian power) / corrected astigmatism X axis of steep meridian = +4.26D Sph/+3.56D Cyl × 90°.
- *Step 5:* MRc is comparable and consistent with ODP.

Example 2

A patient with left eye MR = –3D Sph/–2D Cyl × 180° for BVD = 12 mm.

Figure 11.3 shows the cornea with its two meridians (K_1 and K_2), and shows the position of the K_{ref} value.
- *Step 1:* The mesopic pupil size is 4.5 mm. TCRP K_1 = 44.5D × 180°, K_2 = 47D × 90° at the 5 mm zone.

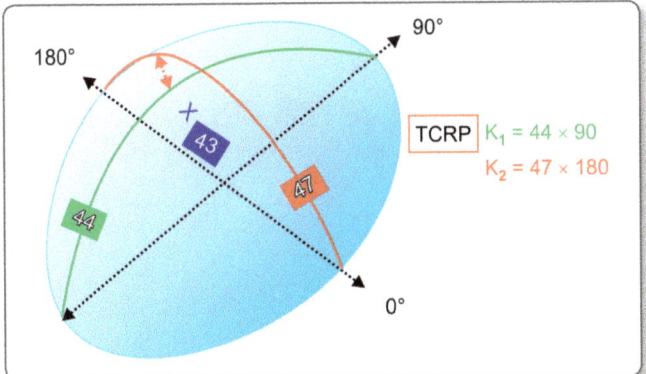

Fig. 11.3: Example 2—meridional power of the cornea.

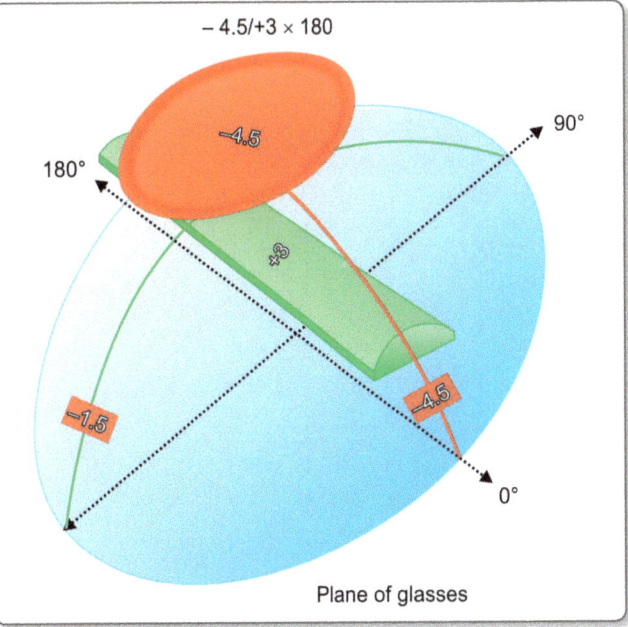

Fig. 11.4: Example 2—meridional power of the manifest refraction at spectacle plane.

- *Step 2:* Corneal astigmatism = $K_2 - K_1$ = 47 − 44 = +3D.
- *Step 3:* The ODP is calculated by using the plus cylinder equation and following the following steps:
  - K_1 is pushed towards K_2 by: $K_2 - K_1$ = 47 − 44 = +3D Cyl.
  - The axis of the +3D Cyl is 90° (K_2 axis).
  - K_2 is pushed to K_{ref} by: $K_{ref} - K_2$ = 43 − 47 = −4D Sph.
  - ODP = −4D Sph/+3D Cyl × 90° in reference to K_{ref} = 43D.
- *Step 4:* The MR is −3D Sph/−2D Cyl × 180°. It is corrected at the corneal plane by meridional correction. Figure 11.4 illustrates the meridional power of MR at the spectacle plane. This MR has a flat meridian = −3.0D (sphere) at the 180° meridian, and a steep meridian = −3D (sphere) + (−) 2D (cylinder) = −5D at the 90° meridian. The MRc is calculated as follows:
  - Corrected flat meridian power = −3/(1 − 0.012 × −3) = −2.9D at the 180° meridian.
  - Corrected steep meridian power = −5/(1 − 0.012 × −5) = −4.7D at the 90° meridian.
  - Corrected astigmatism: corrected flat − corrected steep = −2.9 − (−4.7) = +1.8D.
  - MRc = sphere (corrected steep meridian)/corrected astigmatism X axis of steep meridian = −4.7D Sph/+1.8D Cyl × 90°.
- *Step 5:* MRc is comparable and consistent with ODP.

Example 3

A patient with keratoconus with right eye uncorrected distance visual acuity (UDVA) = 0.3 decimal, spectacle CDVA = 0.7 decimal and MR = −3D Sph/−3D Cyl × 95° for BVD = 12 mm. Figure 11.5 is the four-composite tomography map of his right eye. Figure 11.6 is the power distribution map.
- *Step 1:* The mesopic pupil size is not available. TCRP K_1 = 40.4D × 165.6°, K_2 = 42.7D × 75.6° at the 5 mm zone.
- *Step 2:* Corneal astigmatism = $K_2 - K_1$ = 42.7 − 40.4 = +2.3D.
- *Step 3:* The ODP is calculated by using the plus cylinder equation and following the following steps:
  - K_1 is pushed toward K_2 by: $K_2 - K_1$ = 42.7 − 40.4 = +2.3D Cyl.
  - The axis of the +2.3D Cyl is 75.6° (K_2 axis).
  - K_2 is pushed to K_{ref} by: $K_{ref} - K_2$ = 43.0 − 42.7 = +0.3D Sph.
  - ODP = +0.3D Sph/ +2.3D Cyl × 75.6°.
- *Step 4:* The MR is −3D Sph/−3D Cyl × 95°. It is corrected at the corneal plane by meridional correction. Figure 11.7 illustrates the meridional power of MR at the plane of glasses. This MR has a flat meridian: −3D (sphere) at the 95° meridian, and a steep meridian: −3D (sphere) + (−) 3D (cylinder) = −6D at the 05° meridian. The MRc is calculated as follows:
  - Corrected flat meridian power = −3/(1 − 0.012 × −3) = −2.9D on 95° meridian.
  - Corrected steep meridian power = −6/(1 − 0.012 × −6) = −5.6D on 05° meridian.
  - Corrected astigmatism: corrected flat − corrected steep = −2.9 − (−) 5.6 = +2.7D.
  - MRc = sphere (corrected steep meridian)/corrected astigmatism X axis of steep meridian = −5.6D / +2.7D × 05.
- *Step 5:* In comparison between ODP and MRc, there is a big difference in sphere, cylindric magnitude, and

Section 3: Understanding Corneal Refraction

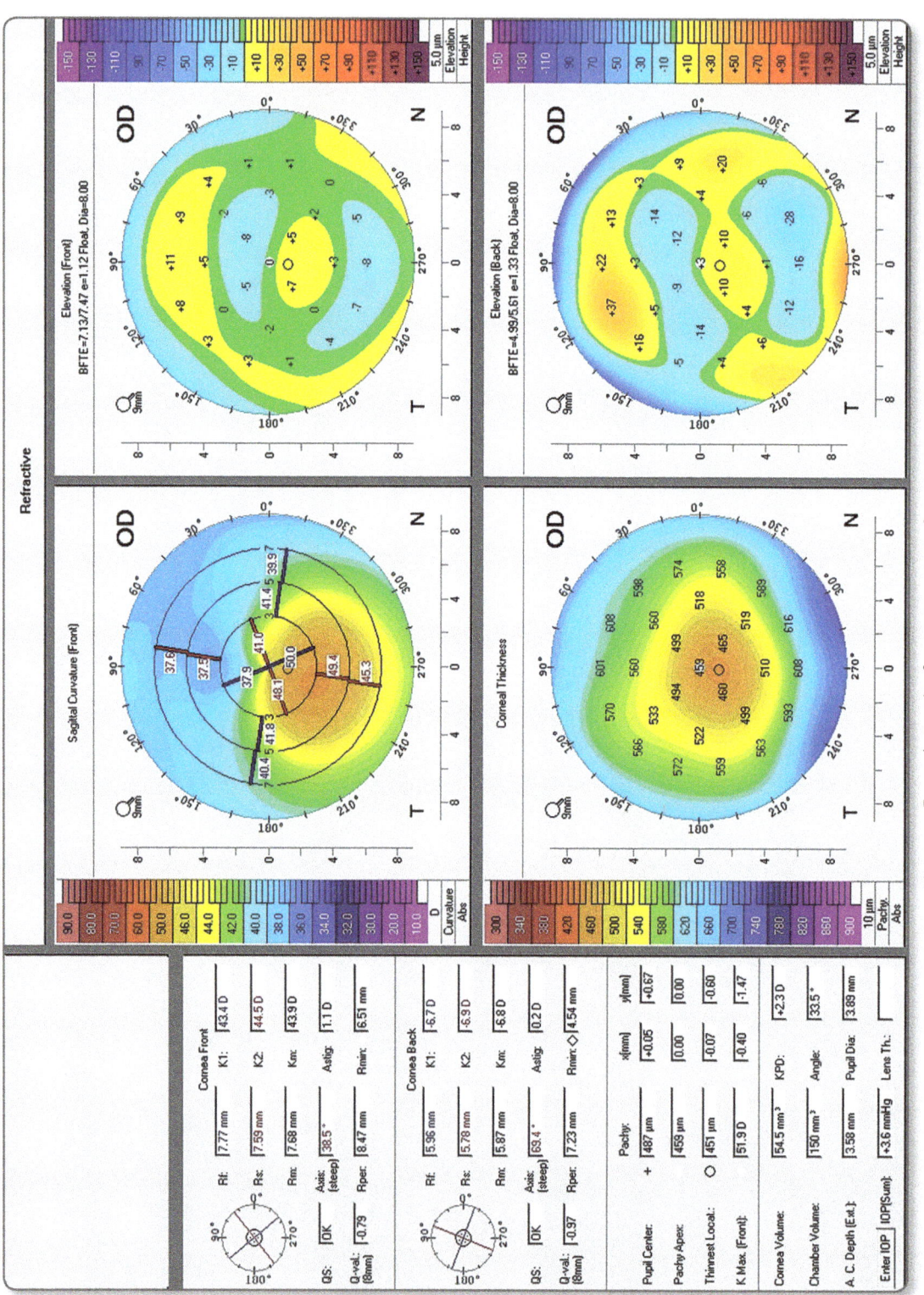

Fig. 11.5: Example 3—the four-composite refractive map.

K-Readings (D) calculated in zones centered on pupil center   (•) Zone ( ) Ring   ( ) Apex (•) Pupil

Zone Diameter		1.0 mm	2.0 mm	3.0 mm	4.0 mm	5.0 mm	6.0 mm	7.0 mm	8.0 mm
Sagittal Front	K1	40.5 (50.4°)	41.2 (164.2°)	41.2 (160.8°)	41.0 (165.7°)	40.8 (168.7°)	40.5 (170.3°)	40.3 (171.2°)	40.0 (171.6°)
	K2	40.9 (140.4°)	41.7 (74.2°)	42.5 (70.8°)	43.3 (75.7°)	43.8 (78.7°)	43.9 (80.3°)	43.7 (81.2°)	43.4 (81.6°)
True Net Power	K1	38.6 (54.5°)	39.5 (2.1°)	39.7 (161.7°)	39.7 (165.3°)	39.6 (167.5°)	39.4 (168.8°)	39.2 (169.8°)	38.9 (170.7°)
	K2	39.0 (144.5°)	39.8 (92.1°)	40.6 (71.7°)	41.5 (75.3°)	42.0 (77.5°)	42.2 (78.8°)	42.1 (79.8°)	41.8 (80.7°)
Tot. Refr. Power	K1	38.8 (59.5°)	39.9 (118.4°)	40.2 (150.3°)	40.4 (161.3°)	40.4 (165.6°)	40.5 (167.5°)	40.5 (168.9°)	
	K2	39.3 (149.5°)	40.1 (28.4°)	41.0 (60.3°)	41.9 (71.3°)	42.7 (75.6°)	43.1 (77.5°)	43.2 (78.9°)	

Fig. 11.6: Example 3—the power distribution map.

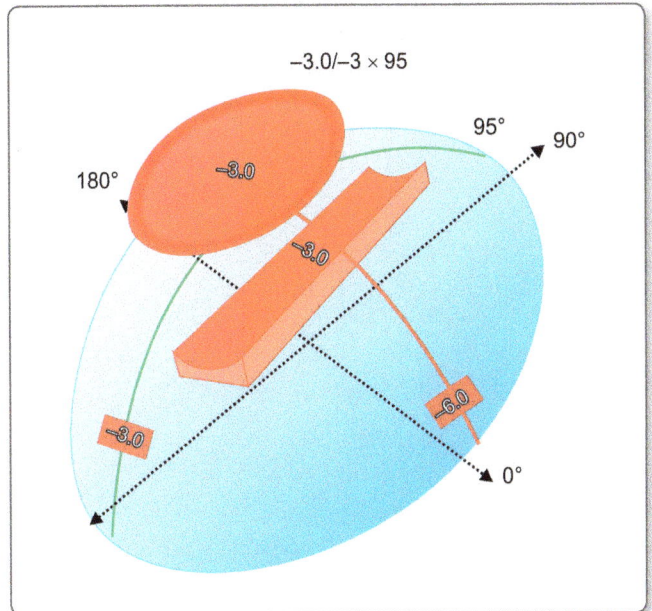

Fig. 11.7: Example 3—meridional power of the manifest refraction at spectacle plane.

cylindric axis. This is not uncommon in moderate and advanced cases of ECDs. This can be explained by the impact of the higher-order aberrations (HOAs) on MR. It is recommended to do cycloplegic refraction (CR) and postmydriatic test (PMT) to refine the MR.

Astigmatic Dissociation

INTRODUCTION

Clinical manifest astigmatism (MA) is measured by subjective refraction, while tomographic astigmatism (TA) is objectively measured by the total corneal refractive power (TCRP), which depends on ray tracing principle, takes into consideration both corneal surfaces and corneal thickness, and uses the true refractive index (1.376) rather than the keratometric index (1.3375). As mentioned in Chapter 11, in case of unavailable measurement of mesopic pupil, the astigmatism in 5 mm zone centered on the pupil center is considered (Fig. 12.1). However, in daily clinical practice, the TCRP is usually not printed. In such cases, the amount of astigmatism given by Sim-Ks on the anterior corneal surface can roughly be considered after deducting the amount of astigmatism of the posterior corneal surface (Fig. 12.2).

Manifest astigmatism occasionally differs from the TA. This is called astigmatic dissociation. It may be either in magnitudes or in axes or both. It is considered as significant, if there is ≥1 D and/or ≥10° difference between MA and TA.

The importance of astigmatic dissociation comes from its effect on decision making in refractive surgery. For instance, in laser vision correction (LVC), if MA is not consistent with the TA, there is a risk of creating irregular astigmatism or inverting corneal astigmatism, and therefore inducing higher-order aberrations (HOAs).

ETIOLOGY

Astigmatic dissociation is caused by:
- Irregular astigmatism.
- Use of contact lenses.
- Misalignment during taking the capture.
- Large angle kappa.
- Tear film disturbance.
- Significant posterior surface astigmatism.
- Corneal opacities.
- Previous corneal surgeries.
- Lenticular astigmatism.

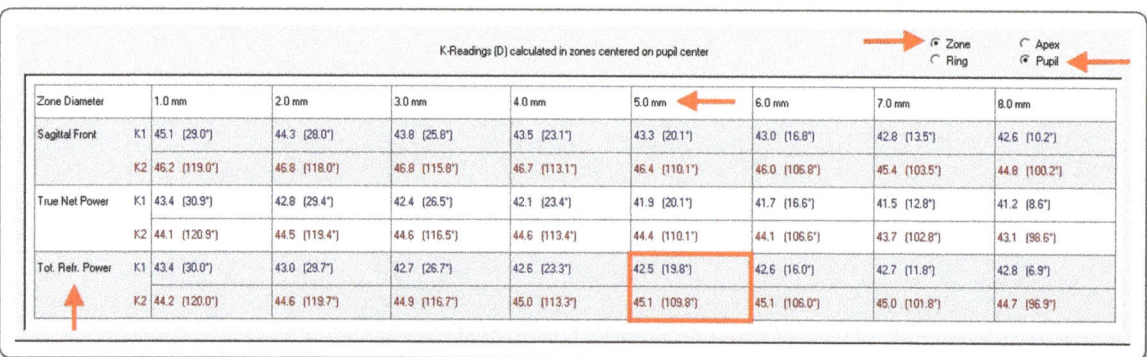

Fig. 12.1: Power distribution. In case of unavailable measurement of mesopic pupil, the 5 mm zone of total corneal refractive power is considered.

- Crystalline lens subluxation.
- IOL tilt, dislocation, or subluxation.
- *Cataract:* All types of cataract cause astigmatic dissociation. In very early cataract, slit lamp biomicroscopy may skip the view. Therefore, in all cases of dissociation, careful dilated crystalline lens examination is necessary, in addition to Scheimpflug image study. Figure 12.3 is an example of an early cataract causing dissociation
- Ocular pathologies affecting the media.
- Bad exposure to the camera because of anatomical factors, such as prominent eyebrows, small eyes, deep-set eyes, nasal bridge or long lashes, or because of tight headscarves.
- Pregnancy.

Most of the mentioned factors are responsible for false positives and false negatives in corneal tomography. They are studied in details in Chapter 16.

TYPES OF DISSOCIATION

There are nine types of astigmatic dissociation:
1. The TA and MA are with-the-rule (WTR) and the magnitude of the former is more than the latter.
2. The TA and MA are WTR, and the magnitude of the former is less than the latter.
3. The TA and MA are against-the-rule (ATR), and the magnitude of the former is more than the latter.
4. The TA and MA are ATR, and the magnitude of the former is less than the latter.
5. The TA is WTR and MA is ATR, and the magnitude of the former is more than the latter.
6. The TA is WTR and MA is ATR, and the magnitude of the former is less than the latter.
7. The TA is ATR and MA is WTR, and the magnitude of the former is more than the latter.
8. The TA is ATR and MA is WTR, and the magnitude of the former is less than the latter.
9. The TA and/or MA are oblique with more than 15° difference between their axes.

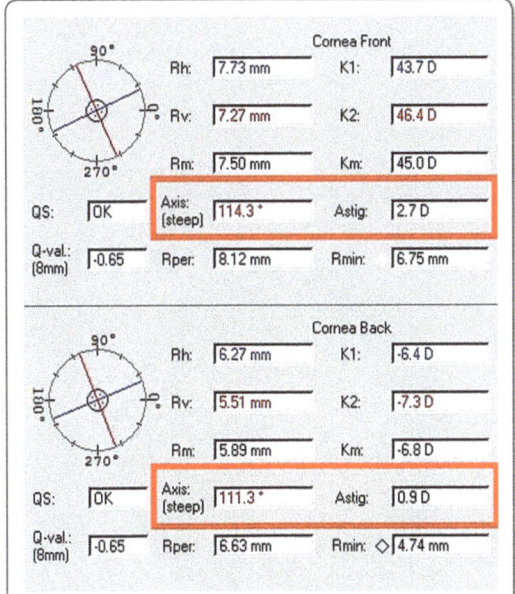

Fig. 12.2: A rough method to calculate cornea astigmatism by deducting the magnitude of the posterior surface from the magnitude of the anterior surface.

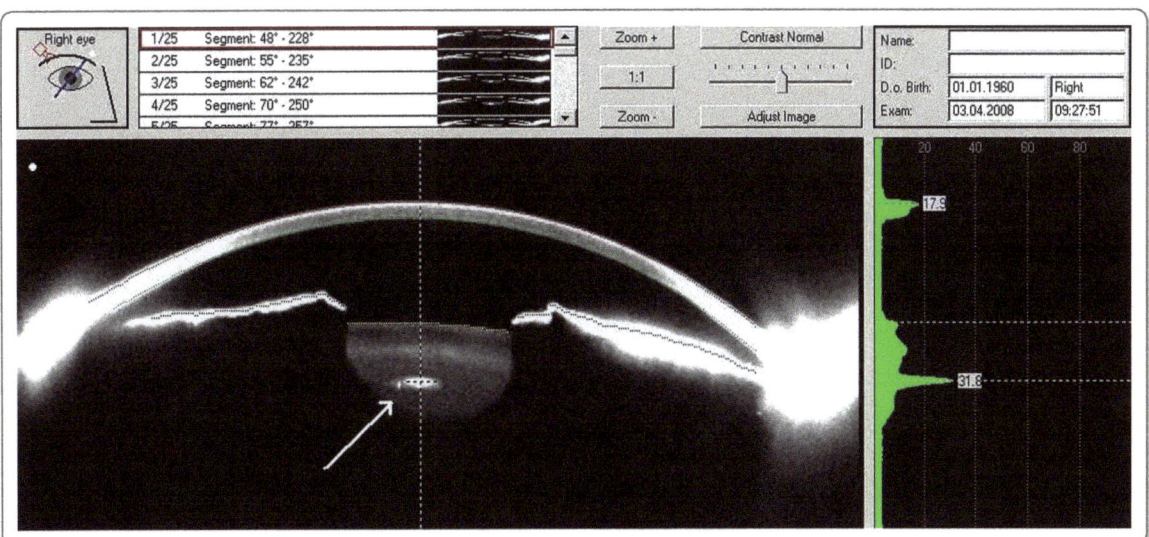

Fig. 12.3: Early cataract resulting in astigmatic disparity.

Table 12.1: Probabilities of astigmatic disparity.

Probability	TA	MA	Amount
1	WTR	WTR	TA > MA
2	WTR	WTR	TA < MA
3	ATR	ATR	TA > MA
4	ATR	ATR	TA < MA
5	WTR	ATR	TA > MA
6	WTR	ATR	TA < MA
7	ATR	WTR	TA > MA
8	ATR	ATR	TA < MA
9	Oblique	Oblique	?

(TA: topographic astigmatism; MA: manifest astigmatism; WTR: with-the-rule; ATR: against-the-rule)

Table 12.1 summarizes the nine probabilities.

To check the MA against the TA and to apply the nine probabilities correctly, the MR is corrected at corneal plane by the following equation:

$$MRc = MR / [1 - (d \times MR)]$$

where "MRc" is the manifest refraction corrected at corneal plane, "d" is back vertex distance (BVD) in meters (usually 0.012 m or 0.015 m).

This formula should be applied on meridional power in the following steps:
- Correct flat meridian power
- Correct steep meridian power
- Corrected astigmatism = corrected steep – corrected flat meridians' power
- MRc = sphere (corrected steep meridian)/corrected astigmatism X axis of steep meridian.

The method is discussed in Chapter 11 in detail.

CLINICAL EXAMPLES

To apply the nine types in clinical practice, nine clinical examples will be studied assuming that the MA was corrected at corneal plain.

To simplify the matter, MA and TA will be myopic.

Example 1

TA is –3D × 180 and MA is –2D × 180 (Fig. 12.4).

Correcting the MA completely leaves a residual TA of about –1D × 180. This will be tolerated by the patient since it is WTR, it is consistent with the preoperative WTR astigmatism, and asymptomatic.

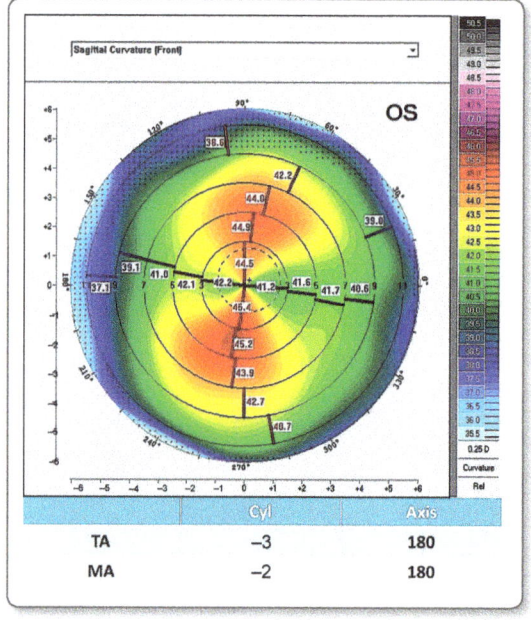

Fig. 12.4: Example 1.
(TA: tomographic astigmatism; MA: manifest astigmatism)

Example 2

TA is –2D × 180° and MA is –3D × 180° (Fig. 12.5).

Correcting the MA completely induces an ATR TA of about –1D × 90°. This will not be tolerated by the patient since it is ATR and not consistent with their preoperative WTR astigmatism even with postoperative uncorrected distance visual acuity (UDVA) 1.0 (Snellen). In such a case, it is recommended to limit the astigmatic correction to the magnitude of the TA with/without compensation by the spherical equivalent (SE). For example, a patient has MR = –2D sph/–3D cyl × 180°, and TA = –2D ×

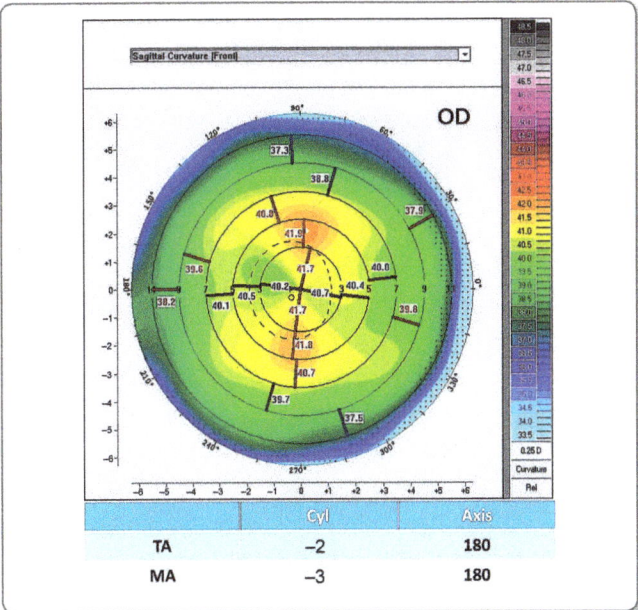

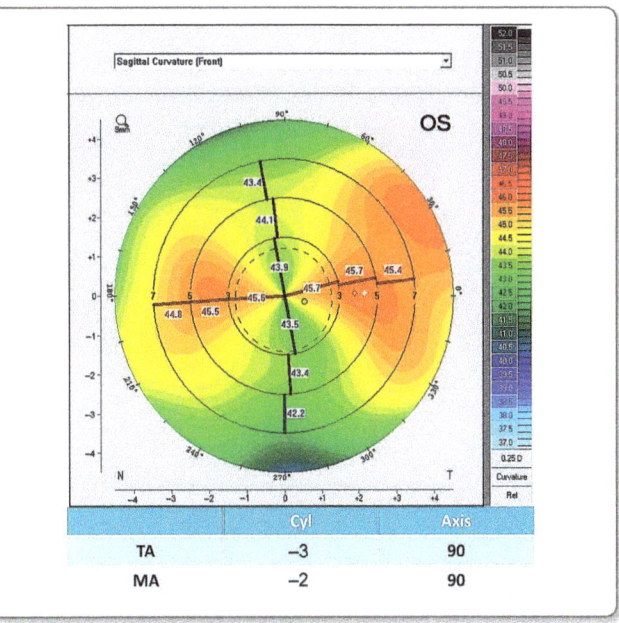

Fig. 12.5: Example 2.
(TA: tomographic astigmatism; MA: manifest astigmatism)

Fig. 12.6: Example 3.
(TA: tomographic astigmatism; MA: manifest astigmatism)

180°. The recommended astigmatic correction is –2D cyl × 180° with a spherical correction ranging between -2D (the original sphere of the patient) and -2.5D (the compensated SE). This depends on testing the CDVA and the red-green duochrome test.

Example 3

TA is –3D × 90° and MA is –2D × 90° (Fig. 12.6).

Correcting the MA completely leaves a residual TA of about –1 × 90°. This will be tolerated by the patient since it is consistent with the preoperative ATR astigmatism.

Example 4

TA is –2D × 80° and MA is –3D × 80° (Fig. 12.7).

Correcting MA completely induces WTR TA of about –1D × 170°. This will be tolerated by the patient since it is WTR although it is not consistent with the preoperative ATR astigmatism. In general, if the expected induced WTR TA is within 1D, it can be tolerable by the patient, otherwise it cannot be. In case of an expected > 1D of induced WTR TA, the magnitude of astigmatic correction should be adjusted so that the expected induced WTR TA will be ≤1D and the remaining untreated astigmatic magnitude can be compensated for by SE. For example, a patient has MR = –2D sph/–4D cyl × 80°, and TA = –2D cyl × 80°. It is

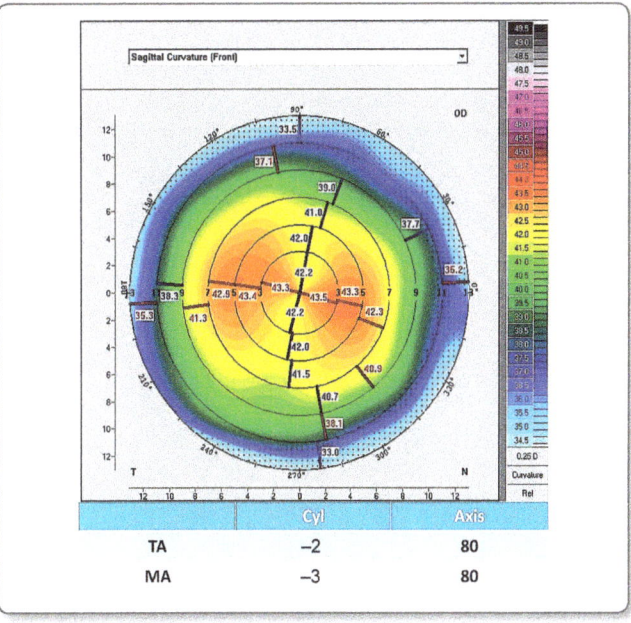

Fig. 12.7: Example 4.
(TA: tomographic astigmatism; MA: manifest astigmatism)

recommended to treat no more than -3D of astigmatism, so that the expected induced TA will be no more than –1D cyl × 170°. Based on that, the spherical correction can range between -2D (the original sphere of the patient) and -2.5D (the compensated SE). This depends on testing the CDVA and the red-green duochrome test.

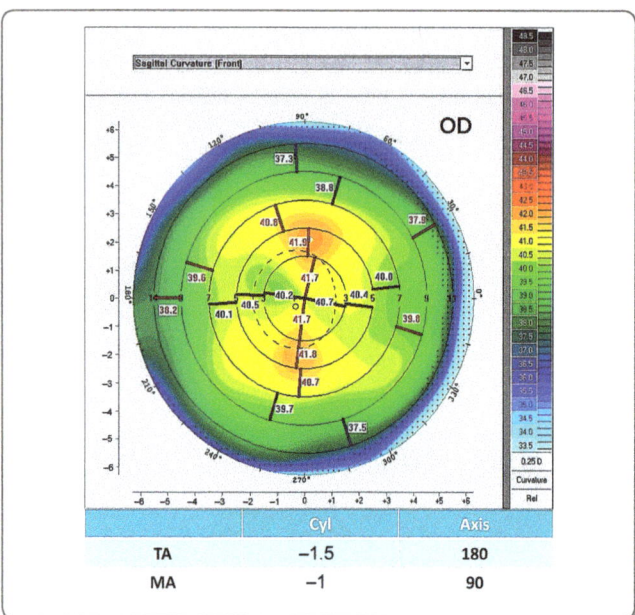

Fig. 12.8: Example 5.
(TA: tomographic astigmatism; MA: manifest astigmatism)

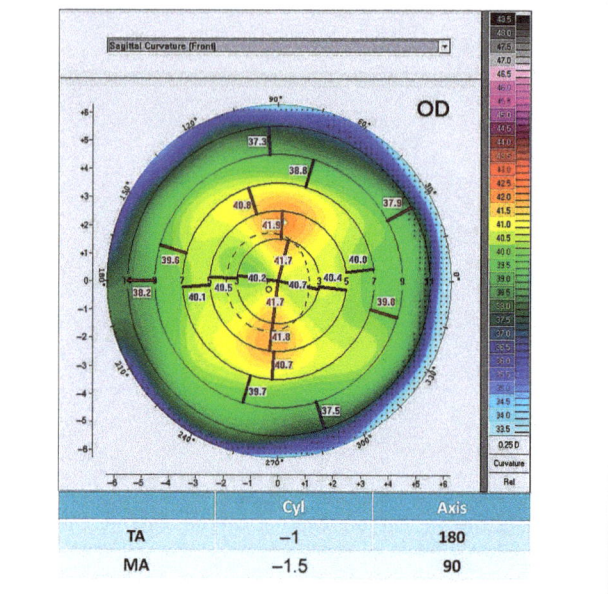

Fig. 12.9: Example 6.
(TA: tomographic astigmatism; MA: manifest astigmatism)

Example 5

TA is –1.5D × 180° and MA is –1D × 90° (Fig. 12.8).

Correcting MA completely induces WTR TA of about –2.5D cyl × 180°! In such a case, it is recommended to recheck the manifest refraction and try to modify it to be with as minimum magnitude of astigmatism as possible. For example, a patient has MR = –2D sph/–0.75D cyl × 90°, CDVA = 0.9 (Snellen), and TA = –1.5D × 180°. It is recommended to recheck the MR, readjust the magnitude of the MA to be as close to 0.0D as possible, and compensate for it by the SE. In this example, the patient may tolerate correction of -2.25D sphere without any cylinder. However, the final decision must depend on testing the CDVA and the red-green duochrome test.

In general, it is unusual to see much difference between MA and TA magnitudes when their axes are completely perpendicular.

Example 6

TA is –1D × 180° and MA is –1.5D × 90° (Fig. 12.9).

What applies on example 5 applies here.

Example 7

TA is –1.5D × 80° and MA is –1D × 170° (Fig. 12.10).

The problem encountered in examples 5 and 6 is exaggerated in this example because the TA is ATR and will be increased by the operation if the MA is completely

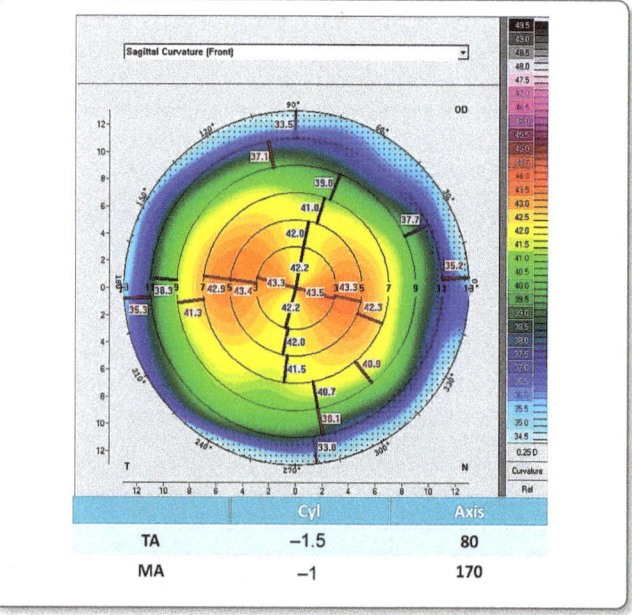

Fig. 12.10: Example 7.
(TA: tomographic astigmatism; MA: manifest astigmatism)

corrected. In such a case, the rule of example 5 should be followed.

Example 8

Tomographic astigmatism is –1D × 80° and MA is –1.5D × 170° (Fig. 12.11).

What applies on example 7 applies here.

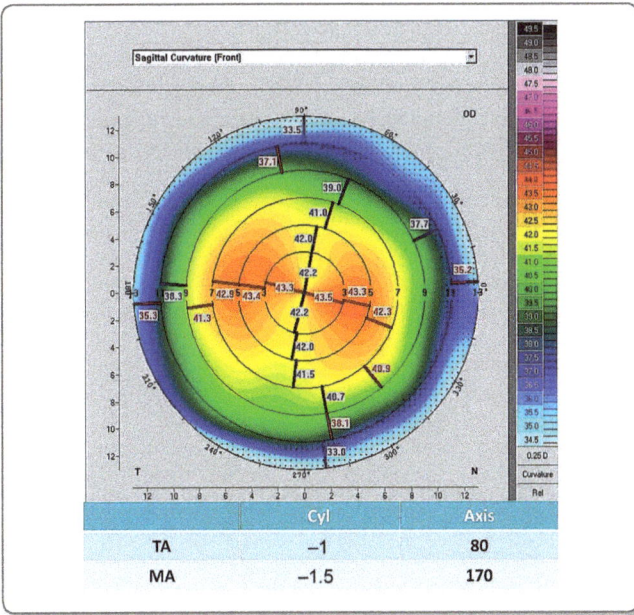

Fig. 12.11: Example 8.
(TA: tomographic astigmatism; MA: manifest astigmatism)

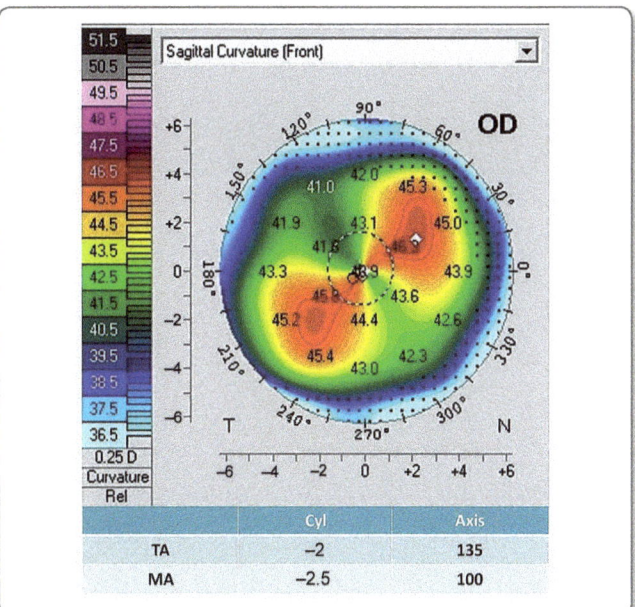

Fig. 12.12: Example 9.
(TA: tomographic astigmatism; MA: manifest astigmatism)

Example 9

Tomographic astigmatism is −2D × 135° and MA is −2.5D × 100° (Fig. 12.12).

It is not uncommon to encounter such an example in clinical practice. Suspicion in cataract or corneal irregularities especially faint scaring is very high. If such causes and other possible causes were excluded, it is wise to take time in thinking about the final correction. Reexamining the patient with fine tuning of the axis and magnitude of the MA is very necessary. If the difference remains, the MA should be chosen and a possible future enhancement should be discussed with the patient.

SUMMARY OF GUIDELINES

In case of astigmatic dissociation:
1. Exclude all possible causes.
2. Imagine what type of corneal astigmatism will be induced if the MA is fully corrected.
3. Do not induce >1D of ATR TA.
4. Try to compensate for the untreated MA by the SE, but the final decision depends of CDVA and the duochrome test.
5. If MA < TA, any residual TA will not affect patient's vision because it is consistent with the preoperative TA.
6. In all cases of significant dissociation, discuss the possibility of a future enhancement with the patient.

SECTION 4

Wavefront Analysis

SECTION OUTLINE

13. Basics of Wavefront Analysis and Measurements
14. Zernike Analysis
15. Fourier Analysis

Basics of Wavefront Analysis and Measurements

CHAPTER 13

PRINCIPLES OF WAVEFRONT AND WAVEFRONT ANALYSIS

The parallel light rays coming from infinity are composed of sinusoidal oscillations. Locations of equal phase within the total array of sinusoidal oscillations form planar wavefronts. A wavefront is a constant phase that is normal to the light rays (Fig. 13.1). When the parallel light rays pass through a perfect refractive surface, they (and the wavefronts) meet precisely at a point known as the focal point "F." Practically, the ideal situation is virtually never encountered because real wavefronts show deviations from a perfect plane after passing through the refractive surface leading to what is known as "wavefront aberrations." The shape of a wavefront passing through a theoretically perfect eye with no aberrations is a flat plane known as "piston" (see below).

The difference (deviation) between the actual wavefront shape and the ideal flat shape represents the amount of aberration in the wavefront as shown in Figure 13.2. The smaller the deviation/aberration, the higher the quality of the refractive system.

Deviations of a real wavefront from an ideal one were mathematically represented by the Dutch physicist Fritz Zernike. Based on the analysis of the scientist Fourier, Fritz Zernike could describe wavefront analysis of ocular refractive surfaces in circle polynomials in the radial (n) and angular (m) directions by using an equation, depending on which, Zernike polynomials are calculated, given indexes

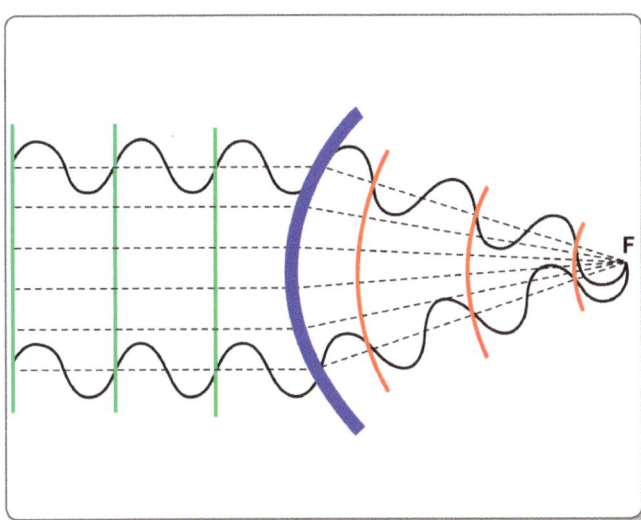

Fig. 13.1: Wavefront principle.

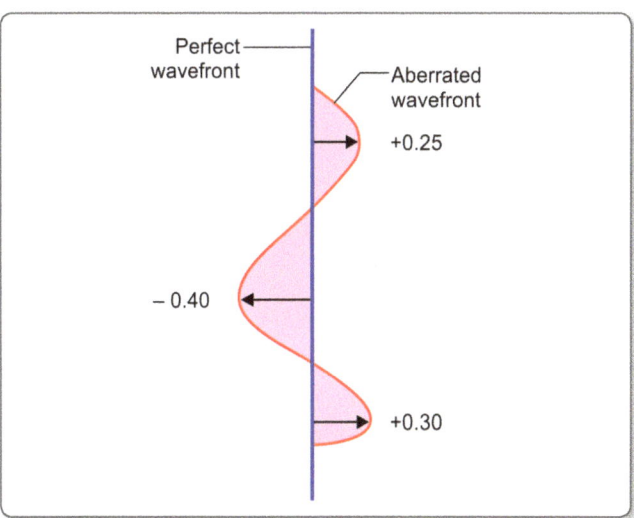

Fig. 13.2: Root mean square measurement of aberrations.

Section 4: Wavefront Analysis

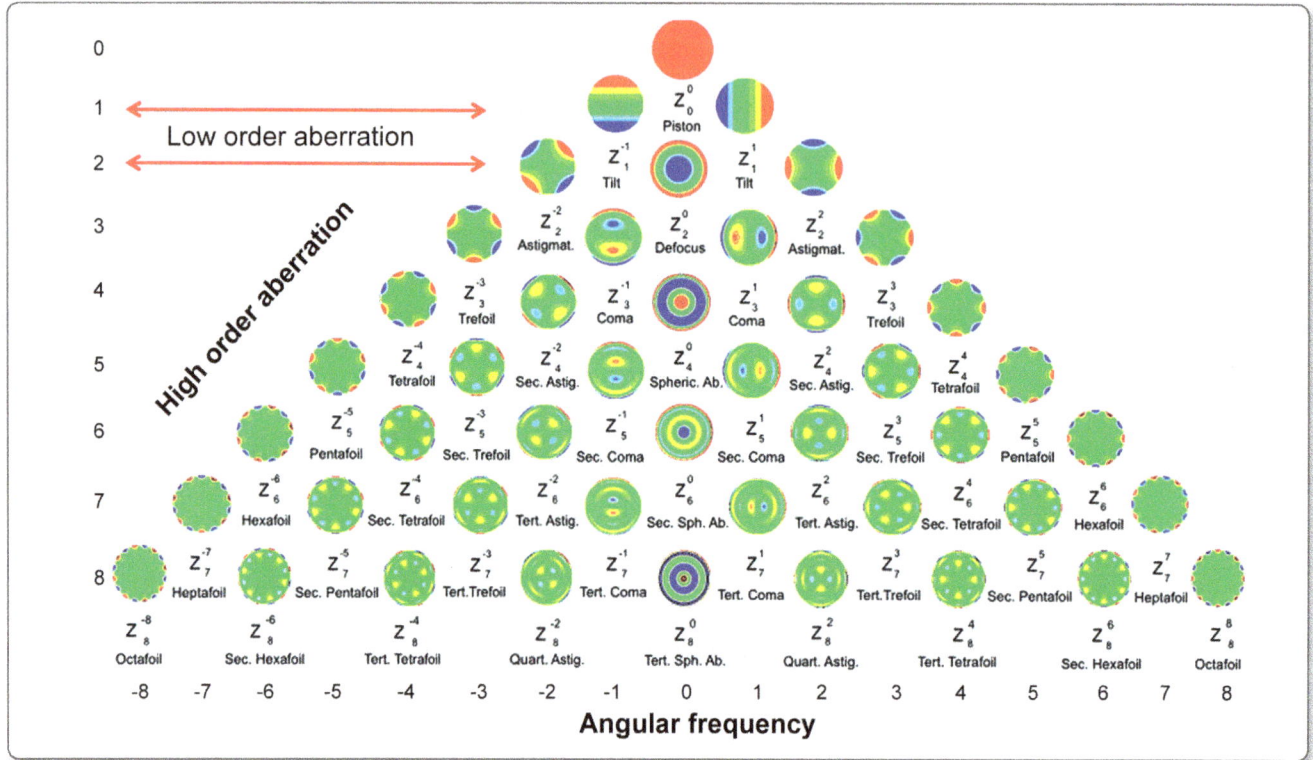

Fig. 13.3: Zernike pyramid.

and expressed as constant, lower-order and higher-order aberrations (Fig. 13.3). Zernike analysis is discussed in detail in Chapter 14.

TYPES OF ABERRATIONS

Based on the origin, eye wavefront aberrations are classified into ocular (or total) and corneal. Based on the composition, the aberrations can be either polychromatic or monochromatic. The former is a function of the refractive indices of colors, while the latter is a function of the profile of the refractive surfaces and is further subclassified into constant, lower-order and higher-order aberrations. Polychromatic aberrations are out of the scope of this book. Monochromatic aberrations are studied in depth in Chapter 14.

MEASUREMENT OF ABERRATIONS

Higher-order aberrations (HOAs) can be measured subjectively and objectively. Subjective measurement is difficult, time consuming and affected by the patient's perception. Corneal wavefront aberrations are objectively measured by corneal tomography, while ocular wavefront aberrations are objectively measured by aberrometers.

Corneal Tomography

Both Scheimpflug-based and scanning slit technologies calculate corneal wavefront aberrations indirectly from the elevation maps.

Aberrometers

Aberrometers measure ocular wavefront aberrations depending on ray tracing technology. Based on the technique used, there are three types of aberrometers:

1. *Outgoing reflective aberrometry*: Used by Hartmann–Shack wavefront sensor.
2. *Ingoing reflective aberrometry*: Used by Tscherning aberroscope, cross-cylinder aberroscope, and the sequential ray tracing technique.
3. *The ingoing feedback aberrometry*: Used in the spatially resolved refractometer. A variant of this technique is the optical path difference method.

Factors Affecting Measurements

There are several factors affecting both human-eye aberrations and their measurement. These factors are:

- *Pupil size*: Pupil size affects the measurement of *ocular* wavefront aberrations. The best functional diameter is 3–3.2 mm. The larger the pupil, the more disturbing the aberrations; at the same time, smaller pupils (<2.5 mm) lead to diffraction which also disturbs image quality. Pupils larger than 6 mm affect quality of vision due to peripheral imperfection. However, measurements are usually affected by large pupil sizes more than smaller ones.
- *Accommodation*: It affects *ocular* aberrations by affecting the amount of defocus, astigmatic aberration and spherical aberration. The latter increases toward negative with accommodation. However, these changes are of small clinical significance in both normal eyes and post-LASIK eyes.
- *Age*: This is discussed in detail later in this chapter.
- *Ocular pathologies*: Any pathology in the optical system certainly induces HOAs, such as cataract, corneal opacities, and vitreous opacities, and leads to erroneous measurements.
- *Previous ocular surgeries*: Such as keratorefractive procedures and intraocular operations.

Measurement Metrics

Wavefront aberrations can be quantified numerically at corneal and pupillary levels, or at retinal level.

Corneal and pupillary level: Objective visual function is measured at corneal level (in corneal wavefront) and pupillary level (in ocular wavefront) by the root mean square (RMS). RMS is an expression of the physical surface or the shape of the wavefront. It expresses the deviation averaged over the entire wavefront in reference to the perfect wavefront as shown in Figure 13.2. The quadratic values are summed and rooted by the following equation (as in the figure example):

$$RMS = \sqrt{[(-0.40)^2 + (+0.25)^2 + (+0.3)^2]} = 0.559\ \mu m$$

RMS is a quantitative representation of the magnitude of wavefront deviation, and it is more accurate in large deviations. It cannot serve as a qualitative representation as different types of aberrations may have equal RMS across the pupil but have different effects on vision; therefore, RMS is unrelated to visual performance. The majority of normal *emmetropic* eyes have total RMS values $\leq 0.4\ \mu m$. In wavefront analysis, RMS is given in two values: (1) total RMS, which is a sum of LOAs and HOAs, and (2) HOA-related RMS. The former is higher than the latter since it includes the effect of refractive errors on the wavefront, but the latter is the one of interest in decision making.

Retinal level: Objective visual function is measured at retinal level by the following metrics, where they are all for ocular wavefront:
- *Point spread function (PSF)*: By definition, PSF is the image that an optical system forms of a point source, which is the most fundamental object. If an optical system were perfect, the image of a point would be a point, but because the optical system of the human eye is not usually perfect, the point is imaged as a spread image. In aberration free optics, the image of a point takes a special shape called "Airy pattern", which is a phenomenon of light diffraction, and, in the human eye, it is the Fraunhofer diffraction pattern of a circular pupil. The amount of diffraction (and therefore the diameter of the Airy disk) enlarges when the diameter of the pupil gets smaller; the ideal pupil diameter for the smallest Airy pattern is 6–7 mm; therefore, PSF and other measurements are usually taken for a standard pupil diameter of 6 mm.

  Measuring PSF helps the physician to see what the patient sees, to simulate potential treatments, and to predict how those treatments would alter the patient's PSF. Additionally, PSF of the total wavefront can give an approximation of the real spherical equivalent refractive error by the expression "Eff Blur," which stands for efficient blur.
- *Strehl ratio (SR)*: Strehl ratio is a measure of optical excellence. It is the simplest meaningful way of expressing the effect of wavefront aberrations on image quality. In other words, this ratio is an expression of the amount of light contained within the Airy disk as a percentage of the theoretical maximum that would be contained within the disk with a perfect optical system. SR = 1 means perfection, and anything less than 1, is less than perfection. Stated roughly, 1 is perfection, 0.8 is okay, 0.9 is good, and 0.95 is extremely good.
- *Modulation transfer function (MTF)*: It is the most widely used scientific method for describing optical system performance. The MTF is a measure of the reduction in contrast from object to image. In other words, it measures how faithfully the optical system reproduces (or transfers) detail from the object to the image produced by the optical system.

  Since the MTF is the ratio of the image modulation to the object modulation in all spatial frequencies, it takes a value ranging from 0 to 1, where 0 stands for imperfection and 1 stands for full perfection.

  The relationship between MTF and spatial frequency is inverse; the higher the spatial frequency, the lower the MTF and the worse the visual acuity. There is also an inverse relationship between MTF and PSF; the narrower the PSF, the higher the MTF and the higher the quality of an optical system.

Moreover, the relationship between MTF and pupil size is also inverse; the larger the pupil, the lower the MTF and the lower the quality of the image.

- *Phase transfer function (PTF)*: It measures the lateral displacement of a sinusoidal image of specific spatial frequency, observed through an aberrated system. It is seldom used in ophthalmology.
- *Optical transfer function (OTF)*: It is a combination of MTF and PTF. Similar to PSF, it describes the response of an imaging system to a point source or point object, but with a greater contrast (increase in the MTF) and sharper definition (reduction in PTF). Like PTF, it is seldom used in ophthalmology.
- *Zernike coefficient (ZC)*: It is an expression of the amount of each individual aberration. Sophisticated equations are used to calculate ZC for each polynomial. Unlike RMS, ZC may take either negative or positive values. Generally speaking, ZC is normal, suspected or abnormal when its value is < 0.25 µm, 0.25–0.5 µm or > 0.5 µm, respectively. Chapter 14 is devoted for Zernike analysis.
- *Fourier analysis*: Fourier analysis is a mathematical method alternative to Zernike polynomials used in analyzing and reconstructing the wavefront of the visual system. Chapter 15 is devoted for Fourier analysis.

CHANGES OF ABERRATIONS WITH AGE

Generally speaking, ocular aberrations change and usually increase with age. These changes are related to the cornea and the crystalline lens.

Corneal Changes with Age

In young eyes, the cornea is typically steeper on the vertical meridian and, therefore, has WTR astigmatism. This tends to reverse with age and, therefore, an older cornea has ATR astigmatism. In general, the cornea tends to be more curved with age. This decrease of radius of curvature is on the account of the anterior corneal surface. The only significant age-related change in corneal aberration is a decrease in the posterior surface asphericity.

Crystalline Lens Changes with Age

Major changes in aberrations are related to aging of the crystalline lens. With age, spherical aberration changes to be less negative or even positive, the RMS increases and contrast sensitivity decreases due to increased scattering.

Corneal/Internal Aberration Compensation

In young eyes, there is a balance of aberrations between cornea and lens. This balance decreases with age to cause positive total spherical aberrations and an increase in coma-like aberrations. The coma-like changes are unexplainable.

CLINICAL APPLICATION OF WAVEFRONT TECHNOLOGY

Prediction of Subjective Refraction

This is known as objective refraction. It is useful in very distorted corneas when subjective refraction is not possible or not valid. However, it is not a straightforward task due to many reasons. First, HOAs have an impact on the manifest spherocylinder refractive error. Second, the eye suffers not only from monochromatic aberrations, but also from polychromatic aberrations. Third, prediction of refraction differs according to the method used and is affected by some factors such as pupil size.

Wavefront in FFKC Detection

Wavefront can be used as a diagnostic measure of ectatic corneal disorders in general, and the detection of FFKC in particular. Some studies found that HOA begin to change either before prominent changes appear on corneal topography and tomography. Main changes can be summarized as follows:

The ZC of *corneal* vertical tilt (ZC_1^{-1}), *corneal* vertical coma (ZC_3^{-1}), and *corneal* horizontal trefoil (ZC_3^3) take significantly more negative values in FFKC.

The ZC of *corneal* total coma RMS starts to increase taking higher values than in normal eyes. No such significant change is found in *corneal* total trefoil.

The ZC *ocular* vertical tilt (ZO_1^{-1}), *ocular* vertical coma (ZO_3^{-1}), and *ocular* horizontal trefoil (ZO_3^3) take significantly high values in FFKC.

No significant change is found either in *ocular* total RMS or trefoil. This might partly be due to internal aberrations compensating for the aberrations generated by the FFKC cornea.

Cutoff points differ between studies due to different devices used in measuring HOA. However, the mentioned HOA and their values can be monitored in suspected cases to document any significant change.

Wavefront-optimized and Wavefront-guided Ablations

While conventional excimer laser ablations typically increase HOAs, both wavefront-optimized (WFO) and wavefront-guided (WFG) ablations tend to induce fewer HOAs and may, in principle, be able to reduce preexisting higher-order optical aberrations.

Intraocular Lens Design

Aspheric IOLs can be designed to compensate for the spherical aberration to optimize the quality of vision after cataract surgery by increasing contrast sensitivity in mesopic conditions.

Presbyopic Treatment

One of the options of presbyopic treatment is asphericity-guided. It is composed of adjusting the Q-value to induce tolerable negative spherical aberrations which increases the depth of focus without compromising the quality and quantity of vision.

CHAPTER 14

Zernike Analysis

INTRODUCTION

Zernike analysis is a mathematical description of wavefront aberrations. Fritz Zernike could describe wavefront aberrations in circle polynomials in the radial (n) and angular (m) directions by using an equation, depending on which, Zernike polynomials are calculated, given indexes and expressed as constant, lower-order aberrations (LOAs) and higher-order aberrations (HOAs) (refer Fig. 13.3). Table 14.1 is Zernike description of aberrations.

Zernike polynomials are expressed in two methods: $Z(n,m)$ or by Z_n^m. The "m" stands for a continuous function that repeats self every 2π radians, and the "n" stands for a radial function that is proportional with the order of the polynomials. To simplify the matter, "m" can be considered as the number of asymmetric meridians, and "n" as the number of slopes along the asymmetric meridians. The "m" is given a –ve sign to indicate vertical aberrations and a +ve sign to indicate horizontal aberrations. Therefore, in Z(5,1) for example, there is only one asymmetric (irregular) meridian (m = 1), the number of slopes on that meridian is 5 slopes (n = 5), and this aberration is horizontal because the sign of "m" is +ve (Fig. 14.1). Another example is Z(4,–2). There are two asymmetric meridians, the number of slopes on each meridian is four slopes, and this aberration is vertical because the sign of "m" is –ve (Fig. 14.2).

Based on that, the nonperiodic types of irregular astigmatism have only one irregular meridian (m = 1), and thus known as irregularly irregular astigmatism, including coma, secondary coma, tertiary coma, etc. They differ from each another by number of slopes on the irregular meridian, so that they take odd numbers, such as Z(3,–1) and Z(3,1) for vertical and horizontal coma, Z(5,–1) and Z(5,1) for vertical and horizontal secondary coma, Z(7,–1) and Z(7,1) for vertical and horizontal tertiary coma, etc. The same can be applied on trefoil (m = 3), pentafoil (m = 5), and heptafoil (m = 7) (refer Fig. 13.3).

On the other hand, the periodic HOAs have two or more irregular meridians, but with regular change in power between them (angular repetition of irregularity), and thus known as regularly irregular astigmatism. They differ from each another by number of irregular meridians and number of slopes on the irregular meridian, but all of them take even numbers, such as Z(4,–2) and Z(4,2) for secondary astigmatism, Z(6,–2) and Z(6,2) for tertiary astigmatism, Z(8,–2) and Z(8,2) for quarterly astigmatism, etc. The same can be applied on tetrafoil (m = 4), hexafoil (m = 6), and octafoil (m = 8) (refer Fig. 13.3).

Moreover, all orders of spherical aberration (SA) are considered as periodic HOAs, but all of them have n = 0, which means that there are no meridians, and have m = 4 (4 slopes all around the circle) for primary SA, m = 6 (6 slopes) for secondary SA, m = 8 (8 slopes) for tertiary SA, etc. (refer Fig. 13.3).

In the following, the principle, description and types of polynomials will be explained in depth.

CONSTANT ABERRATIONS

Constant aberrations exist in all optical systems. They occupy the zero order and the first order of the Zernike pyramid.
- *Zero order*: It is known as Piston or Reference point (Fig. 14.3). It is given the symbol Z(0,0), which means: no meridians and no slopes; it is just a planner pattern.
- *First order*: It is known as tilt or prism. It is a flat deviation in the direction that a beam of light propagates. It is

Chapter 14: Zernike Analysis

Table 14.1: Zernike description of aberrations.

Coefficient	Index Z(n, m)	Order	Description
0	Z(0,0)	Zero	Piston
1	Z(1,−1)	First	Vertical tilt
2	Z(1, 1)	First	Horizontal tilt
3	Z(2,−2)	Second	Vertical astigmatism
4	Z(2,0)	Second	Defocus
5	Z(2,2)	Second	Horizontal astigmatism
6	Z(3,−3)	Third	Vertical trefoil
7	Z(3,−1)	Third	Vertical coma
8	Z(3,1)	Third	Horizontal coma
9	Z(3,3)	Third	Horizontal trefoil
10	Z(4,−4)	Fourth	Vertical tetrafoil
11	Z(4,−2)	Fourth	Secondary vertical astigmatism
12	Z(4,0)	Fourth	Spherical aberration
13	Z(4,2)	Fourth	Secondary horizontal astigmatism
14	Z(4,4)	Fourth	Horizontal tetrafoil
15	Z(5,−5)	Fifth	Vertical pentafoil
16	Z(5, −3)	Fifth	Secondary vertical trefoil
17	Z(5,−1)	Fifth	Secondary vertical coma
18	Z(5,1)	Fifth	Secondary horizontal coma
19	Z(5,3)	Fifth	Secondary horizontal trefoil
20	Z(5,5)	Fifth	Horizontal pentafoil
21	Z(6,−6)	Sixth	Vertical hexafoil
22	Z(6,−4)	Sixth	Secondary vertical tetrafoil
23	Z(6,−2)	Sixth	Tertiary vertical astigmatism
24	Z(6,0)	Sixth	Secondary spherical aberration
25	Z(6,2)	Sixth	Tertiary horizontal astigmatism
26	Z(6,4)	Sixth	Secondary horizontal tetrafoil
27	Z(6,6)	Sixth	Horizontal hexafoil

caused by decentered optics. It is given the symbol Z(1,−1) for vertical and Z(1,1) for horizontal, which means only one meridian with only one slope (Fig. 14.4).

Constant aberrations are not taken into consideration when measuring the aberrations to avoid over estimation.

LOWER-ORDER ABERRATIONS

Lower-order aberrations are aberrations that occupy the second order of the pyramid. They include two components of astigmatism and a spherical blur component or defocus. LOAs are usually associated with the spherocylindrical refractive errors and can be corrected with glasses. In the general population, LOAs constitute approximately 80–90% of all aberrations.

Second order: It contains defocus and astigmatic aberration.

- *Defocus*: It is the translation along the optical axis away from the plane or surface of best focus. In general, defocus reduces the sharpness and contrast of the image. In the human eye, spherical refractive errors are associated with defocus; in myopia the focal point lies in front of the retina, whereas in hypermetropia it lies behind it. Defocus is given the symbol Z(2,0), which means no meridians but two slopes (Fig. 14.5). Defocus increases with larger pupil size as shown in Figure 14.6.

Section 4: Wavefront Analysis

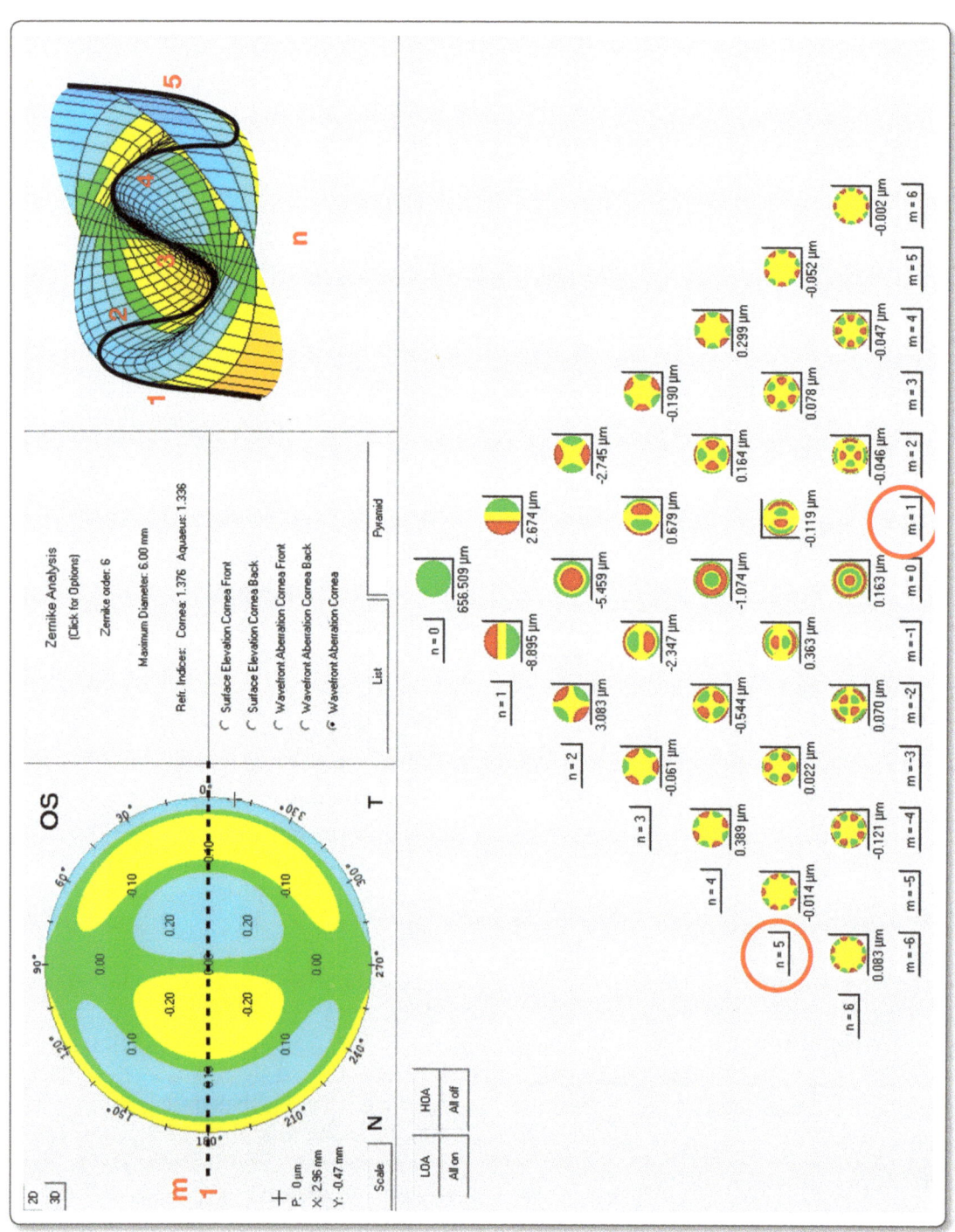

Fig. 14.1: Representation of the Z(5,1) higher-order aberration.

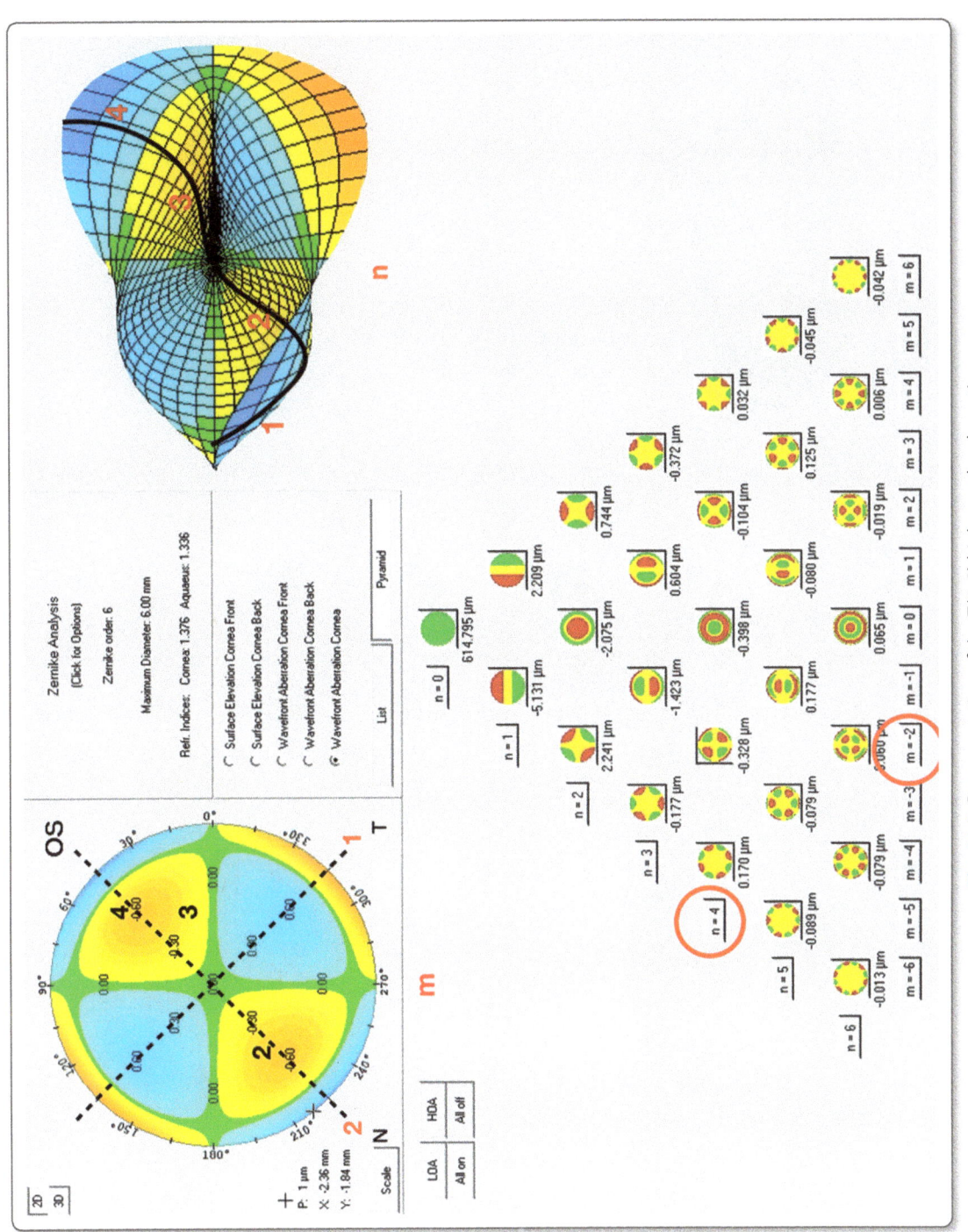

Fig. 14.2: Representation of the Z(4,-2) higher-order aberration.

Section 4: *Wavefront Analysis*

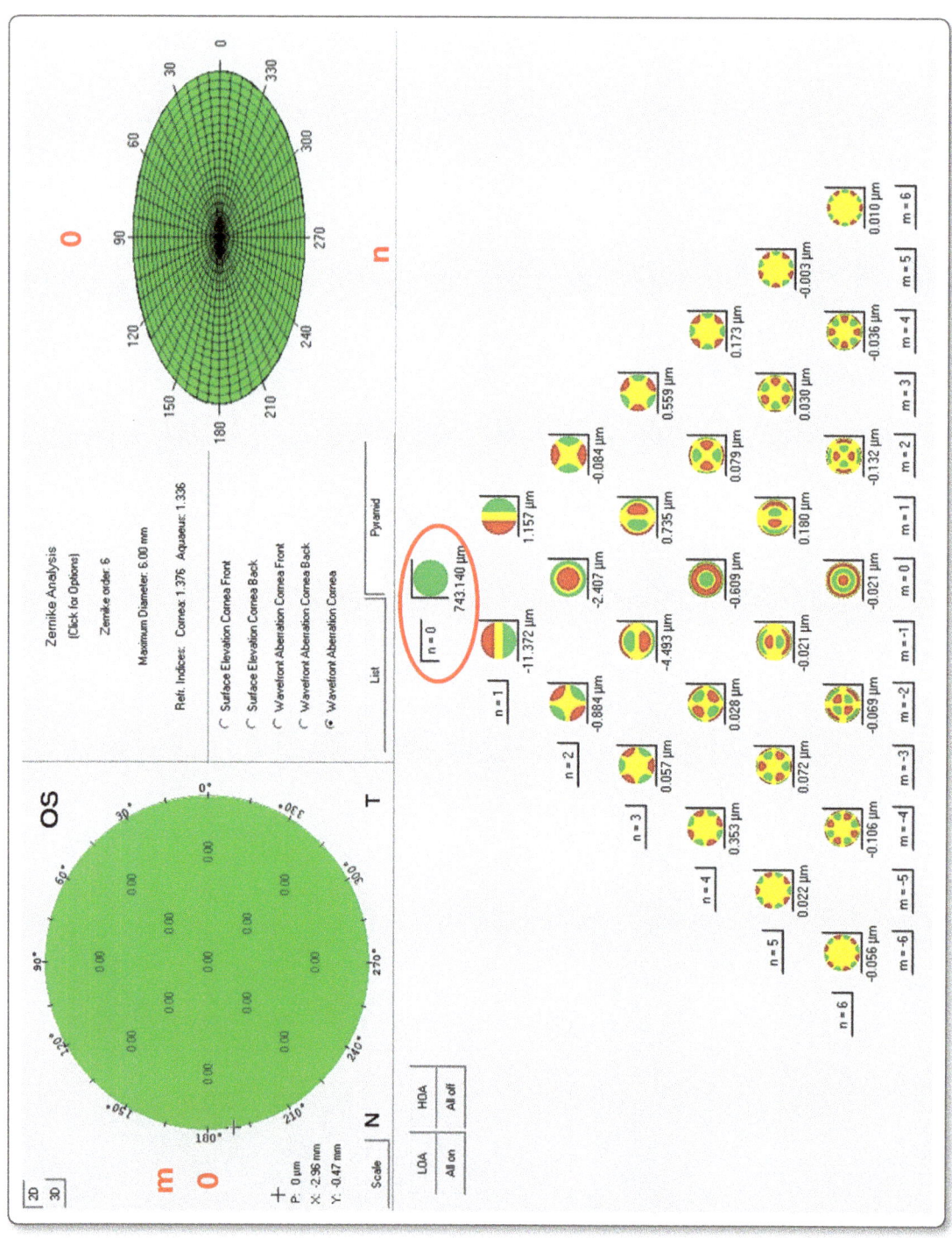

Fig. 14.3: Piston.

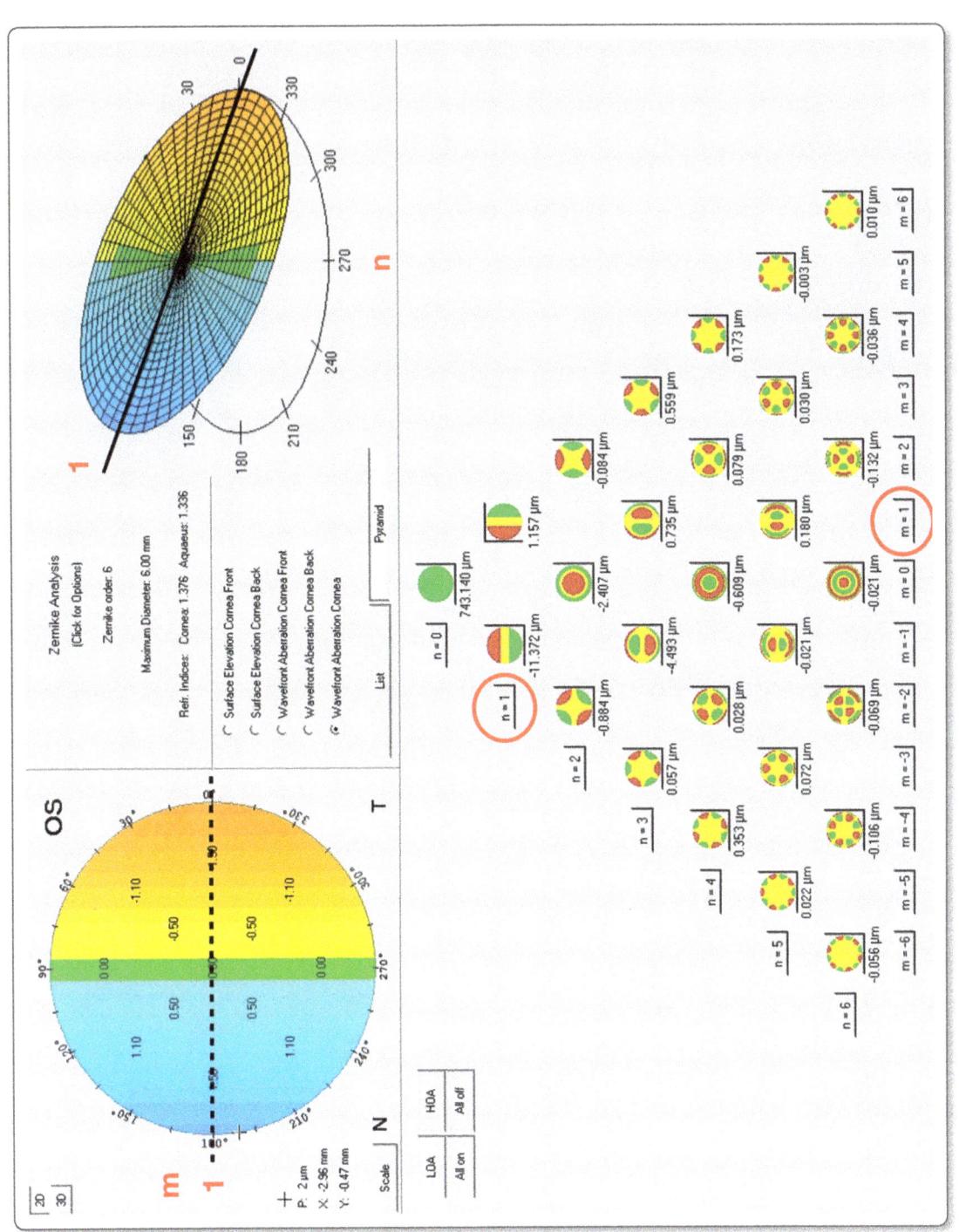

Fig. 14.4: Tilt or prism.

Section 4: *Wavefront Analysis*

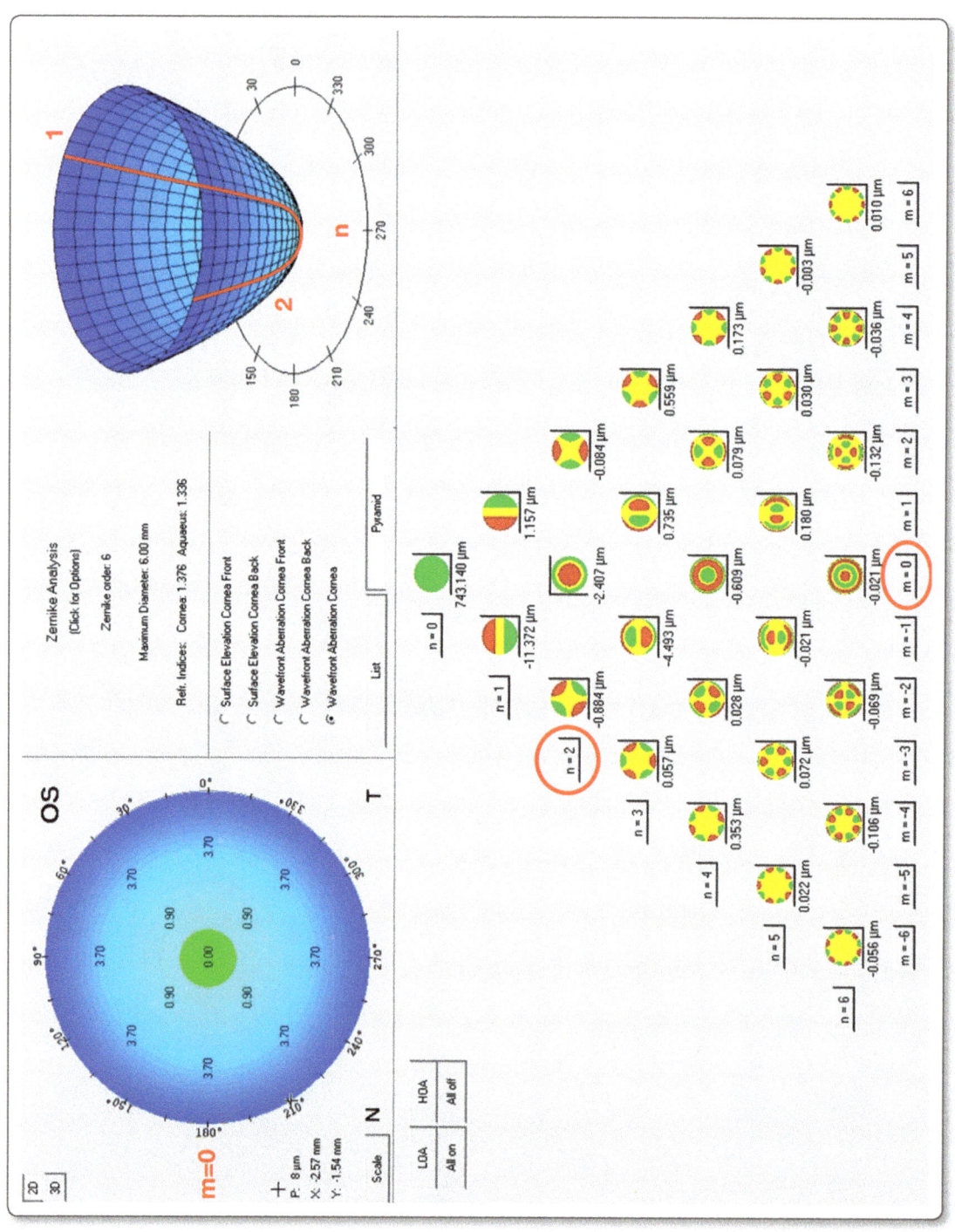

Fig. 14.5: Defocus.

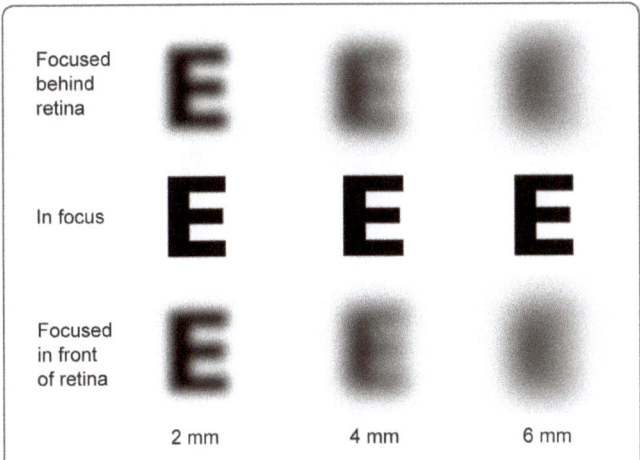

Fig. 14.6: The relation between defocus and pupil size.

- *Astigmatic aberration*: In the human eye, regular astigmatism is associated with lower-order astigmatic aberration. It is given the symbol Z(2,–2) for vertical and Z(2,2) for horizontal, which means two meridians with two slopes on each of them (Fig. 14.7).

HIGHER-ORDER ABERRATIONS

Higher-order aberrations constitute about 15% of the total aberrations. They have more complex geometrical forms and start at the third order in Zernike polynomials. They may or may not be associated with refractive errors. However, they affect the objective and subjective measurements of refractive errors, for example coma affects astigmatism and SA affects the sphere. HOAs cannot be corrected with conventional optics. They need special designs of contact lenses or glasses, or may be treated by photorefractive surgery or special designs of phakic IOLs.

The impact of HOAs on vision quality depends on various factors, including the underlying cause, amount and type of HOAs, pupil size and light conditions. They usually cause haloes (Fig. 14.8), glare (Fig. 14.9), ghost images (Fig. 14.10), starburst (Fig. 14.11) patterns and monocular diplopia especially in low lighting conditions and during night driving. People with larger pupil sizes generally may have more visual symptoms related to HOAs, particularly in low lighting conditions. But even people with small or moderate pupils can have significant visual symptoms when the HOAs are caused by conditions such as corneal scars or cataracts. Also, specific types and orientation of HOAs have been found in some studies to affect vision quality of eyes with smaller pupils. Large amounts of certain HOAs can have a severe, even disabling, impact on vision quality.

Some of the HOAs have terms such as coma, trefoil, and SA, but many more of them are identified only by mathematical expressions to have an order. Order refers to the complexity of the shape of the wavefront emerging through the pupil; the more complex the shape, the higher the order of aberration. However, in clinical practice, optical analysis is only considered important to the sixth order, and by some researchers up to the fourth order.

Third Order Aberrations

They are trefoil and coma.
- *Trefoil (Fig. 14.12)*: It is also known as triangular astigmatism. The term came from the *Trifolium* plant (Clover) that has compound trifoliate leaflets. The eye with a *trefoil* aberration receives a point of light like a Mercedes-Benz symbol (Fig. 14.13). Peripheral vision is usually affected more than central vision. Additionally, the trefoil affects both sphere and astigmatism measurements. In Zernike polynomials, trefoil is given the symbol Z(3,–3) for vertical and Z(3,3) for horizontal, which means three meridians with three slopes on each of them.
- *Coma (Fig. 14.14)*: It is the most HOA affecting central vision. It is defined as a variation of magnification (refractive power) in one meridian over the entrance pupil. Coma causes the light source to be seen like a comet (has a tail) as shown in Figure 14.15. The coma results from central and paracentral asymmetry in ocular optical components, which affects central vision, such as in keratoconus, decentered post-LVC zone and decentered IOL. Additionally, the coma affects the measurement of astigmatism. In Zernike polynomials, coma is given the symbol Z(3,–1) for vertical and Z(3,1) for horizontal, which means one meridian with three slops on it.

Fourth Order Aberrations

They are SA, secondary astigmatism, and tetrafoil.
- *SA (Fig. 14.16)*: SA results from abnormal Q-value. It usually affects peripheral vision, affects measurements of sphere and results in halos around oncoming lights. Figure 14.17 is a simulation of the scene of light source seen by an eye with SA. SA can either be positive or negative. The positive type is encountered in oblate optics, while the negative type is encountered in prolate and hyperprolate optics (refer Fig. 5.5). The human eye is designed to compensate for the positive SA by two mechanisms: corneal and lenticular. Corneal mechanism

Section 4: Wavefront Analysis

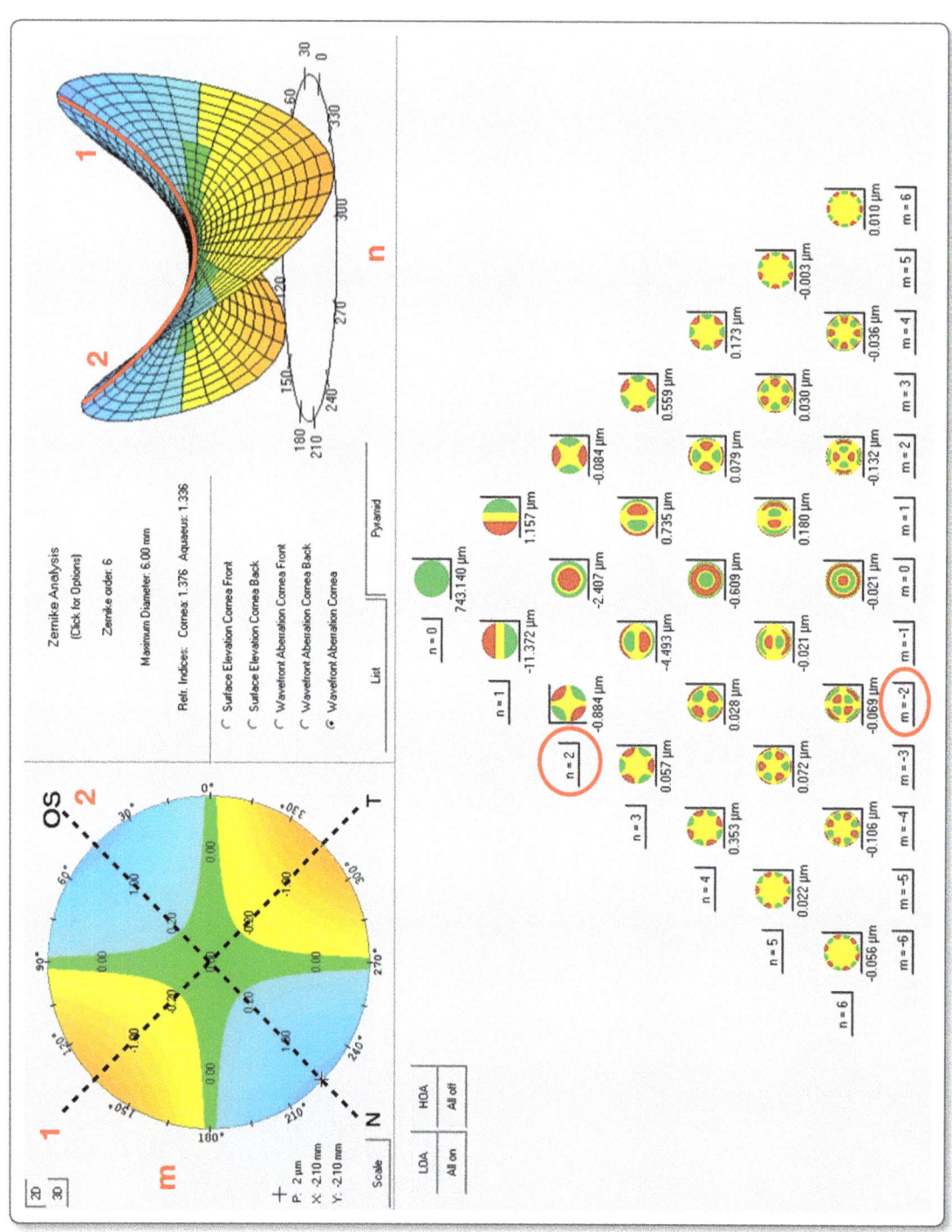

Fig. 14.7: Astigmatic lower-order aberration.

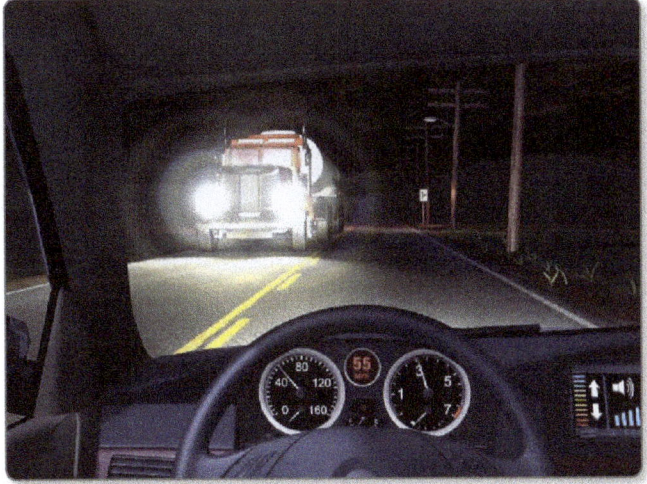

Fig. 14.8: Halos.

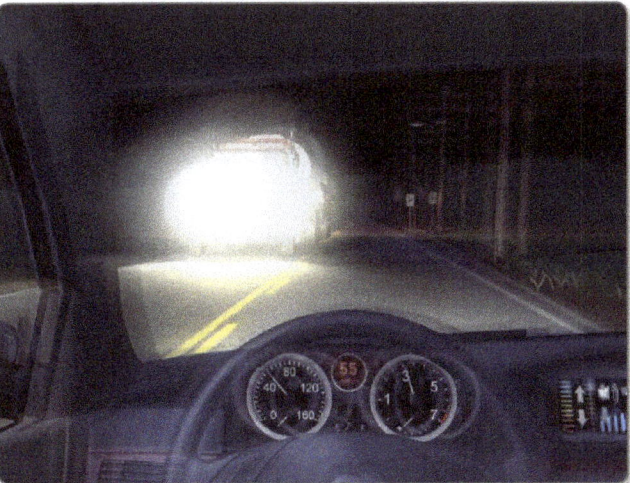

Fig. 14.10: Ghost images.

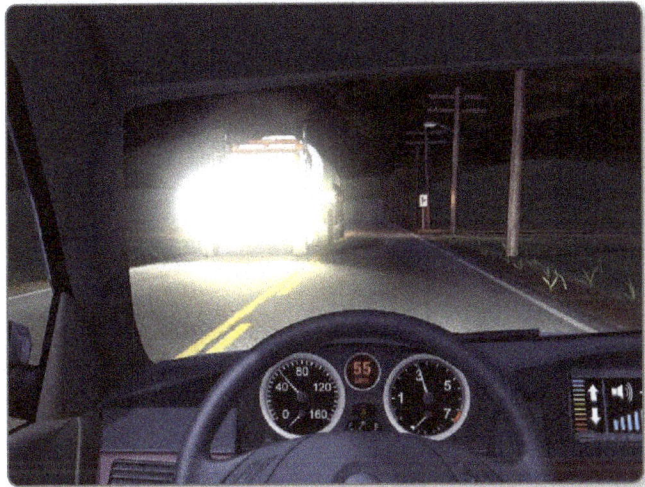

Fig. 14.9: Glare.

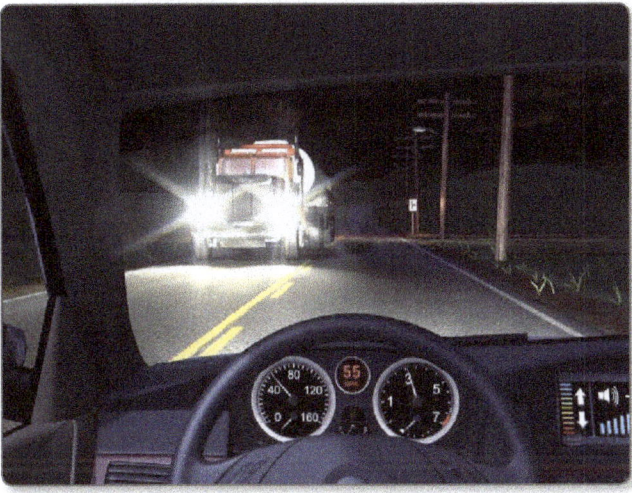

Fig. 14.11: Starburst.

consists of the prolate shape of the cornea. Lenticular mechanism consists of the virtue of the curvature of its front and back surface as well as the refractive index difference between the central area and periphery. SA usually becomes more positive after conventional corneal surgery for myopia, and less positive or negative after hypermetropic corneal surgery. This results from the small optical zone size and the suboptimal asphericity of the postoperative anterior corneal profile. In Zernike polynomials, SA is given the symbol $Z(4,0)$.

- *Secondary astigmatism (Fig. 14.18)*: It is given $Z(4,-2)$ for the vertical and $Z(4,2)$ for the horizontal subtypes. It has two regular irregular meridians with four slopes on each meridian. This aberration affects mid peripheral vision and measurements of astigmatism.
- *Tetrafoil (Fig. 14.19)*: It is given $Z(4,-4)$ and $Z(4,4)$ for the vertical and horizontal subtypes, respectively. It has four regular irregular meridians with four slopes on each meridian. This aberration affects peripheral vision and measurements of both sphere and astigmatism.

Fifth Order and Higher

Starting from the fifth order descending progressively in the analysis of the aberrations in the pyramid, each of the above aberrations presents its secondary, tertiary component, which is a variation in shape of the primary based on number of meridians and number of slopes. However, the rate of the fifth and the higher levels is usually low and their role in the visual performance degradation is usually small, but can become significant in some special conditions such as irregular scarring, incisional surgery, and penetrating keratoplasty.

Section 4: Wavefront Analysis

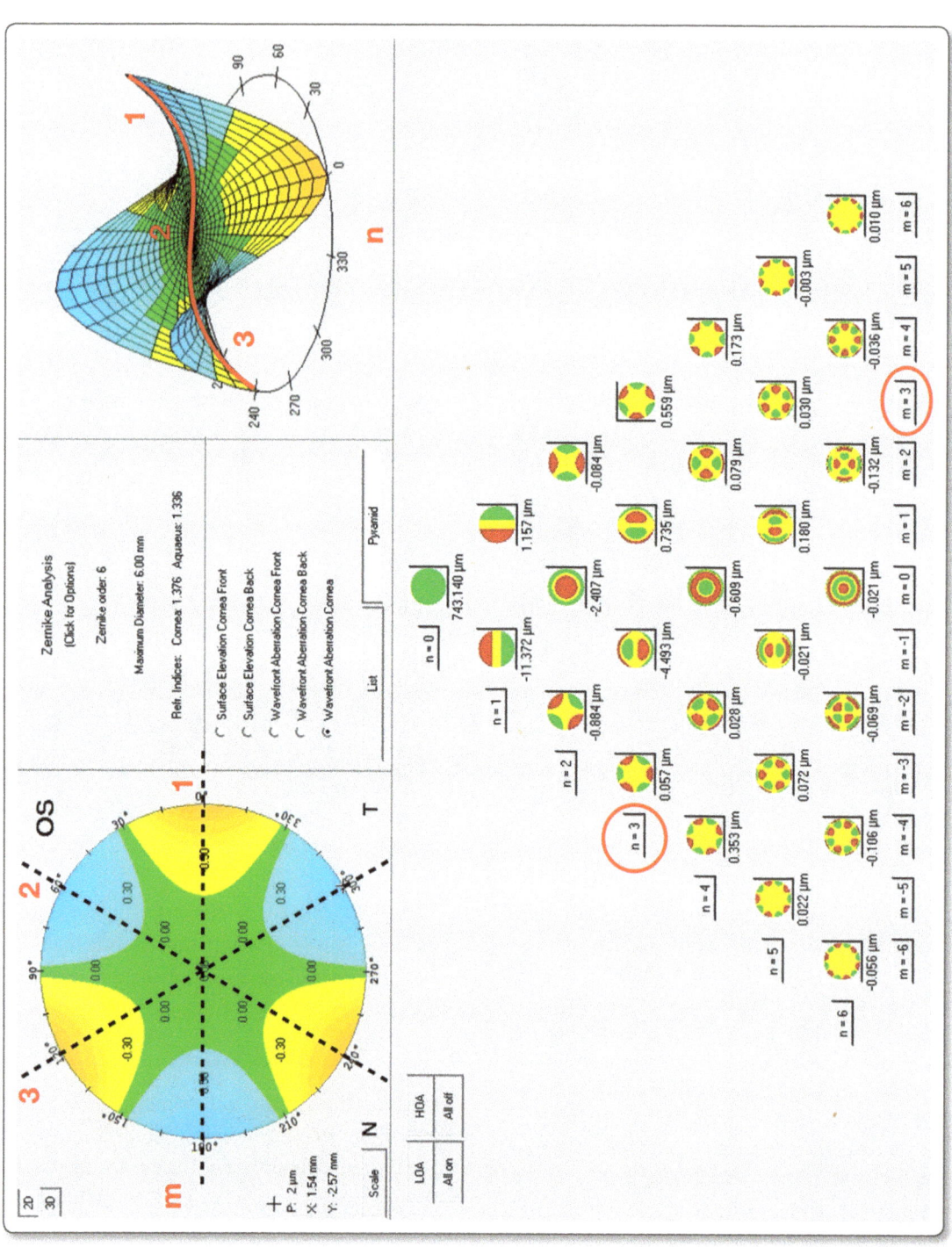

Fig. 14.12: Trefoil.

Chapter 14: *Zernike Analysis*   **133**

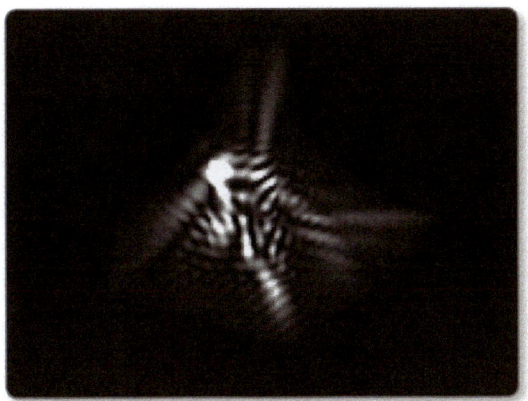

Fig. 14.13: Mercedes-Benz image resulting from trefoil aberration.

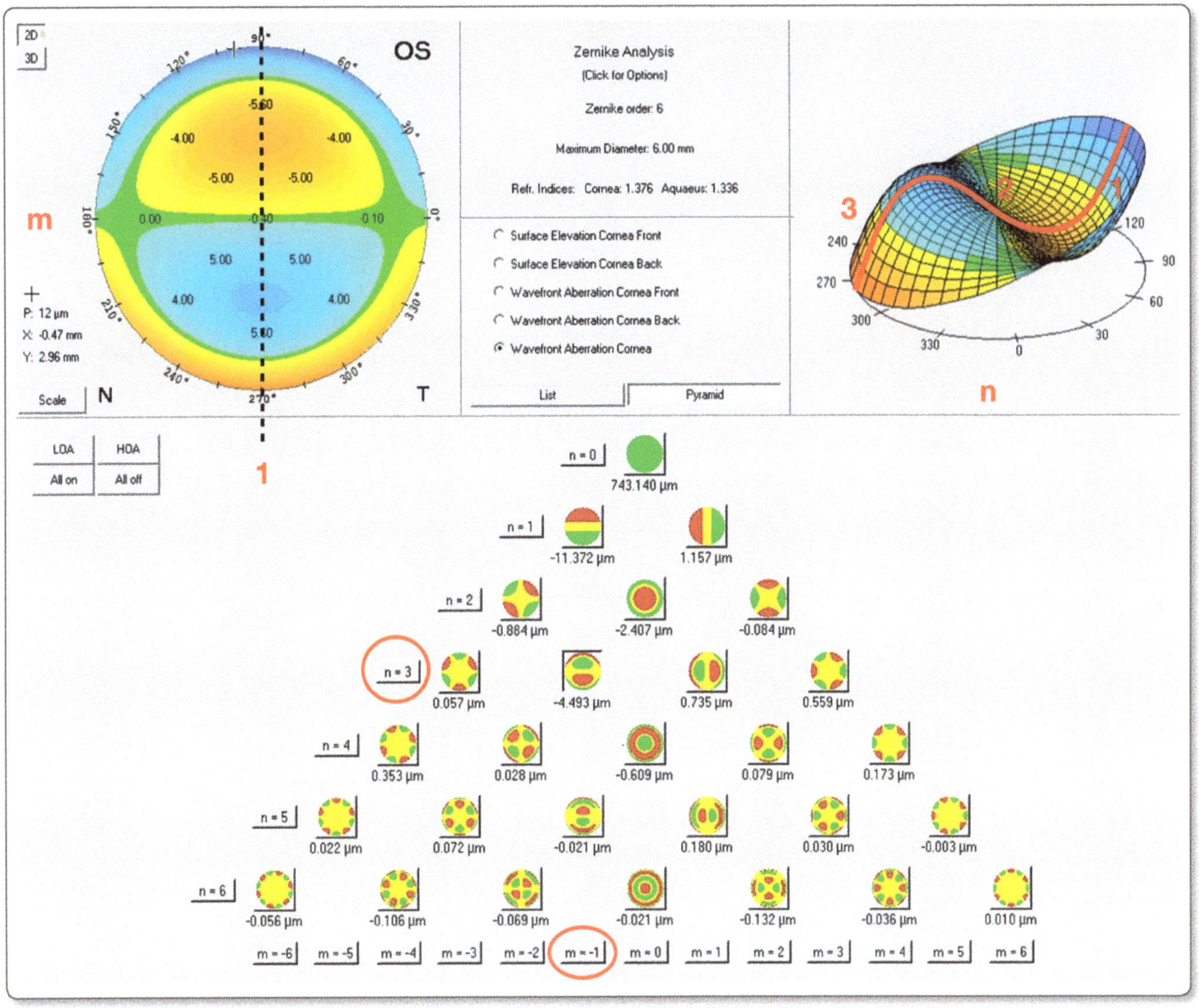

Fig. 14.14: Coma.

134 *Section 4: Wavefront Analysis*

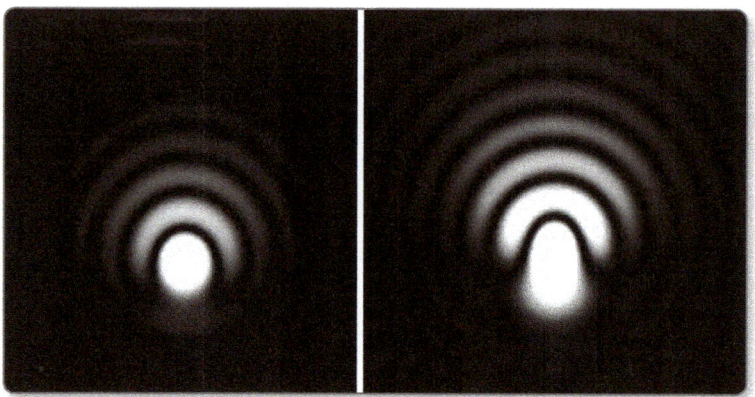

Fig. 14.15: Comet resulting from coma aberration.

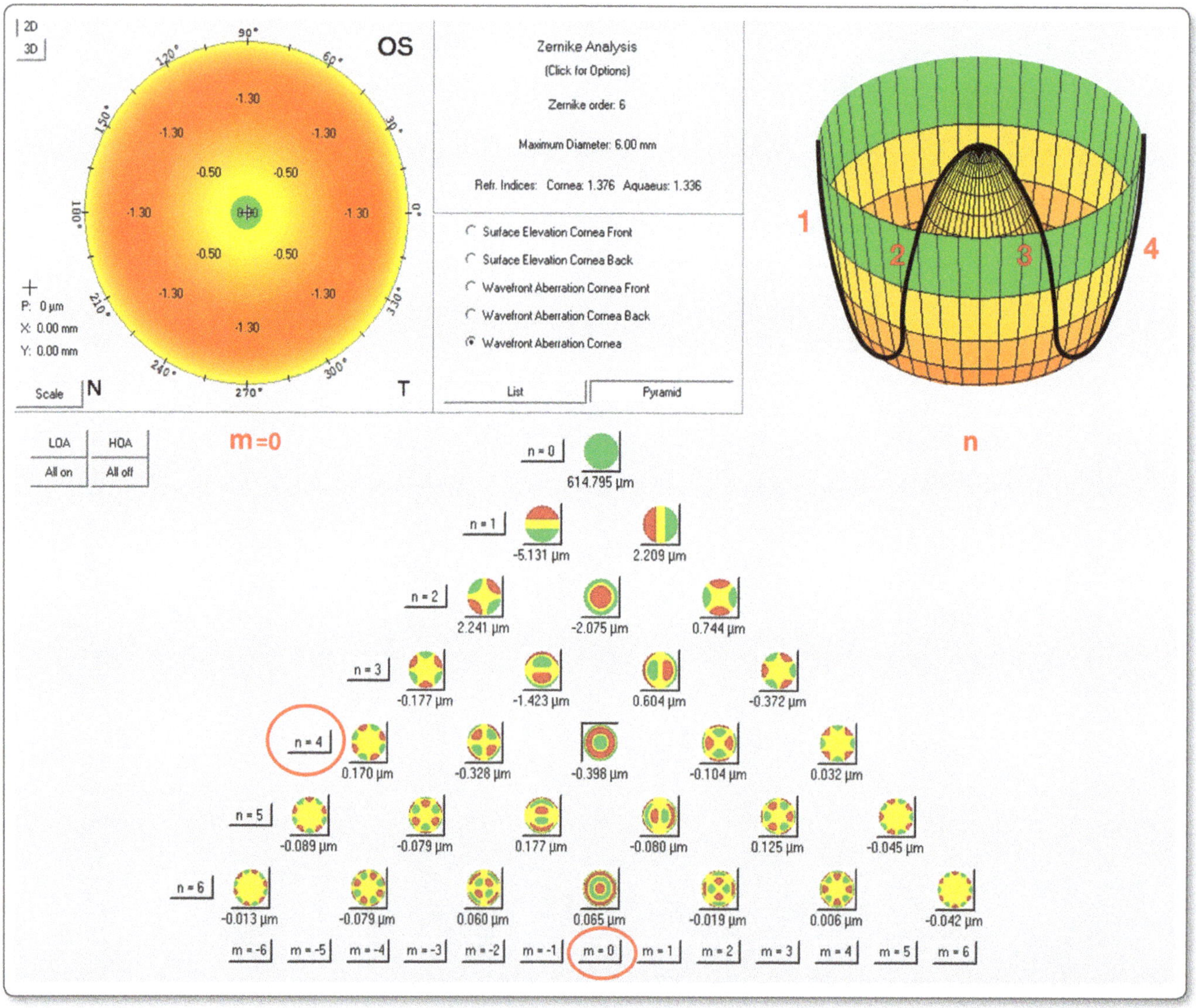

Fig. 14.16: Spherical aberration.

Chapter 14: Zernike Analysis

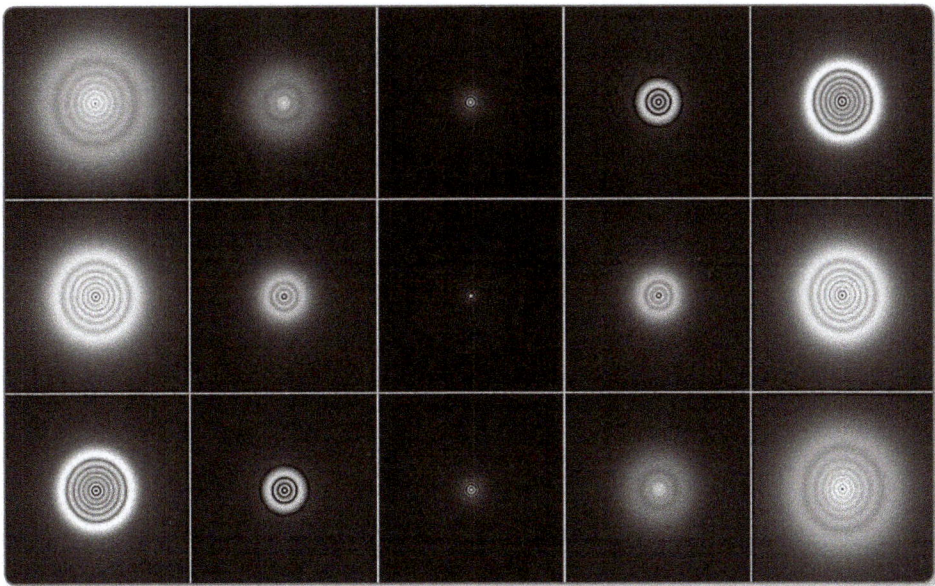

Fig. 14.17: Halos resulting from spherical aberration.

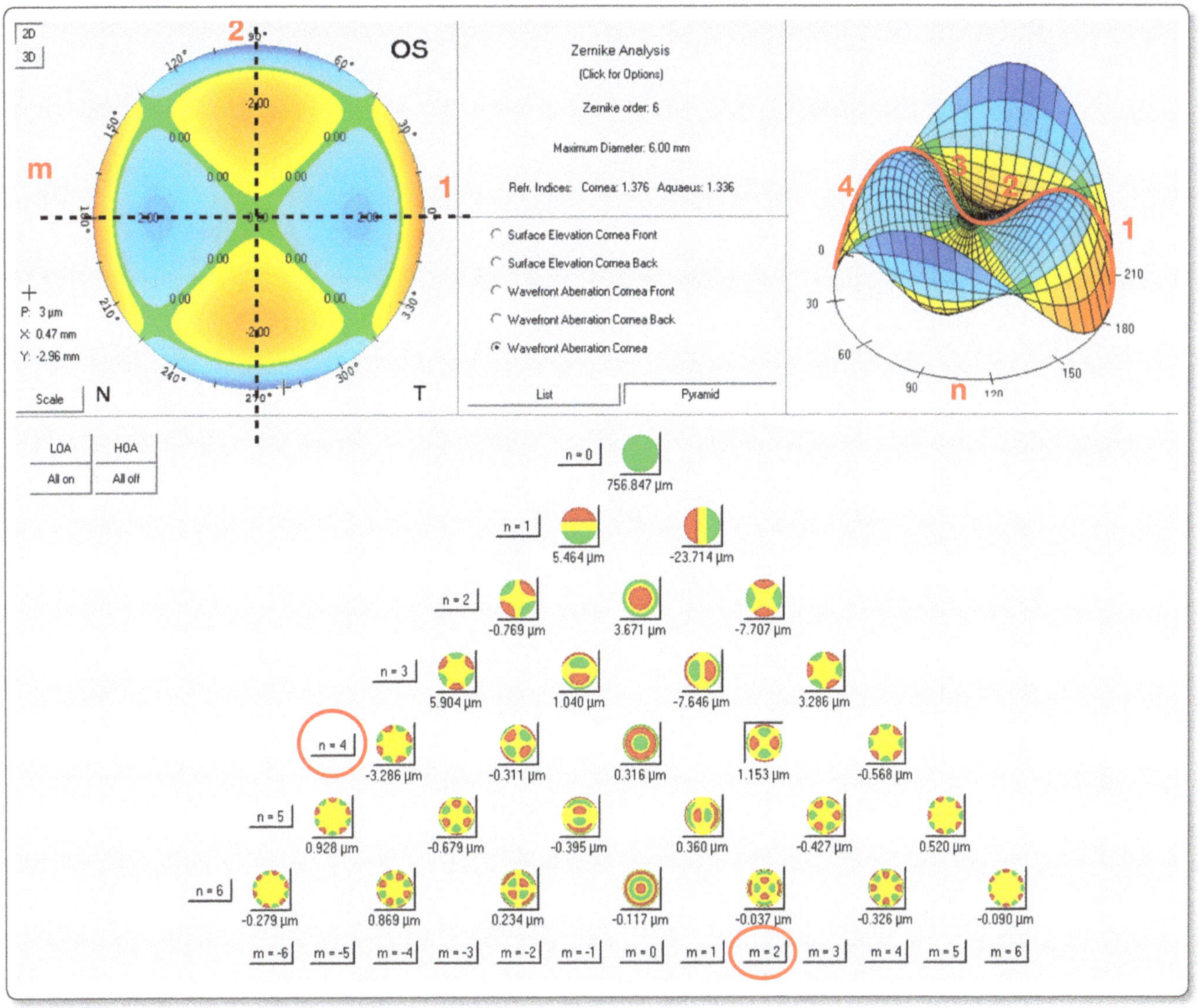

Fig. 14.18: Secondary astigmatism.

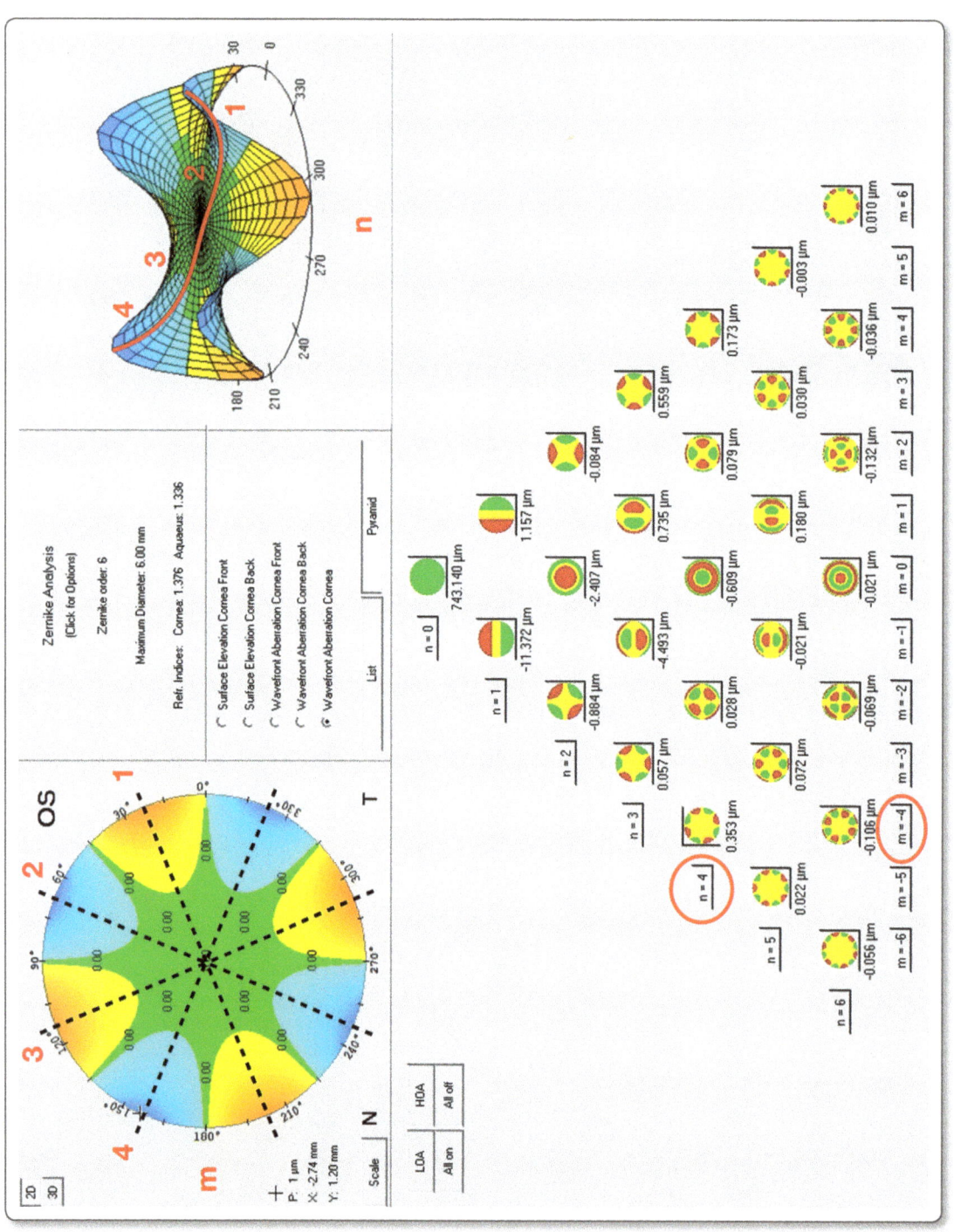

Fig. 14.19: Tetrafoil.

Fourier Analysis

INTRODUCTION

Fourier analysis is a mathematical method alternative to Zernike polynomials used in analyzing and reconstructing the wavefront of the visual system. It is also known as Fourier transform and is named after the French mathematician Joseph Fourier. It is the analysis of a periodic function into its simple sinusoidal or harmonic components, whose sum forms a Fourier series. It is mostly used to deconstruct corneal wavefront scans by decomposing the image into spatial frequency components where the composite corneal wavefront is deconstructed into the following components (Fig. 15.1): spherical component (corneal sphere), decentration (corneal coma), regular astigmatism (corneal astigmatism), and irregularities (residual higher-order aberrations (HOAs).

Fourier analysis is superior to Zernike polynomials because the polynomials have the following limitations:
- They can be used only in circular patterns, such as circular pupils. If the pupil is elliptical, the data outside the circle are not valid.
- They approximate the wavefront error of the eye/cornea by averaging and smoothening. They limit the data resolution in eyes with high amounts of irregular astigmatism. However, Zernike smoothing of the data could be beneficial on occasion, especially where irregular data could be artifactual, e.g. due to dry eye rather than the physical corneal shape.
- The data lose fidelity beyond the ninth order and more, and noise rather than information is introduced beyond the tenth order.
- They are unable to describe the aberrations generated by straight line irregularities, such as those resulting from flap striae and cap amputations.

FOURIER ANALYSIS OF CORNEAL WAVEFRONT

Figure 15.1 represents Fourier analysis of corneal wavefront into four components. A case of keratoconus was chosen to highlight the importance of the analysis.
- *Spherical component (Fig. 15.2)*: This map represents the potential sphere of the cornea. Objective corneal dioptric power (ODP) is discussed in Chapter 11. When comparing the central K in this map with the K_{ref} = 43 D, the reader can imagine the potential spherical power of this cornea. In our example, the difference is 43 − 58 = −15.3 D. There are two boxes at the bottom of the map: (1) spherical Rmin, representing the steepest radius of curvature in this map, and (2) spherical ECC, representing the mean numerical eccentricity of the spherical component. From the latter, the reader can calculate corneal asphericity based on this map. $Q = -e^2$, so in our example, $Q = -(1.28)^2 = -1.64$, which means that the cornea is hyperprolate.
- *Decentration (Fig. 15.3)*: This map represents decentration of corneal optics which is translated as coma, secondary coma, tertiary coma, etc. The important clinical application of this map is in topography-guided treatment.
- *Regular astigmatism (Fig. 15.4)*: This map represents regular astigmatism component. There are two boxes at

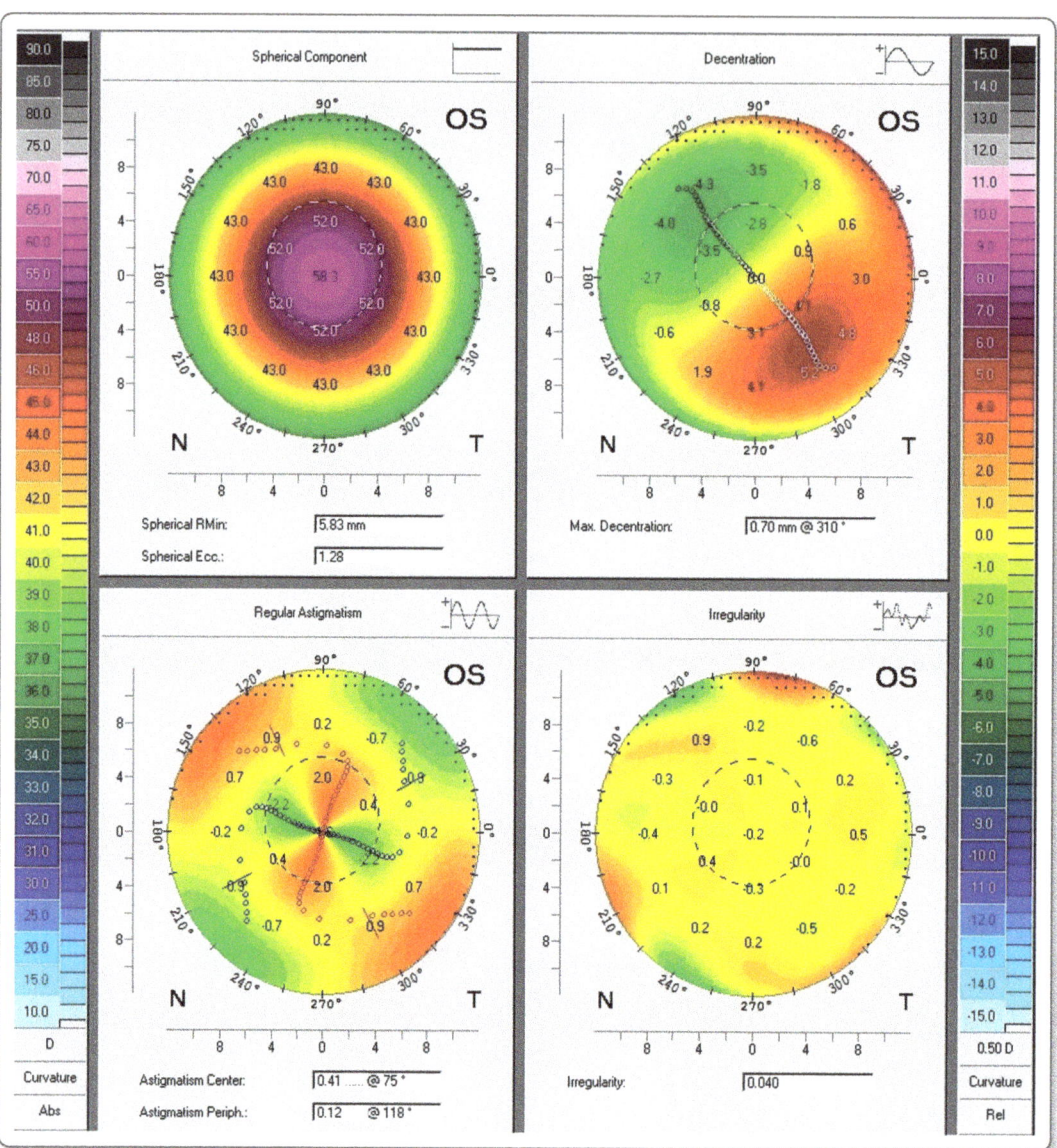

Fig. 15.1: Fourier analysis of corneal wavefront into four components.

the bottom of the map: (1) astigmatism center, showing the amount and axis of corneal astigmatism within the central 3 mm zone, and (2) astigmatism periph, showing the amount and axis between 6 mm and 9 mm zones. There are two clinical applications of this map:

1. The central astigmatism in this map is usually more consistent with the subjective refraction than the Sim-K astigmatism. In other words, in cases of distorted corneas and nonoptimal corrected vision, the amount and axis of astigmatism in this map can be considered as an initial step in subjective refraction, just like when considering corneal astigmatism of total corneal refractive power as discussed in Chapter 11.

2. Whenever there is a dissociation in axis between central and peripheral astigmatism, a significant higher-order astigmatism exists, such as astigmatism from the order of secondary, tertiary, quarterly, etc. In our case, there is a significant dissociation, which can be identified by three elements:

   i. A difference between central and peripheral axes more than 15°.

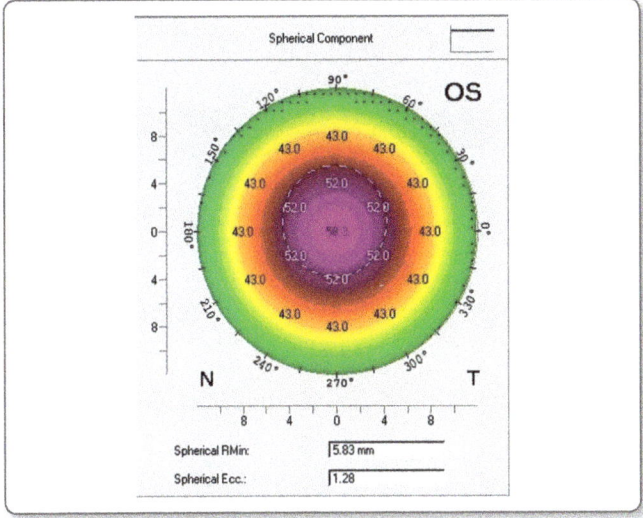

Fig. 15.2: Spherical component in Fourier analysis.

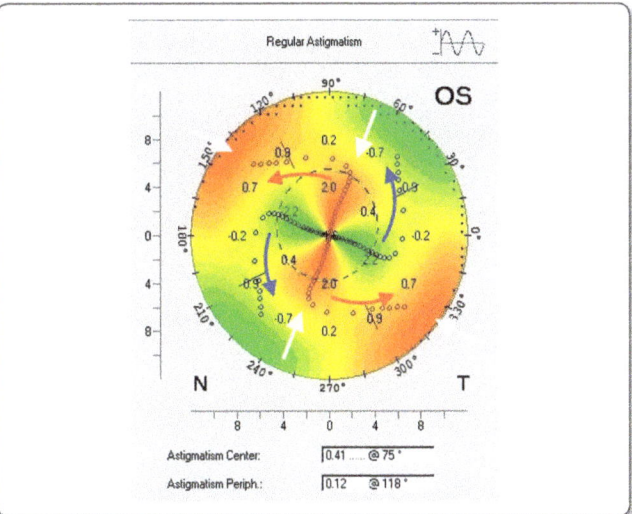

Fig. 15.4: Regular astigmatism component in Fourier analysis.

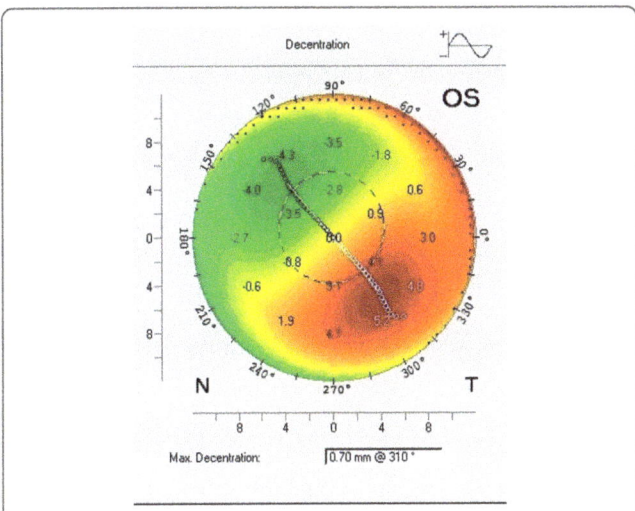

Fig. 15.3: Decentration component in Fourier analysis.

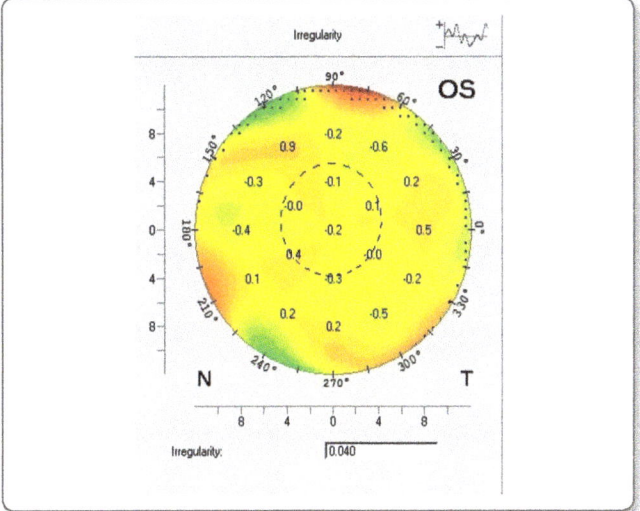

Fig. 15.5: Irregularity component in Fourier analysis.

    ii. The vortex distribution of the circles on the map (red and blue arrows).
    iii. The astigmatic pattern of the map shows peripheral steep and flat areas that do not correspond to the central symmetric bowtie (white arrows).

- *Irregularity (Fig. 15.5)*: This map represents other HOAs from the Foil family (trefoil, tetrafoil, pentafoil, hexafoil, etc.).

Figure 15.6 is Fourier analysis of a normal cornea for comparison.

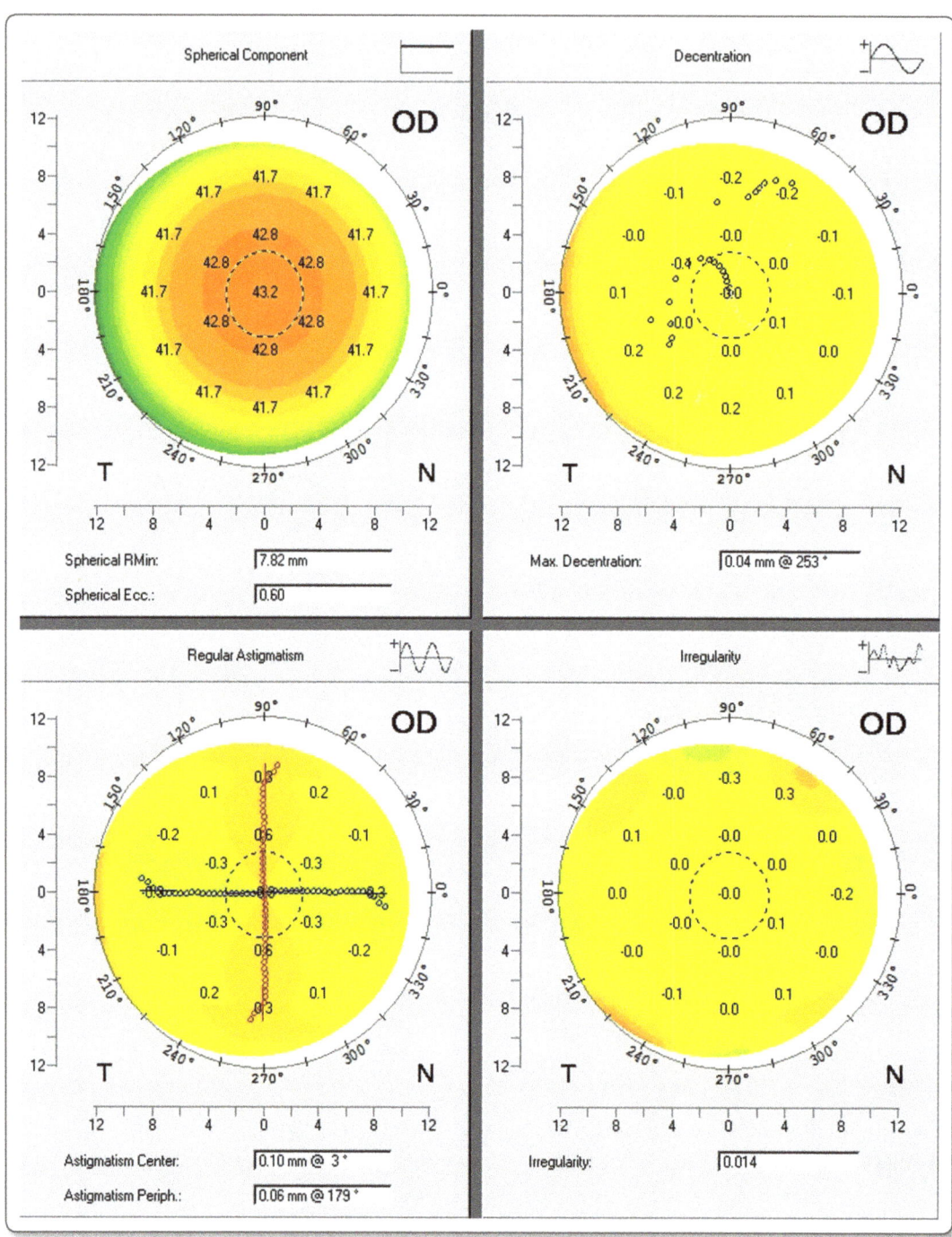

Fig. 15.6: Fourier analysis of a normal cornea.

SECTION 5

A Systematic Interpretation of Corneal Tomography

SECTION OUTLINE

16. Factors of False Findings
17. Enantiomorphism
18. Practical Subjective Scoring System

Factors of False Findings

INTRODUCTION

There are several factors that have an impact on the reliability of corneal tomography. They are responsible for false positives (false *abnormal* findings) and false negatives (false *normal* findings). These factors should be recognized and ruled out before interpreting the tomography. False positives may lead to overestimation and exclusion of proper candidates for refractive surgery, while false negatives may lead to underestimation and inclusion of improper candidates. In addition, diagnosis of some diseases rely on accurate findings in corneal tomography, therefore any false findings will mislead the diagnosis and therefore treatment decision.

CONTACT LENSES

Soft Contact Lenses

Long usage of soft contact lenses (CLs) can induce topographic patterns of corneal steepening (hot spot) and relatively increased myopia (myopic shift) (Fig. 16.1). These changes cease gradually after cessation of the lenses over a period of 5-6 weeks. Corneal steepening may induce false astigmatism, or may change the value and/or the axis of the existing astigmatism.

Visual acuity is also affected by the extended wear of soft CLs. In most cases, there is a significant improvement in the uncorrected distance visual acuity (UDVA) 5 weeks after cessation of CLs in comparison with the immediate measurement after taking off the lenses. This corresponds to the improvement found in regularity and radial symmetry in the topographic image, in addition to tear film quality.

Central corneal thickness increases after discontinuation of soft CLs in 90% of cases. The average increase is about 20 μm. On the other hand, corneal thickness increases in the very center of the hot spot induced by the lenses. That is because CLs have rest points on the surface of the cornea, which is believed to cause focal epithelial hyperplasia because of continuous rubbing effect of the lenses. This epithelial hypertrophy appears as a hot spot, which is different from that induced by ectatic corneal diseases (ECDs) by two features: in the former, the cornea shows thickening at the hot spot rather than the thinning that is usually seen with the latter, and the corresponding posterior elevation values are usually normal contrary to ECDs. Based on these two features, CL effect may mimic keratoconus suspect (KCS). Chapters 19 and 22 are devoted to the definitions of ECDs and entities mimicking them.

Rigid Gas Permeable Contact Lenses

Corneal warpage induced by rigid gas permeable (RGP) lenses presents as central corneal flattening and decreased myopia (hypermetropic shift), and in case of CL decentration, the pattern may be misinterpreted as an ectatic hot spot. These changes may take longer period than soft CLs to disappear. The period may last for 9-12 weeks. In some cases, relative steepening with increased myopia may occur after discontinuing the RGP lenses. Changes in corneal astigmatism after discontinuing the RGP lenses are generally less significant when compared with soft CLs.

Visual acuity is also affected by the use of the RGP lenses. A significant improvement in the UDVA is encountered 12 weeks after cessation of the RGP lens in comparison with the immediate measurement after taking off the lenses. This

Section 5: *A Systematic Interpretation of Corneal Tomography*

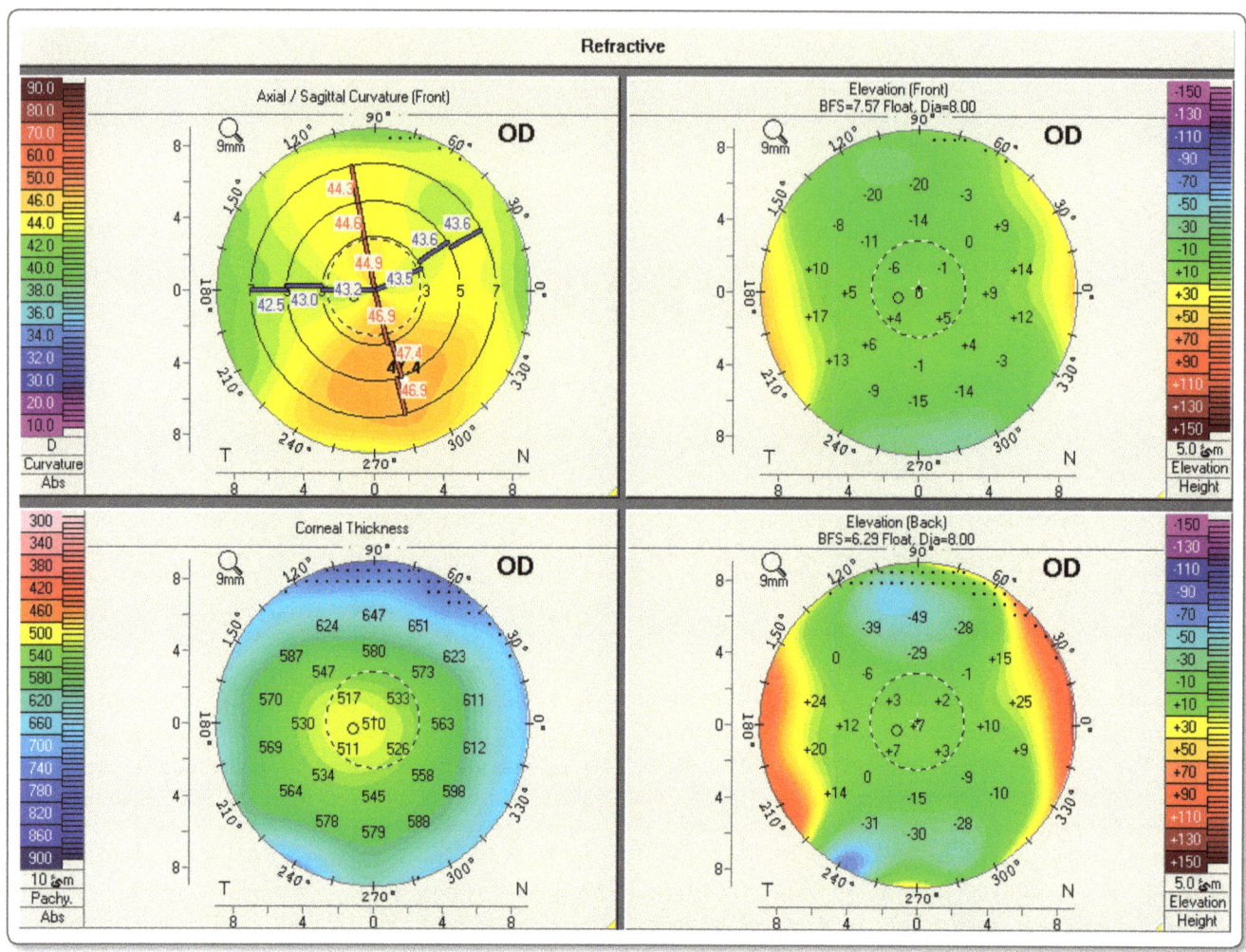

Fig. 16.1: Hot spot induced by soft contact lens.

corresponds to the improvement in regularity and radial symmetry in the topographic image, in addition to tear film quality.

Central corneal thickness increases after discontinuation of the RGP lenses in 90% of cases. The average increase is about 15 μm.

The RGP lenses also affect the shape and the severity of corneas with ECDs. Figures 16.2A to C show the anterior curvature map of a keratoconic cornea immediately (field A) and 16 days (field B) after removal of the RGP lens. Field C shows the difference: the curvature values at cone apex increased by more than 3.5 D.

MISALIGNMENT

Loss of fixation or misalignment during capturing the cornea is one of the main factors for false findings. Both patient and examiner may be responsible for misalignment. Misalignment may cause false positives and false negatives.

Types of Misalignment

- *Patient's error misalignment*: This occurs when the patient does not fixate properly on the target. This error is called misalignment by rotation. Of course, this appears clearly to the examiner, but instead of asking the patient to refixate and align properly, the examiner tries to overcome this problem by realigning the camera on the displaced pupil!
- *Examiner's error misalignment*: The patient here aligns properly on the fixation point, but the examiner doesn't adjust the camera properly on patient's pupil. This error is called misalignment by translation.

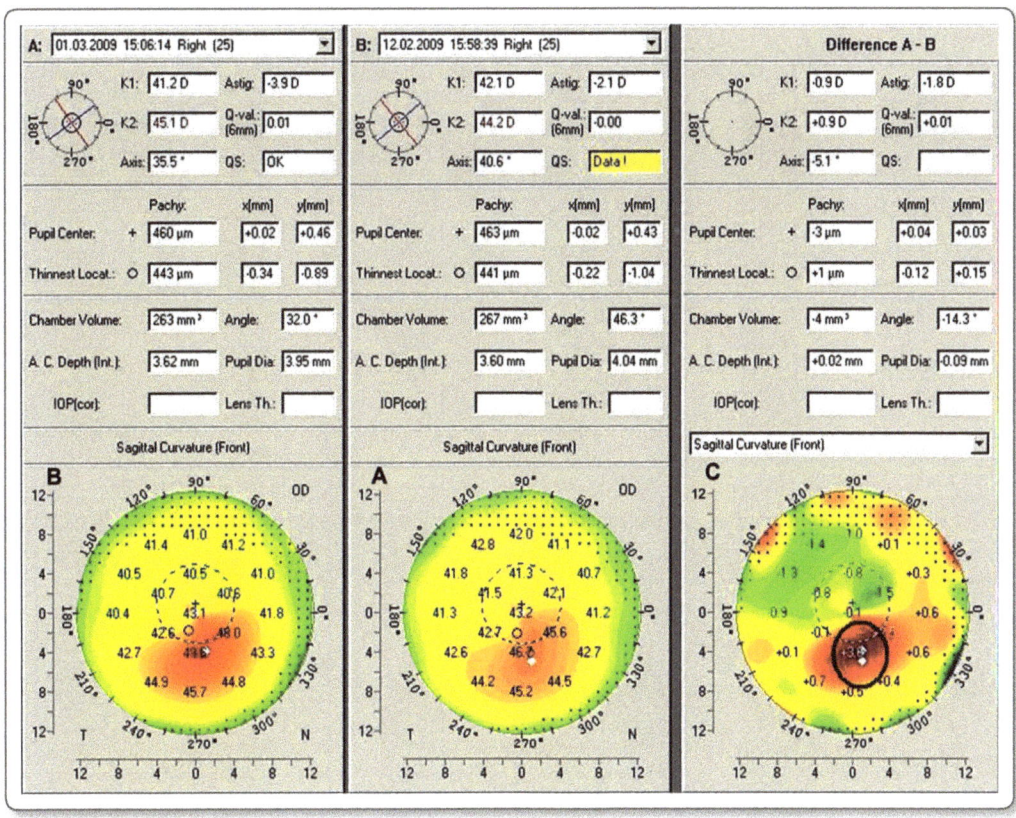

Figs. 16.2A to C: The two-difference map of a keratoconic eye showing the flattening effect of an RGP lens. (A) Immediately after removal of the lens; (B) 16 days after removal of the lens; and (C) The change in curvature over the 16-day period. The K-reading at cone apex increased by more than 3.5 D over the 16-day period.

Effect of Misalignment

All tomographic maps are affected by misalignment. Figure 16.3 is a four-composite map of an eye that was fixating downward during the capture. Figure 16.4 is the four-composite map of the same eye after teaching the patient the proper fixation. Notice how misalignment may be responsible for false keratoconus features.

1. *Changes in the curvature maps*: Figures 16.5 and 16.6 are illustrations of changes occurring in the symmetric bowtie (SB) due to misalignment. It is clear that the bowtie will change depending on the direction of gaze. Therefore, *not* every asymmetric bowtie or skewed patterns are *abnormal*; they may result from misalignment. This is called "false positives."

   Figure 16.7 is an example of "false negative." The real pattern is SB/SRAX. Assuming that this is the left eye and the patient was fixating temporally, the pattern will appear as SB. In addition, if the SRAX of the real SB/SRAX was insignificant (<22°), and the patient was fixating nasally, the SRAX would become significant.

   Moreover, K-readings including Kmax and average K, axis and magnitude of astigmatism, and inferior superior and nasal temporal symmetry will change.

   Based on the above illustrations, the reader can imagine how other patterns will change giving a variety of classified and unclassified patterns that can be misinterpreted.

2. *Changes in the elevation maps*: Similar to the curvature maps, symmetric patterns on the elevation maps convert into asymmetric patterns and vice versa. In addition, normal values usually convert into abnormal values. This is obvious when looking at Figures 16.3 and 16.4.

3. *Changes in the thickness map*: The normal concentric shape will change into dome pattern or horizontal displacement pattern. X and Y coordinate of the thinnest location (TL) will show abnormal values in case of false positives or will show normal values in case of false negatives. This is obvious when looking at Figures 16.3 and 16.4.

4. *Changes in the spatial thickness profile*: Misalignment may affect the average progression more than the

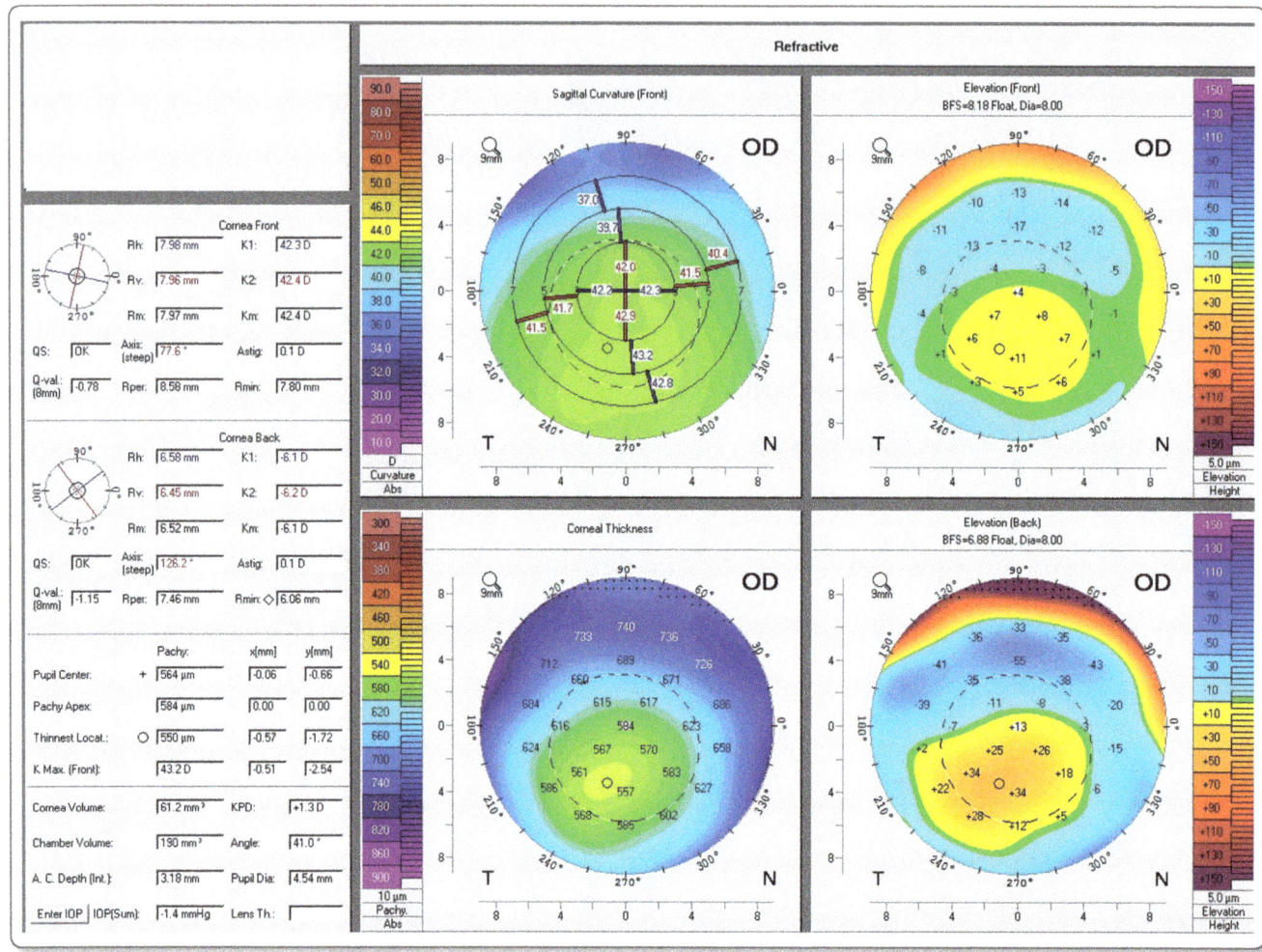

Fig. 16.3: Misalignment. The four-composite refractive map of an eye fixating downward during capturing the cornea.

pattern of the red curve. Figure 16.8 is the spatial profile in misalignment situation, while Figure 16.9 is in proper fixation situation. Notice the change in average.

Clues of Misalignment

The following clues should be inspected before interpreting any tomographical capture:
- *Quality specification (QS)*: If it is abnormal (yellow or red), the capture should be repeated. However, being (white OK) is *not* a clue of a good capture. Look at Figure 16.3, there is a gross misalignment while the QS is white OK!
- *Km stability*: Usually, three captures should be taken in a session. The three captures should be compared in terms of average K (Km) on anterior corneal surface. If there is > 0.3 D change between any two captures, they should be repeated.
- *Astigmatic dissociation*: It is defined by > 1 D and/or >10° difference between manifest astigmatism (MA) and tomographic astigmatism (TA) taken from the total corneal refractive power (TCRP). One of the causes is misalignment.
- *Unusual pupil center coordinates*: If X and/or Y of entrance pupil center are ≥ 0.2 mm.
- *Unusual TL coordinates*: If X and/or Y of TL are ≥ 0.2 mm.
- *Intereye asymmetry*: If there is a difference ≥ 0.1 mm between the two eyes:
  1. In X and/or Y of entrance pupil center.
  2. In X and/or Y of TL.
- Asymmetric patterns on the curvature, elevation or pachymetry maps.

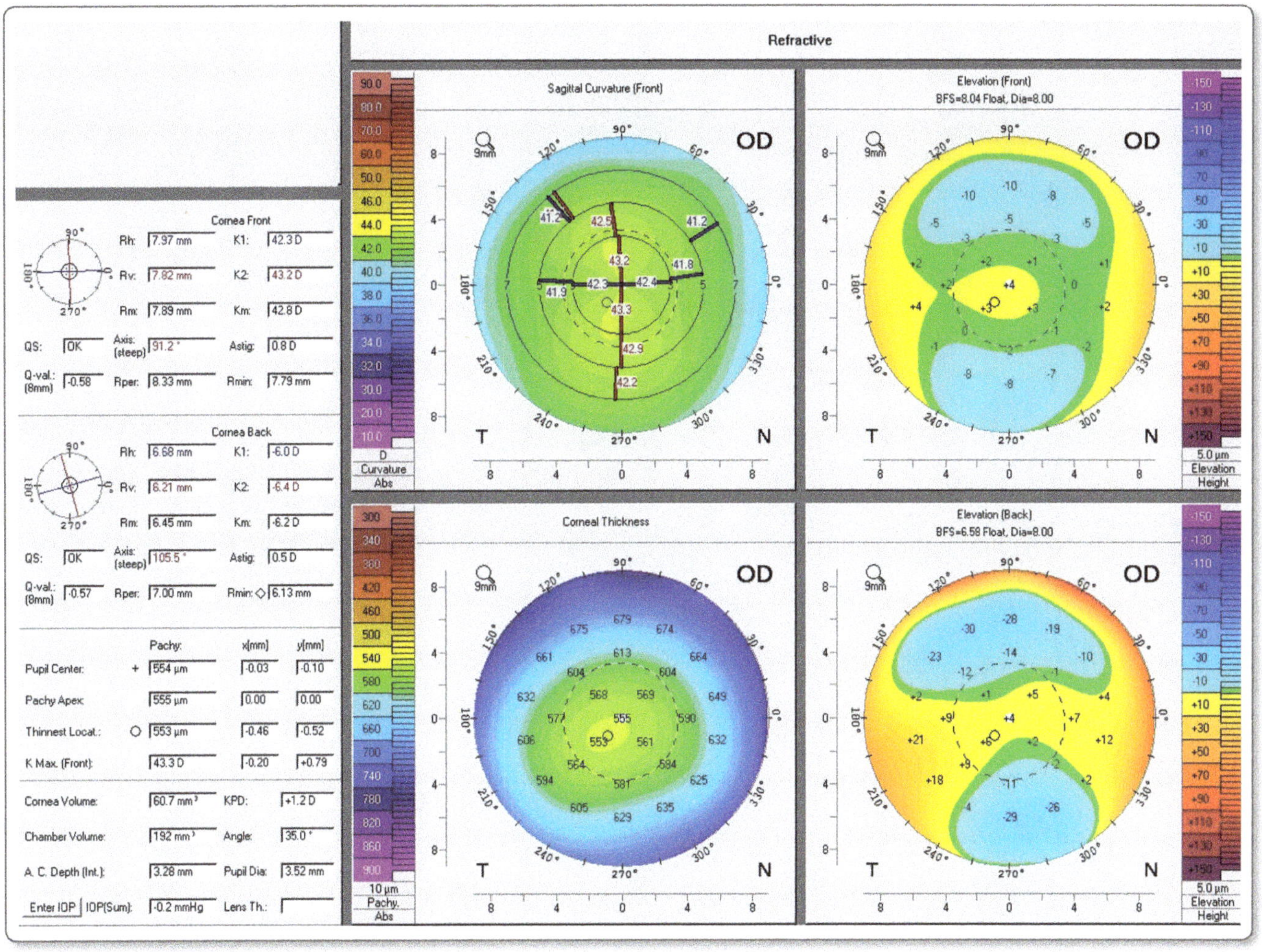

Fig. 16.4: Misalignment. The four-composite refractive map of the same eye in Figure 16.3 after realignment.

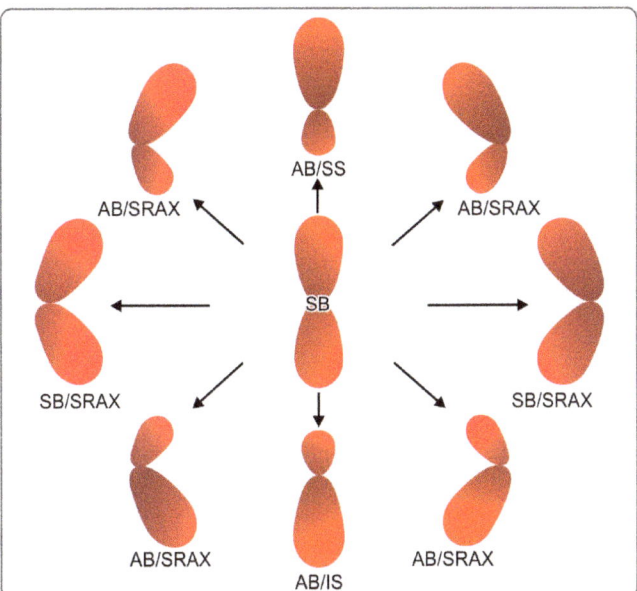

Fig. 16.5: Effect of misalignment and large angle kappa on the presentation of a true vertical symmetric bowtie (SB).

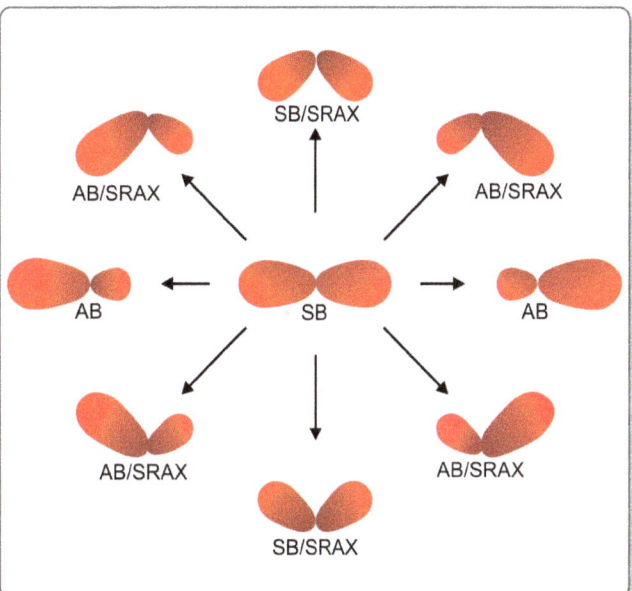

Fig. 16.6: Effect of misalignment and large angle kappa on the presentation of a true horizontal symmetric bowtie (SB).

Section 5: A Systematic Interpretation of Corneal Tomography

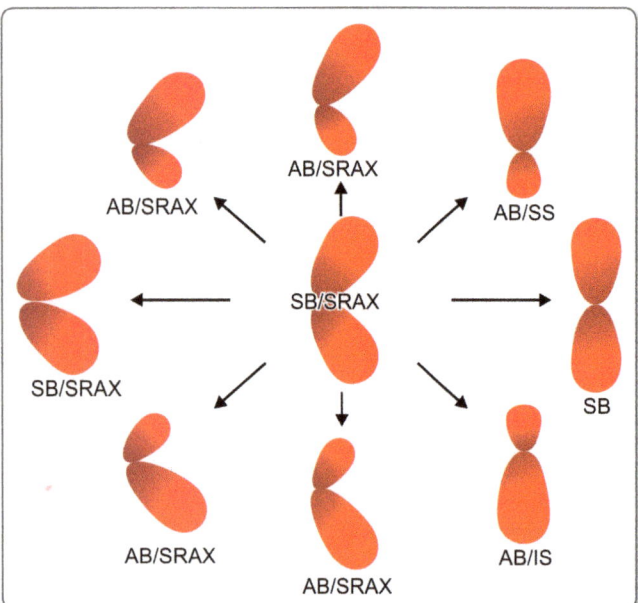

Fig. 16.7: Effect of misalignment and large angle kappa on the presentation of a true vertical symmetric bowtie with skewed radial axis index (SB/SRAX).

LARGE ANGLE KAPPA OR LAMBDA

The definition of these two angles is mentioned in Chapter 1. The effect of large angles is similar to misalignment. The only difference is: when repeating the captures and the case is large angles, the X and Y of entrance pupil center coordinates will not change or the change will be < 0.1 mm.

TEAR FILM DISTURBANCE

Tear Film Deficiency

Dry eye affects the integrity of the epithelium. This causes surface irregularities, changes in K-readings and hot spot formation as shown in Figure 16.10. These changes improve or disappear after a proper treatment (Fig. 16.11). Since Placido disk measures the anterior corneal surface, particularly the tear coat of the cornea, it is much more affected than Scheimpflug imaging with tear film deficiency.

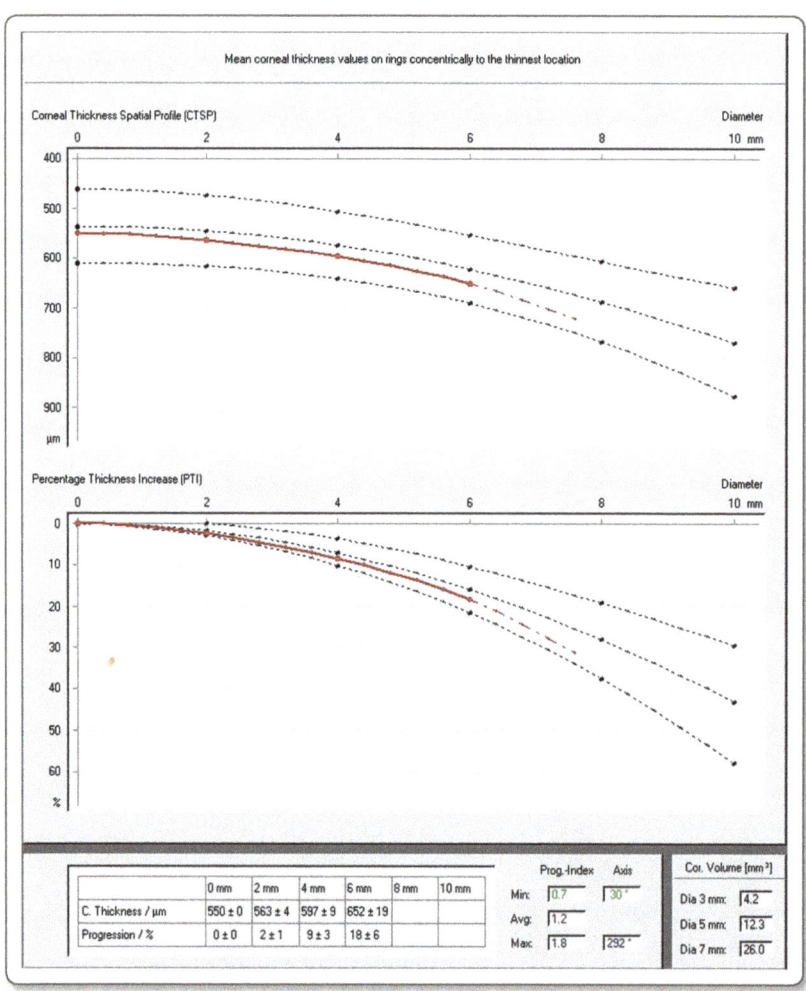

Fig. 16.8: Misalignment. The thickness profiles of the same eye in Figure 16.3 in misalignment situation.

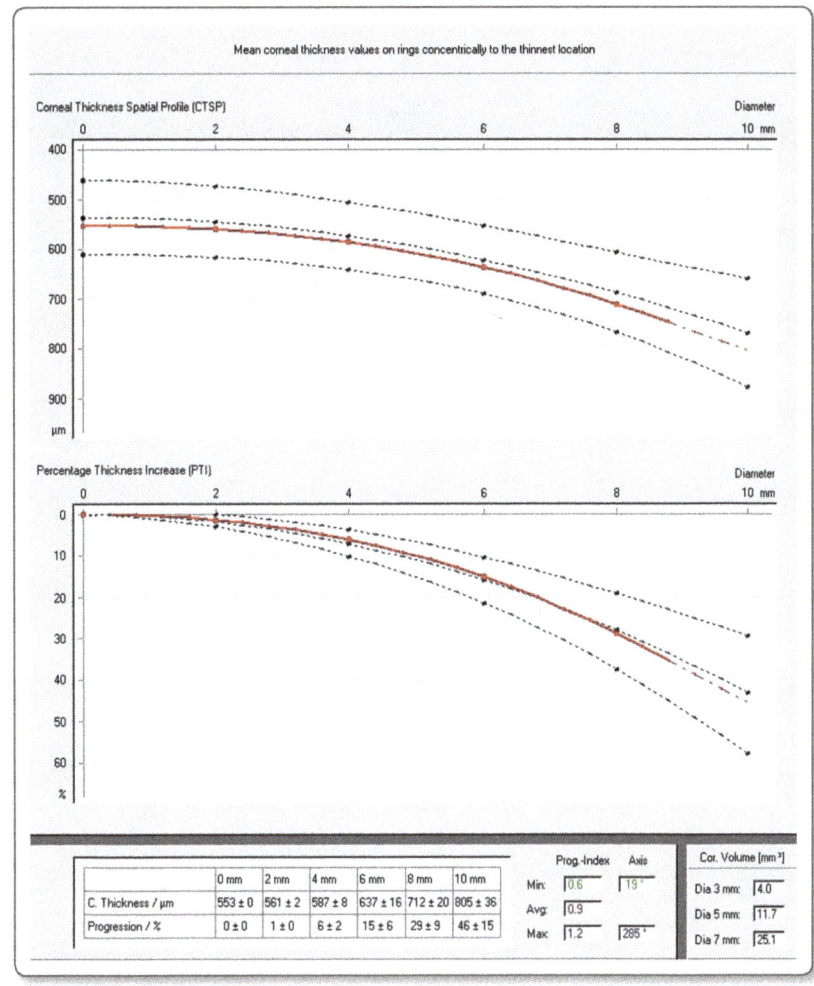

Fig. 16.9: Misalignment. The thickness profiles of the same eye in Figure 16.3 in realignment situation.

Tear Film Excess

Excessive tear film meniscus is a factor of false hot spot formation. The excessive tear meniscus on the lower lid margin takes a concave shape followed by an upper convex corneal surface (Fig. 16.12). This would be interpreted by the computer as a hot spot as shown in Figure 16.13A. Figure 16.13B is the same cornea after wiping; notice the disappearance of the hot spot.

POSTERIOR SURFACE ASTIGMATISM

Posterior corneal surface is toric and has a higher toricity than the anterior corneal surface in some radii. The astigmatism on the posterior surface has an impact on the total corneal astigmatism, therefore neglecting it has led to miscalculations of intraocular lenses, particularly the toric types of lenses. New formulas take into consideration this astigmatism for better measurements. In addition, unusual posterior surface astigmatism (>−0.5 D) leads to astigmatic dissociation. The average amount of posterior surface astigmatism is −0.3 D, while it exceeds −0.5 D in 9% of normal eyes.

CORNEAL OPACITIES AND PATHOLOGIES

Corneal opacities, haze, loss of transparency, degenerations and dystrophies are a major source of corneal irregularities, false findings and hot spot formation (refer Figs. 8.7 to 8.12).

PREVIOUS CORNEAL SURGERIES

Corneal surgeries are:
- Laser vision correction (LVC).
- Cataract surgeries.
- Corneal grafts.
- Radial keratotomy (RK).
- Astigmatic keratotomy (AK) and limbal relaxing incisions (LRIs).

Section 5: A Systematic Interpretation of Corneal Tomography

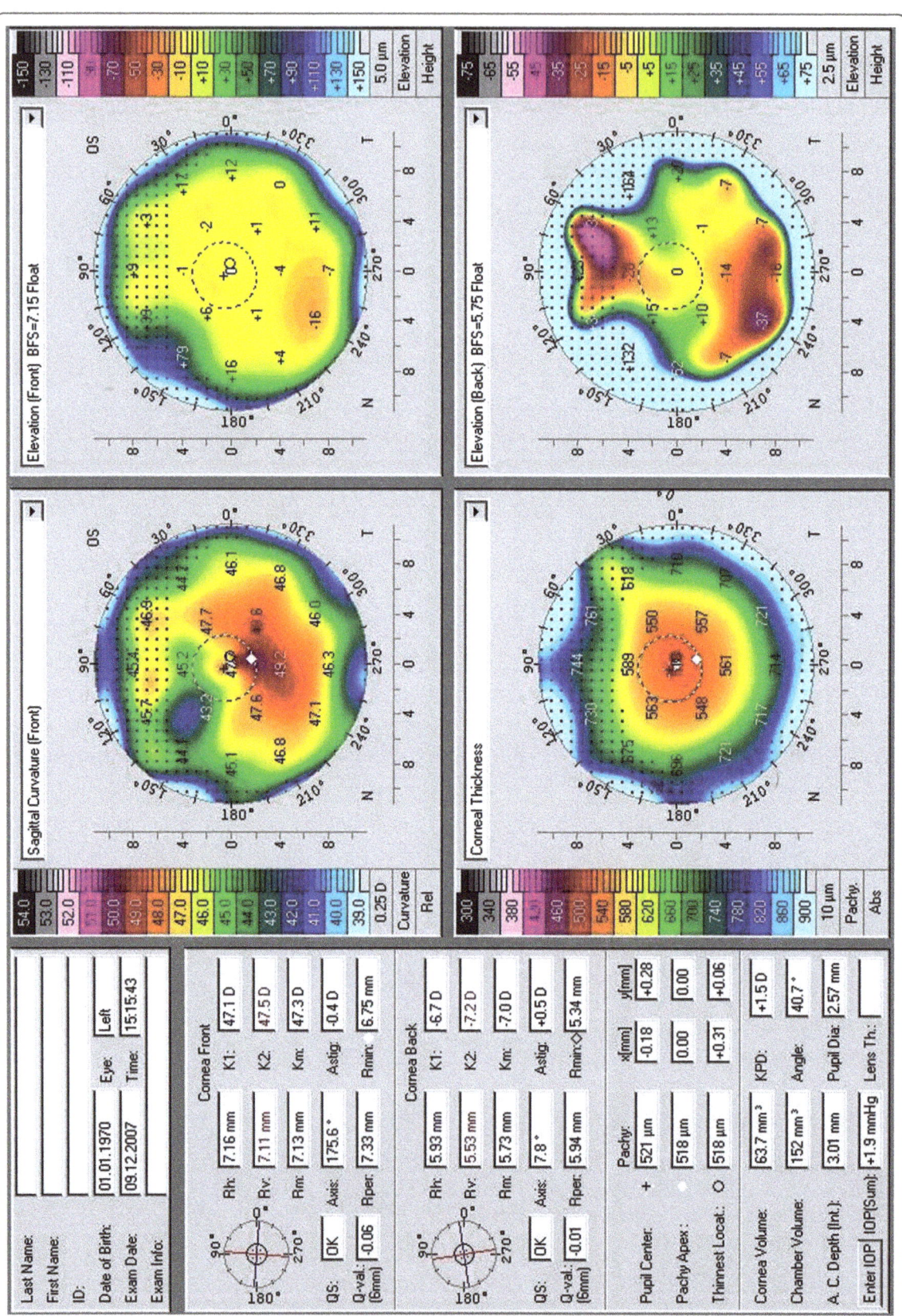

Fig. 16.10: Dry eye. The four-composite refractive map before treatment.

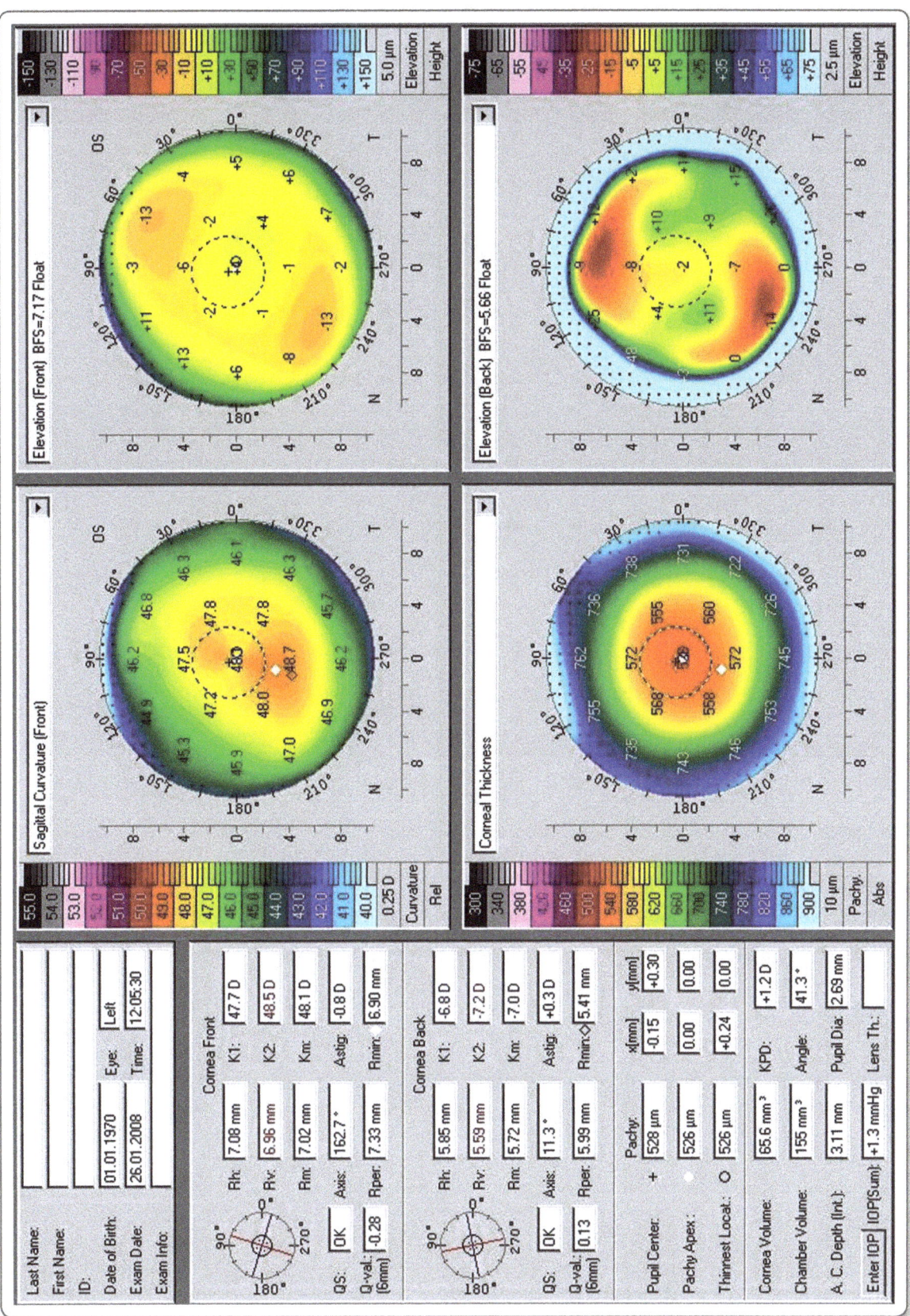

Fig. 16.11: Dry eye. The four-composite refractive map after treatment.

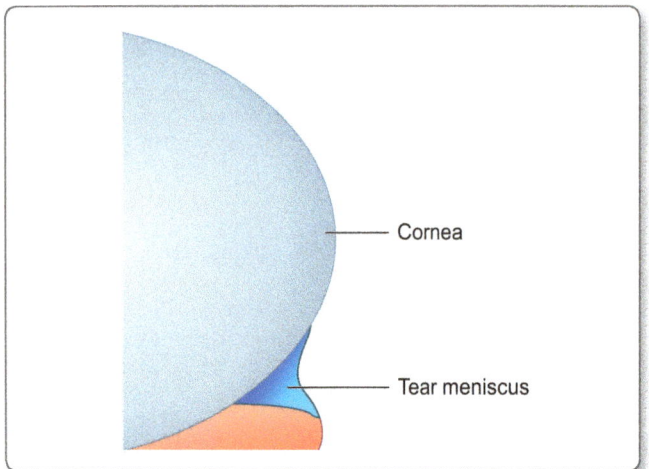

Fig. 16.12: Effect of excess tears on tomography.

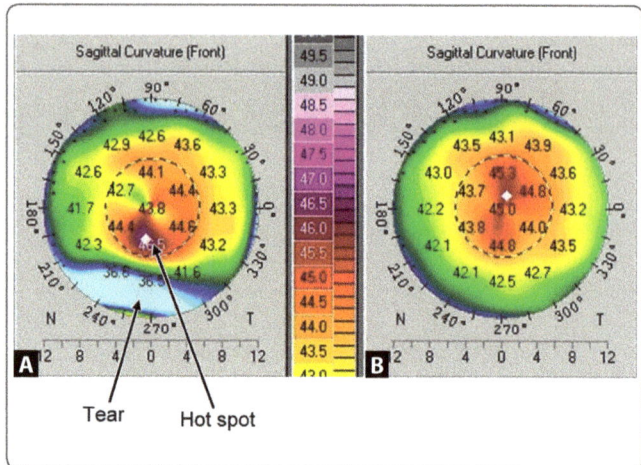

Figs. 16.13A and B: Excess tears. The presence and absence of a hot spot in excess tear situation (A) and normal situation (B).

Careful history taking is a key point in the work up for refractive surgery. Previous corneal surgeries are important sources for corneal irregularities, false findings or hot spot formation. They affect by the following mechanisms:
- Tear film disturbance.
- Distortion due to sutures.
- Distortion due to postoperative flap complications.
- Light scattering due to interface complications or surface haze.
- Irregular RK incisions and incisions extending into the optical zone.
- Irregular or asymmetric AK incisions or LRIs.
- Corneal instability due to RK.
- Abnormal corneal response, leading to decentered, irregular or small postoperative optical zones. These may occur due to improper laser ablation as well.
- Postoperative ectasia.

BAD EXPOSURE TO THE CAMERA

During taking the capture, the eye should properly be exposed to the camera to avoid any missing data and therefore extrapolation. Bad exposure to the camera can result from anatomical features, patient noncooperation or tight headscarves.

Anatomical Features

They include prominent eyebrows, small palpebral fissures, small eyes, deep-set eyes, nasal bridge, and long lashes.

These features can be overcome by adjusting patient's face in compensating positions. For example, if the cause is prominent nasal bridge, the face can be turned to left to capture the right eye and vice versa.

Patient Noncooperation

Frequent blinking, moving the eyes, and following the camera are common in noncooperative patients. Good patient education would overcome this. In addition, it is very important to treat the causes of frequent blinking such as dry eye. It is strongly recommended *to avoid* using anesthesia drops to overcome frequent blinking.

Tight Headscarves

Headscarves may obscure the camera especially from the temporal sides.

PREGNANCY

During pregnancy, a temporary increase in corneal curvature and corneal thickness is usually encountered. They are related to hormonal changes. This is why a pregnant woman is not a good candidate for refractive surgery. When a female with keratoconus becomes pregnant, there is a risk of progression and hence the need for follow up. Chapter 21 is devoted to progression criteria of ECDs. These criteria may be masked by the usual changes in curvature and thickness during pregnancy. This is why physicians should be reluctant to perform any treatment during or directly after pregnancy and wait until corneal curvature stabilizes.

CHAPTER 17

Enantiomorphism

INTRODUCTION

Enantiomorphism is the phenomenon in which there is a mirror symmetry between the two eyes in both tomographic shapes and values. Figures 17.1 and 17.2 are the four-composite maps of right eye (OD) and left eye (OS), respectively, of a refractive surgery candidate. The reader can notice how OD is a mirror shape of OS. Figures 17.3 to 17.6 demonstrate single map comparisons.

This phenomenon was studied in terms of intereye symmetry to discriminate between normal and keratoconic corneas and define a numeric scoring system of similarity that outlines the normal range of asymmetry between right and left eyes. Table 17.1 is a summary of one of the suggested scoring systems.

Aside from numeric scoring systems, enantiomorphism is very important in terms of studying tomographical patterns. When some irregularities exist in both corneas in a mirror shape, they may be considered as normal. These irregularities are:

- When the horizontal component of angle kappa is large:
  - Symmetric bowtie with skewed radial axis index (SB/SRAX).
  - Horizontal displacement of the thinnest location (TL).
  - Skewed hourglass.
- When the vertical component of angle kappa is large:
  - Inferior steep (IS).
  - Asymmetric bowtie inferior steep (AB/IS).
  - Vertical displacement of the TL.
  - Skewed hourglass.
- When both components of angle kappa are large:
  - Asymmetric bowtie with skewed radial axis index (AB/SRAX).
  - Vertical-horizontal displacement of the TL.
  - Skewed hourglass.

In other words, when the mentioned mirror-shaped irregularities are encountered in the two eyes, large angle kappa should be considered as it may be the cause. Figures 17.7 and 17.8 represent a case of enantiomorphism with large angle kappa (large pupil center coordinates in the Pentacam system). Notice the SB/SRAX, skewed hourglass and the horizontal displacement of the TL.

Table 17.1: Intereye corneal asymmetry score.*	
Scoring criteria	Positive (+1 point) if intereye difference
Mean anterior keratometry (K_m anterior)	≥ 0.3 D
Mean posterior keratometry (K_m posterior)	≥ 0.1 D
Thinnest pachymetry	≥ 12 μm
Front elevation at thinnest location	≥ 2 μm
Back elevation at thinnest location	≥ 5 μm

*Score of 3 is observed in up to 6 to 11% of healthy patients, whereas a score of 4 is found in less than 4% of patients without keratoconus. A score of 5 should be considered highly abnormal (1% or less of non-keratoconic patients).

Source: Galletti JD, Ruiseñor Vázquez PR, Minguez N, et al. Corneal asymmetry analysis by pentacam Scheimpflug tomography for keratoconus diagnosis. J Refract Surg. 2015;31(2):116-23.

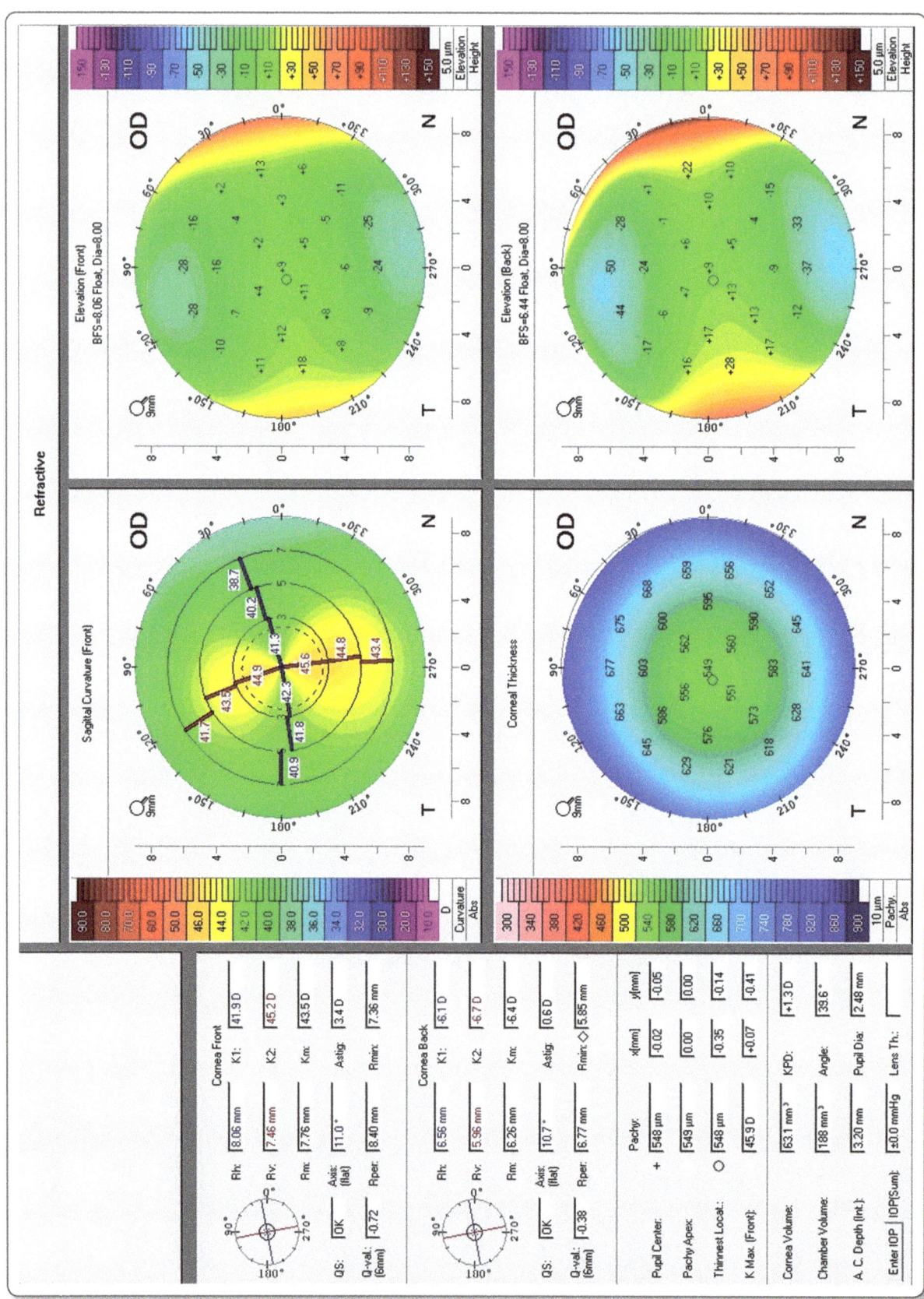

Fig. 17.1: Enantiomorphism. OD of a refractive surgery candidate. It is a mirror shape of OS in Figure 17.2.

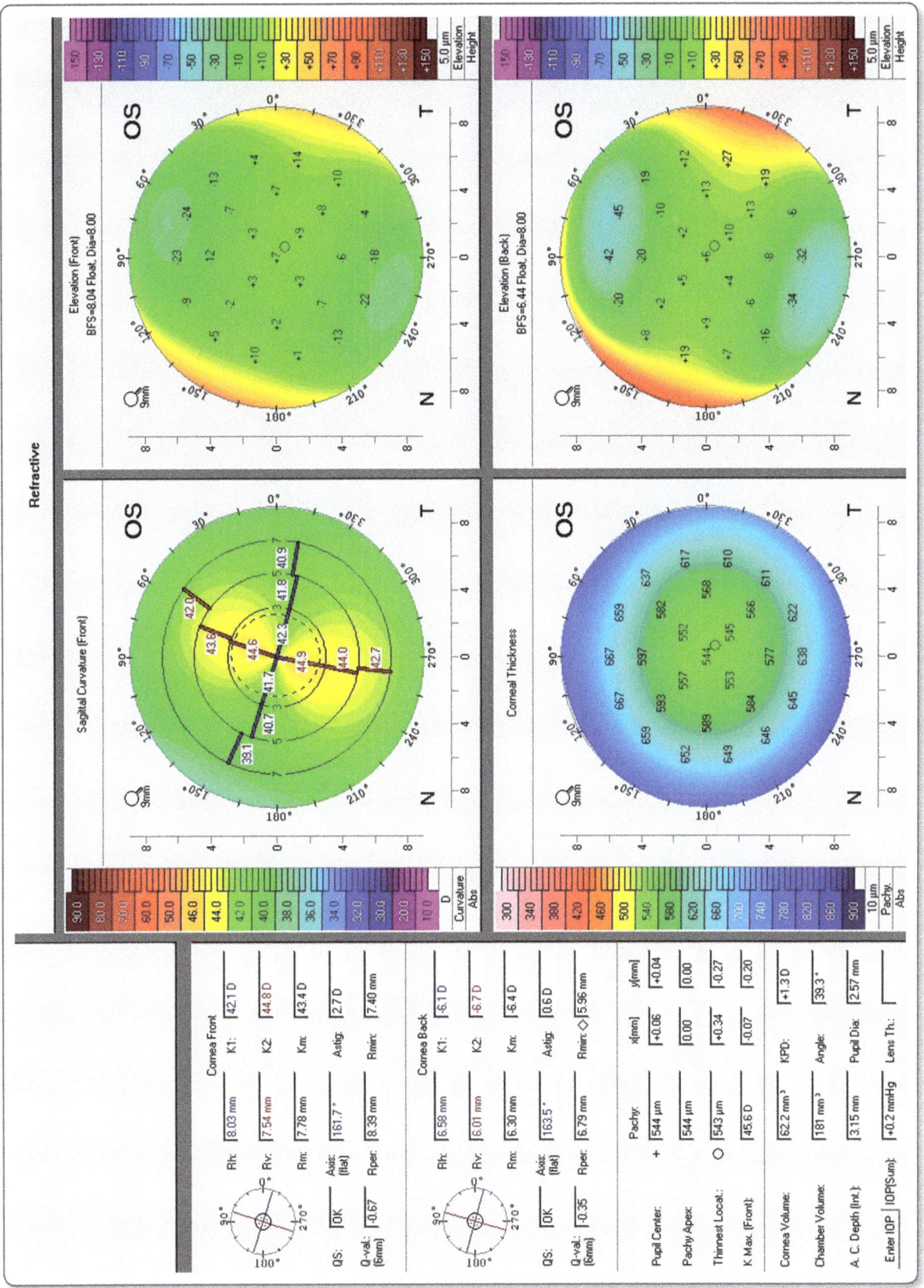

Fig. 17.2: Enantiomorphism. OS of a refractive surgery candidate. It is a mirror shape of OD in Figure 17.1.

Section 5: *A Systematic Interpretation of Corneal Tomography*

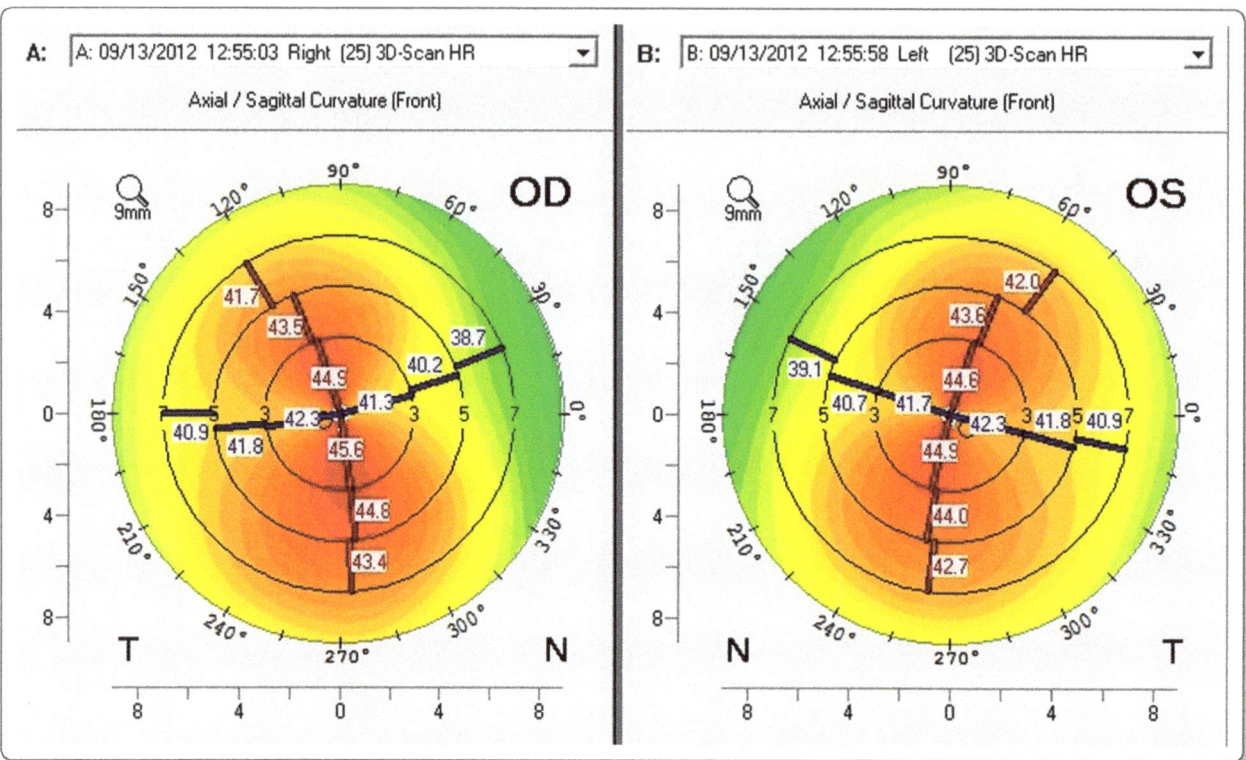

Fig. 17.3: Enantiomorphism in curvature maps.

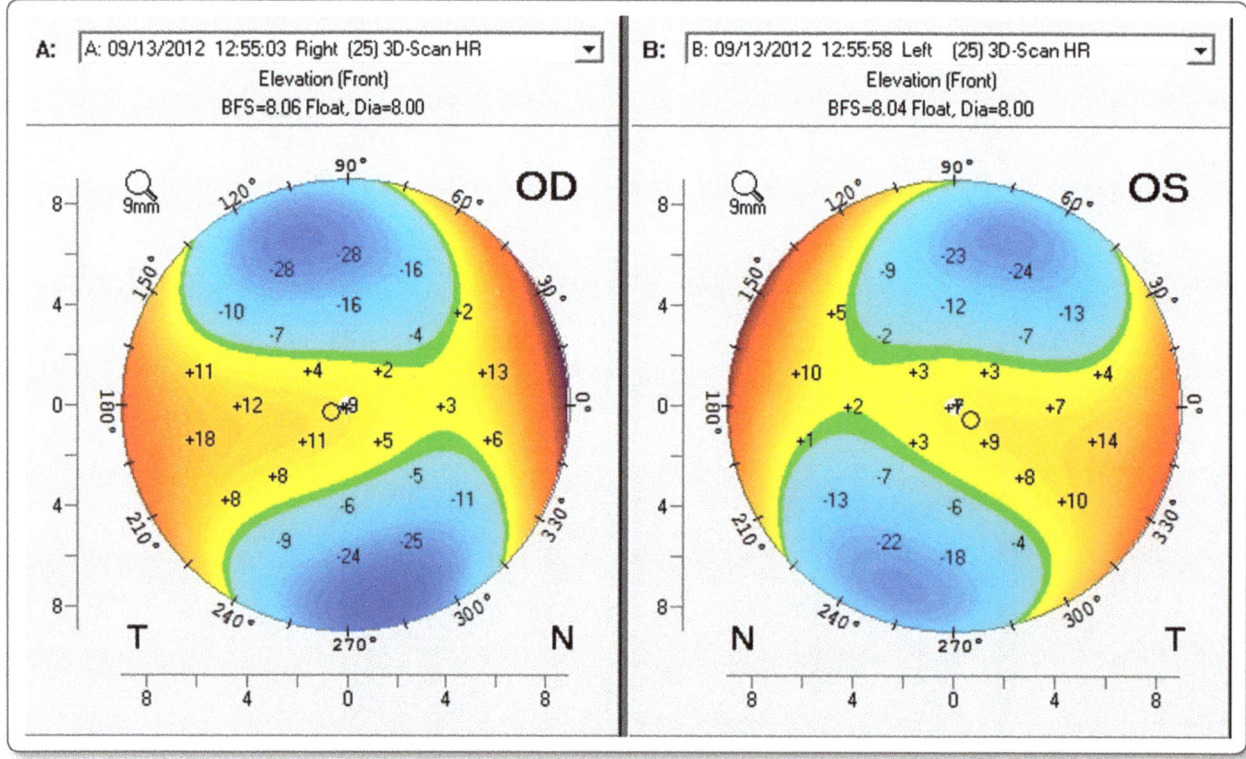

Fig. 17.4: Enantiomorphism in anterior elevation maps.

Chapter 17: Enantiomorphism

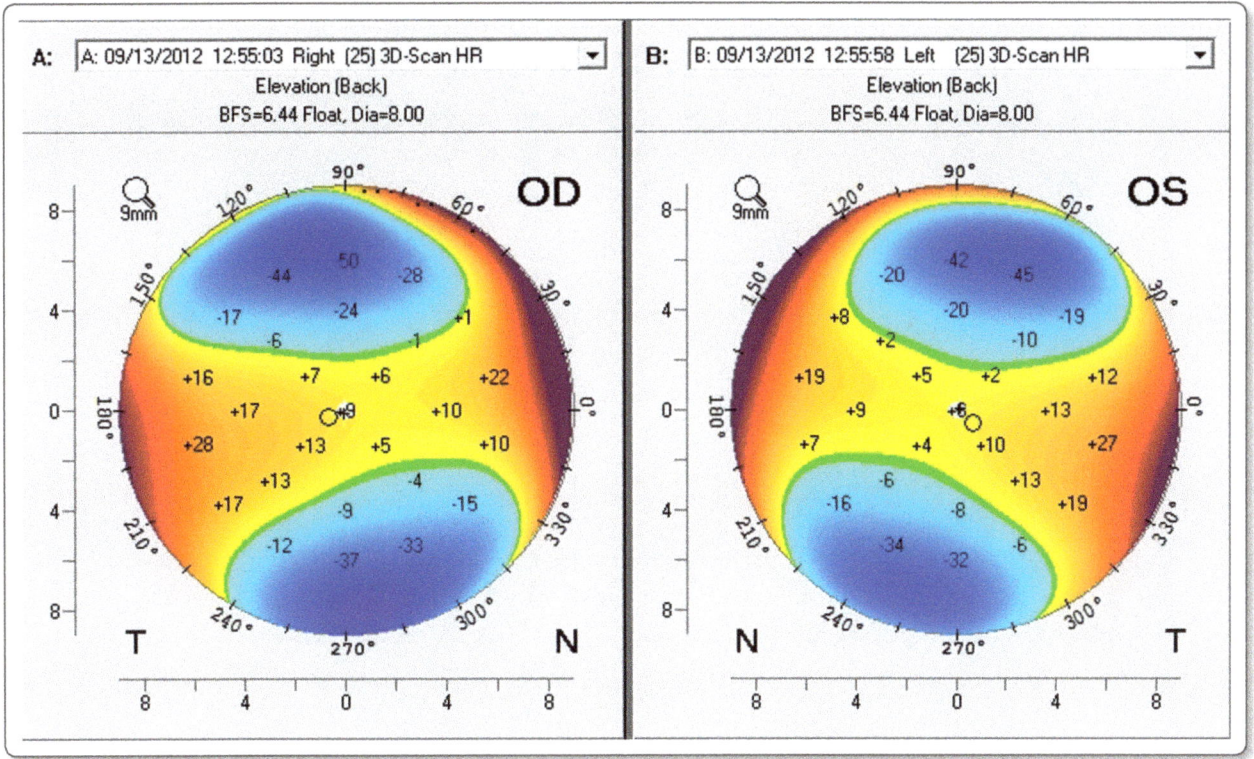

Fig. 17.5: Enantiomorphism in posterior elevation maps.

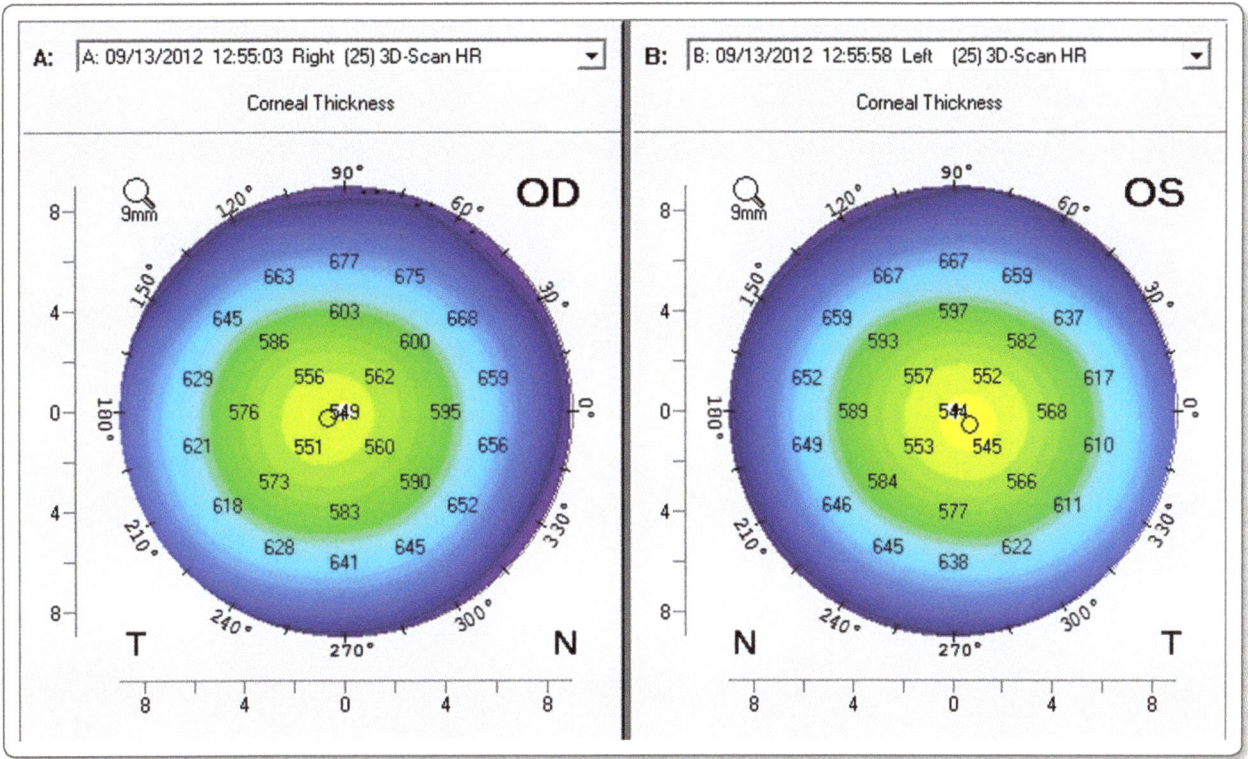

Fig. 17.6: Enantiomorphism in thickness maps.

Section 5: A Systematic Interpretation of Corneal Tomography

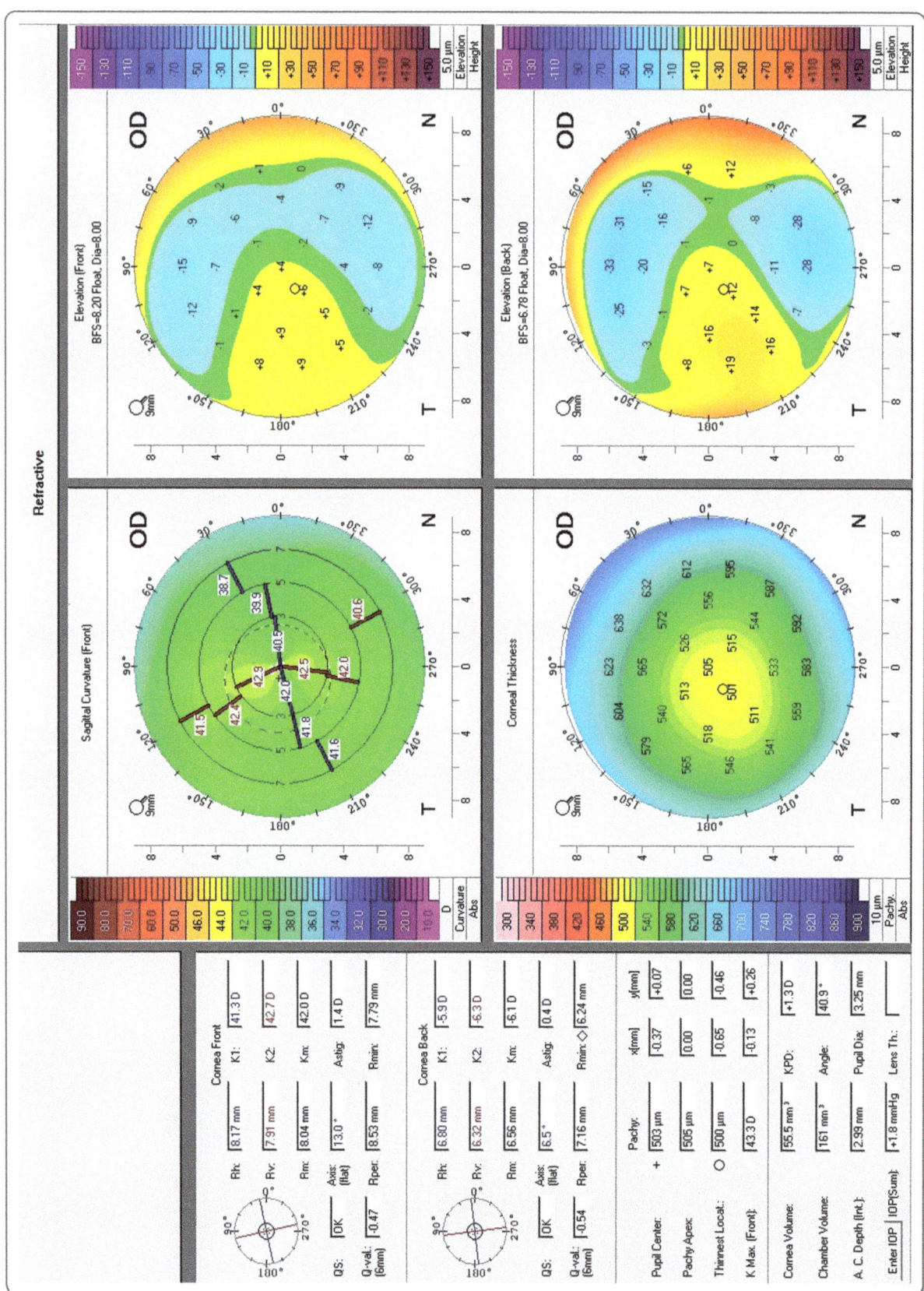

Fig. 17.7: Enantiomorphism in case of large angle kappa. The four-composite refractive map of OD.

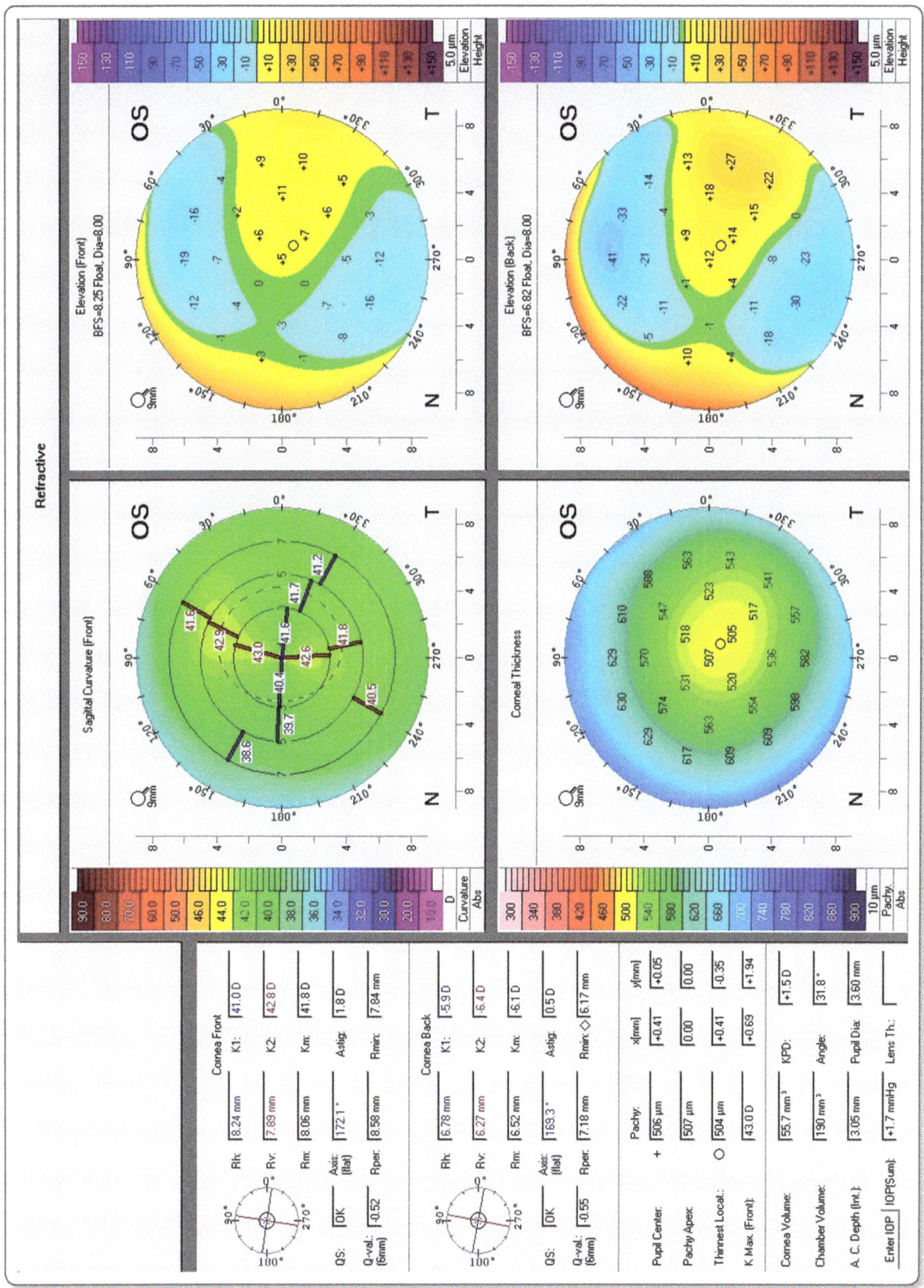

Fig. 17.8: Enantiomorphism in case of large angle kappa. The four-composite refractive map of OS.

Practical Subjective Scoring System

INTRODUCTION

Skillful interpretation of tomography is based on subjective and objective evaluation. Depending on objective indexes generated by machines is helpful as a step, but not the only step. In addition, skillful interpretation of tomographical data is the keystone of subjective evaluation.

In order to simplify decision making, I recommend a systematic methodology that consists of a concise 10-step algorithm and a final classification of moderate and high-risk factors. The reader will notice that there is no "low-risk factors" in my algorithm because this term can only be given to completely normal corneas because refractive surgery is not risk free.

My algorithm is prone to overestimation and excessive exclusion of good candidates. This would occur if the steps for obtaining good-quality images were not followed. Therefore, the responsibility starts from the technician who captures the cornea. In this chapter, image quality control will be explained before discussing the system.

IMAGE QUALITY CONTROL

Purpose

Obtaining reliable images is important for the following reasons:
- Candidate selection for refractive surgery.
- Evaluation of ectatic corneal diseases (ECDs).
- Postoperative follow-up.
- Observing the progression of ECDs.
- Researches.

Steps

It is recommended to follow the following steps as a checklist:

1. *Settings*: See the screening guidelines in Chapter 3.
2. Contact lenses should be stopped at least 1 week in advance. This is one of the responsibilities of the call center before arranging an appointment.
3. Good and detailed history taking including pregnancy, lactation, and previous eye surgeries.
4. Slit-lamp biomicroscopy to rule out dry eye, corneal opacities and other pathologies.
5. Educate the patient before capturing the cornea.
6. Exclude factors of bad exposure to the camera (Chapter 16).
7. Take three captures for each cornea.
8. Check QS, anterior Km, X and Y of pupil center and thinnest location. Compare both eyes.
9. Repeat the captures in case of bad QS (yellow and red), misalignment clues or any abnormal pattern on any map (Chapter 16).
10. In case of repeatable bad QS, such as in corneal opacities, very distorted corneas in ECDs, or after operations, do the following:
    - Click on QS box to display the items (Fig. 18.1).
    - Select the captures with least extrapolation and data gaps.
    - Write a note to the physician explaining that.

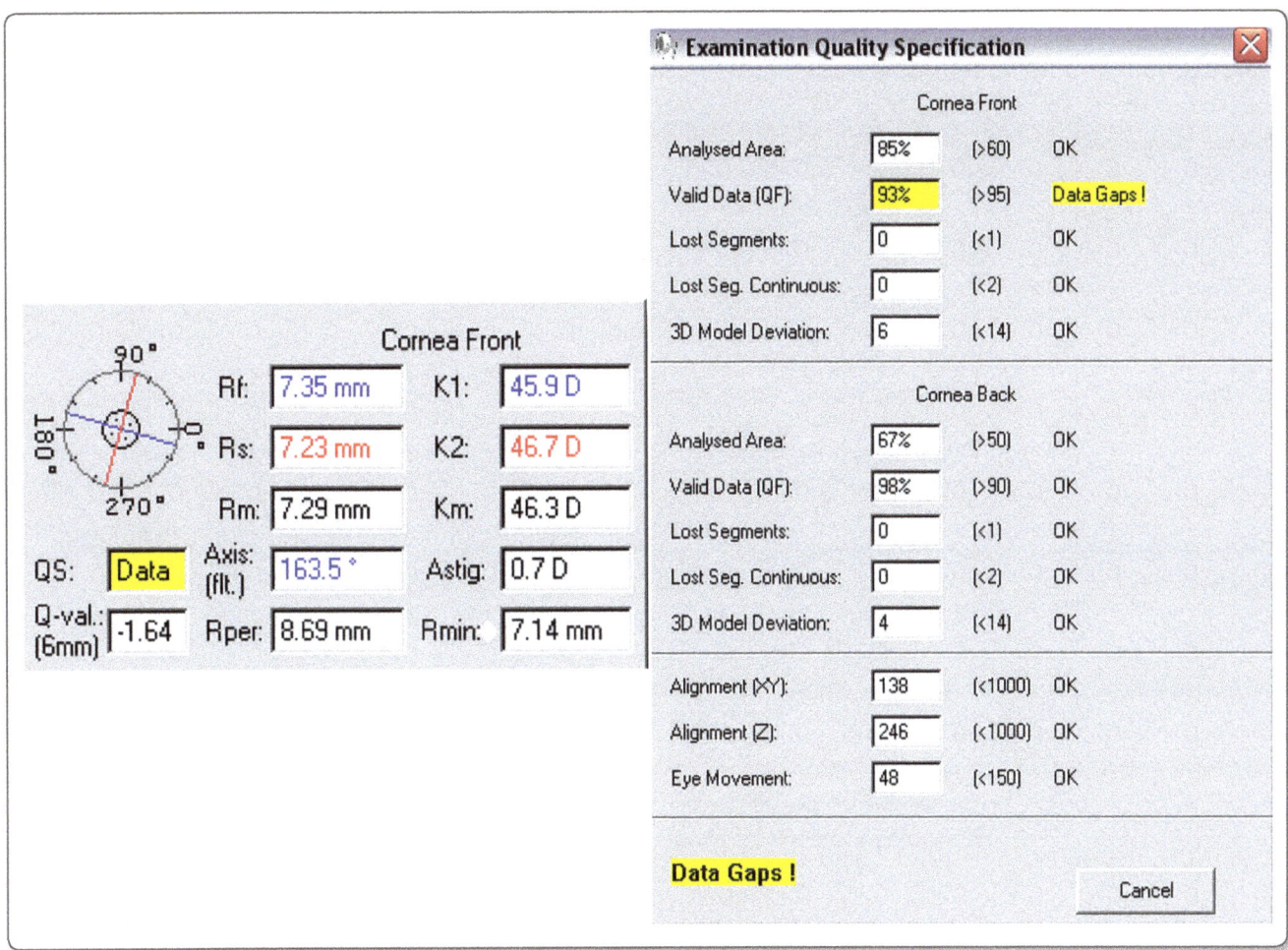

Fig. 18.1: Quality specification.

PRACTICAL SUBJECTIVE SCORING SYSTEM (PS3)

After obtaining good, reliable and reproducible images, PS3 is ready to be applied. The PS3 consists of two steps, (1) an overview step and (2) a detailed step. The overview step aims at having an idea about the captured cornea. The detailed step aims at classifying the cornea into low, moderate or high risk in terms of laser vision correction (LVC).

Overview Step

It consists of having a look at Belin–Ambrósio Display (BAD) and Belin ABCD Keratoconus Staging. The former is discussed in detail in Chapter 7 and the later is discussed in detail in Chapter 20. Whenever there are a yellow or red flags on the BAD, or Grade 1 and above on the ABCD system, the physician should be cautious and pay more attention to the second detailed step.

Detailed Step

This step consists of a 10-step algorithm: (1) Anterior Km (average central Sim-K), (2) thinnest location, (3) astigmatic study, (4) anterior sagittal map, (5) anterior elevation map, (6) posterior elevation map, (7) corneal thickness map, (8) corneal thickness profiles, (9) relative pachymetry, and (10) intereye asymmetry.

1. Anterior Km:
   - Normal: < 48 D.
   - Moderate risk: 48–50 D.
   - High risk: >50 D.
2. Thinnest location:
   - Normal: >500 µm.
   - Moderate risk: 470–500 µm.
   - High risk: <470 µm.
3. Astigmatic study: Compare manifest astigmatism with corneal astigmatism taken from total corneal refractive

Section 5: A Systematic Interpretation of Corneal Tomography

Table 18.1: Practical subjective scoring system.

Parameters	Low risk (normal)	Moderate risk	High risk
Anterior Km (D)	> 48	48 – 50.00	> 50.00
Thinnest location (μm)	> 500	470 – 500	< 470
Astigmatic study	< 1 D, <10°	≥ 1D, ≥ 10°	-
Anterior sagittal map	• A with normal Km • B with insignificant inferior superior difference • C with SRAX < 22° • C with SRAX ≥ 22° but < 1 D corneal astigmatism	• A with moderate Km • B with significant inferior superior difference and normal Km • B with significant inferior superior difference and moderate Km	• A and B with high Km • C with SRAX ≥ 22° and ≥ 1.0 D • D
Elevation maps	• < 8 μm anterior, < 18 μm posterior in myopic eyes • < 7 μm anterior, < 28 μm posterior in hypermetropic eyes	-	• ≥ 8 μm anterior, ≥ 18 μm posterior in myopic eyes • ≥ 7 μm anterior, ≥ 28 μm posterior in hypermetropic eyes
Corneal thickness map	Concentric pattern	Dome pattern	Bell and Globus pattern
Thickness profiles	Gradual slope with average < 1.20	Gradual slope with average ≥ 1.20 S after 6 mm	Quick slope S before 6 mm Inverted slope
Relative thickness map	≥ -8% (more positive)	<−8% (more negative)	
Intereye asymmetry	Score 1–3	Score 4	Score 5
Laser vision correction (LVC) decision	No LVC: One high risk factor or two moderate risk factors in one eye		
	Surface ablation: One moderate risk factor in one or both eyes		
	All LVC types: Neither high nor moderate risk factors in both eyes		

power at a mesopic pupil zone (if not available, consider the 5 mm zone) centered with the pupil (Chapter 12).
  - Normal: Difference in magnitude < 1 D and/or difference in axis < 10°.
  - Moderate risk: Difference in amount ≥ 1 D and/or difference in axis ≥ 10°.
  - No high risk.
4. Anterior sagittal map:
  - Normal:
    ♦ Group A and Km < 48 D.
    ♦ Group B and (I-S < 1.5 D or S-I < 2.5 D) and Km < 48 D.
    ♦ Group C and SRAX < 22°.
    ♦ Group C and SRAX ≥ 22° but corneal astigmatism < 1 D.
  - Moderate risk:
    ♦ Group A and Km 48 to 50 D.
    ♦ Group B and (I-S ≥ 1.5 D or S-I ≥ 2.5D) but Km < 48 D.
    ♦ Group B and (I-S < 1.5 D or S-I < 2.5 DD) and Km 48 to 50 D.
  - High risk:
    ♦ Group A and B and Km > 50 D.
    ♦ Group C and SRAX ≥ 22° and corneal astigmatism ≥ 1 D.
    ♦ Group D.
5-6. Anterior and posterior elevation maps: Elevation corresponding to the thinnest location:
  - Normal:
    ♦ <8 μm anterior, < 18 μm posterior in myopic eyes.
    ♦ <7 μm anterior, < 28 μm posterior in hypermetropic eyes.
  - No moderate risk.
  - High risk:
    ♦ ≥ 8 μm anterior, ≥ 18 μm posterior in myopic eyes.
    ♦ ≥ 7 μm anterior, ≥ 28 μm posterior in hypermetropic eyes.
7. Corneal thickness map:
  - Normal: Concentric pattern.
  - Moderate risk: Dome shape.
  - High risk: Bell and globus shapes.

8. Corneal thickness profiles:
   - Normal: Gradual slope with average < 1.2.
   - Moderate risk:
     - Gradual slope with average ≥ 1.2.
     - S after 6 mm.
   - High risk:
     - Quick slope.
     - S before 6 mm.
     - Inverted slope.
9. Relative pachymetry
   - Normal: ≥ -8% (e.g –2%).
   - Moderate risk: < -8% (e.g -12%).
   - High risk: No high risk.
10. Intereye asymmetry.

The tomography of both corneas should be studied and compared. A normal cornea does not mean the other cornea is normal. On the other hand, an abnormal cornea indicates that both corneas are abnormal even with the other cornea being apparently normal. Table 17.1 in Chapter 17 demonstrates the intereye corneal asymmetry score.
- Normal: Score 1–3.
- Moderate risk: Score 4.
- High risk: Score 5.

DECISION TREE BASED ON PS3

Table 18.1 is a summary of low, moderate, and high-risk factors based on PS3.
- *No LVC*: One high risk or two moderate risk factors in one eye.
- *Surface ablation*: One moderate risk factor in one or both eyes.
- *All LVC types*: Neither high nor moderate risk factors in both eyes.

SECTION 6

Corneal Tomography in Ectatic Corneal Diseases

SECTION OUTLINE

19. Tomographic Characteristics of Ectatic Corneal Diseases
20. Grading Systems of Ectatic Corneal Diseases
21. Progression Criteria
22. Entities Misdiagnosed as Ectasia

Tomographic Characteristics of Ectatic Corneal Diseases

INTRODUCTION

Ectatic corneal diseases (ECDs) are the main source of irregular astigmatism. They can be categorized into (Table 19.1):
- *Established ectasia*: Keratoconus (KC), pellucid marginal degeneration (PMD), pellucid-like keratoconus (PLK), keratoglobus (KG), and postlaser vision correction (post-LVC) ectasia.
- *Paraectasia*: Forme fruste keratoconus (FFKC) and keratoconus suspect (KCS).
- *Corneas with high potential*: Posterior KC, apparently normal corneas, and unclassified abnormal corneas.

To define ECDs properly, readers are recommended to review normal and abnormal tomographic patterns (Chapters 5 to 8), the effect of angle kappa and misalignment (Chapter 16), and enantiomorphism phenomenon (Chapter 17).

Table 19.1: Ectatic corneal diseases and abnormal corneas.

Established ectasia	
Established ectasia	• Keratoconus • Pellucid marginal degeneration • Pellucid-like keratoconus • Keratoglobus • Post-LVC ectasia.
Paraectasia	• Forme fruste keratoconus • Keratoconus suspect.
Corneas with high potential	• Posterior keratoconus versus subclinical keratoconus • Apparently normal cornea • Unclassified abnormal corneas.

(LVC: laser vision correction)

TOMOGRAPHIC DEFINITION OF ECTATIC CORNEAL DISEASES

Established Ectasia or Ectatic Corneal Diseases per se

- *Keratoconus*: It is characterized by a combination of an abnormal anterior curvature map and an abnormal posterior elevation map. This is regardless of the pachymetry map as KC may be encountered in thick corneas (Fig. 19.1), while thin corneas may be normal (Fig. 19.2).
- *Pellucid marginal degeneration (Fig. 19.3)*: It is described by a combination of a crab-claw pattern on the anterior curvature map and an abnormal posterior elevation map. Since the crab-claw pattern is not diagnostic of PMD, the "bell sign" on the pachymetry map is the hallmark of PMD that differentiates it from PLK. PMD and KC are considered as different clinical presentations of the same ECD.
- *Pellucid-like keratoconus (Fig. 19.4)*: There are patterns of KC that are associated with the crab-claw shape. These patterns are not associated with the "bell sign". These patterns can be given the term "pellucid-like keratoconus

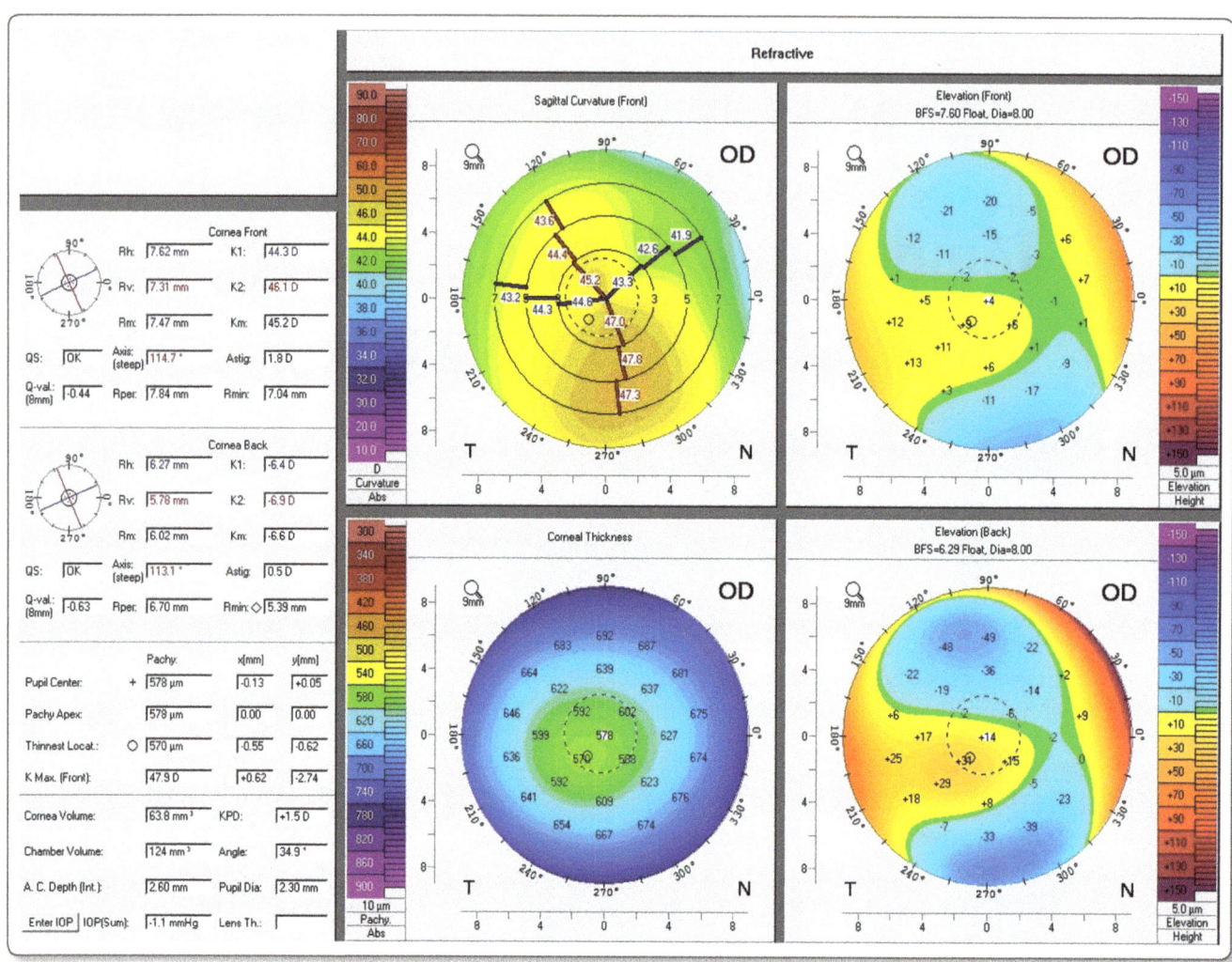

Fig. 19.1: Keratoconus with normal thickness.

or PLK". In some cases, PLK can be an early stage of PMD. In other words, if PLK is diagnosed, it should be monitored as it may convert into PMD.

- *Keratoglobus (Fig. 19.5)*: It is characterized by a generalized steepening in the anterior curvature map and a generalized thinning extending to the limbus.
- *Post-LVC ectasia (Fig. 19.6)*: It usually occur post-LASIK and rarely post-PRK. It may take the pattern of any ECD.

Paraectasia

It includes FFKC and KCS. These two terms are the most debatable ones. Belin and associates described KCS as those patients who do not exhibit frank disease, but have either a strong family history of ectatic disease or demonstrate one or more known associated parameters (i.e. corneal thickness, anterior and posterior elevation, and biomechanical changes) that are significantly outside the normal range but do not meet the criteria of ECD. Klyce and associates differentiated between FFKC and KCS. They stated that in a unilateral KC, the fellow eye that has no clinical findings of any sort except for certain topographic changes should carry the diagnosis of FFKC, while KCS should be a term reserved for corneas with very specific topographic changes in patients who do not have KC in both eyes.

I believe that these two terms can better be described by an abnormal anterior curvature map with a normal posterior elevation map (Fig. 19.7), and Klyce's definition can be used to differentiate between them. Because this entity is a curvature abnormality, Belin Ambrósio display (BAD) cannot detect it. Figure 19.8 is the BAD of the same eye in Figure 19.7. The reader can notice that the BAD is normal.

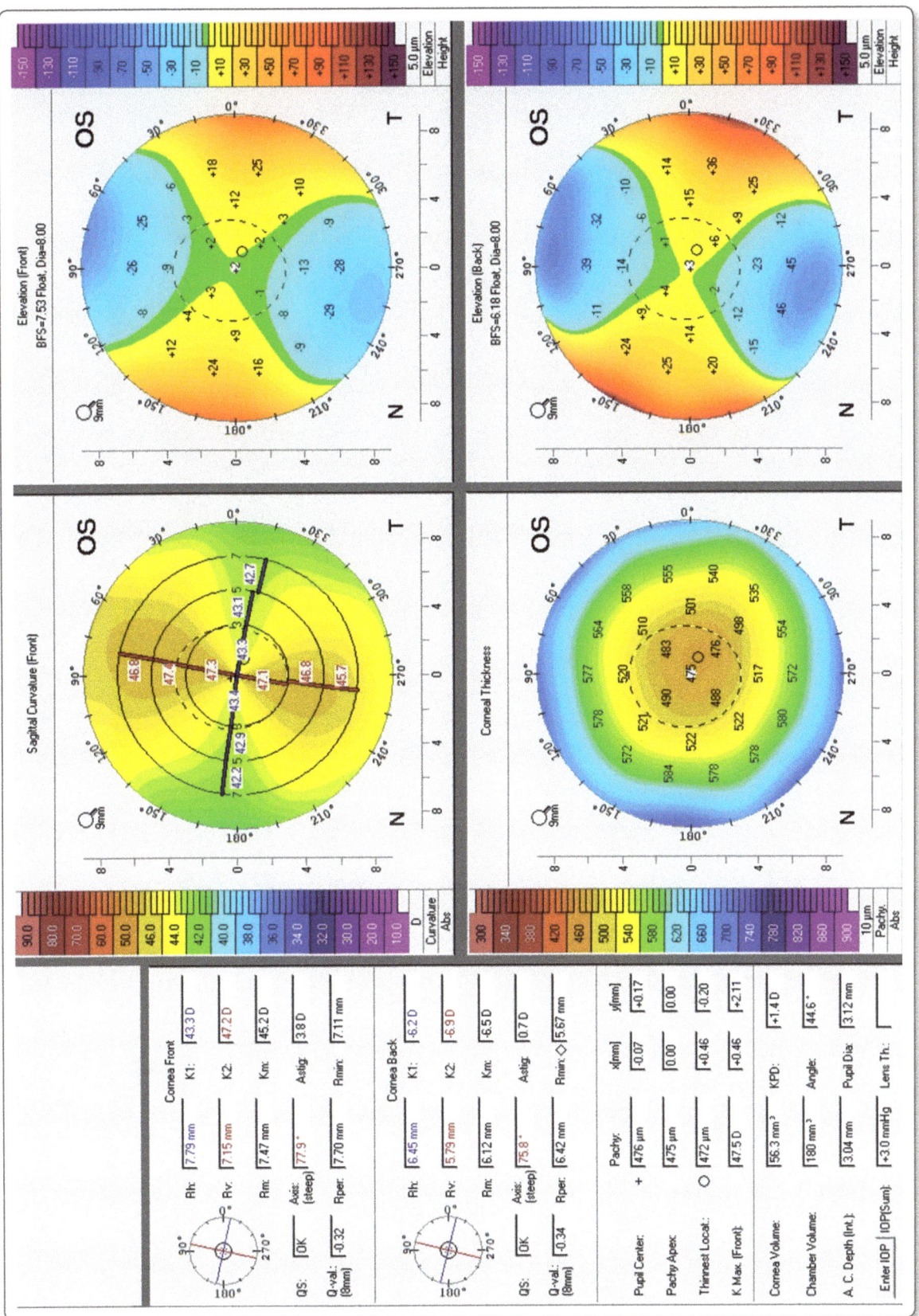

Fig. 19.2: Normal thin cornea.

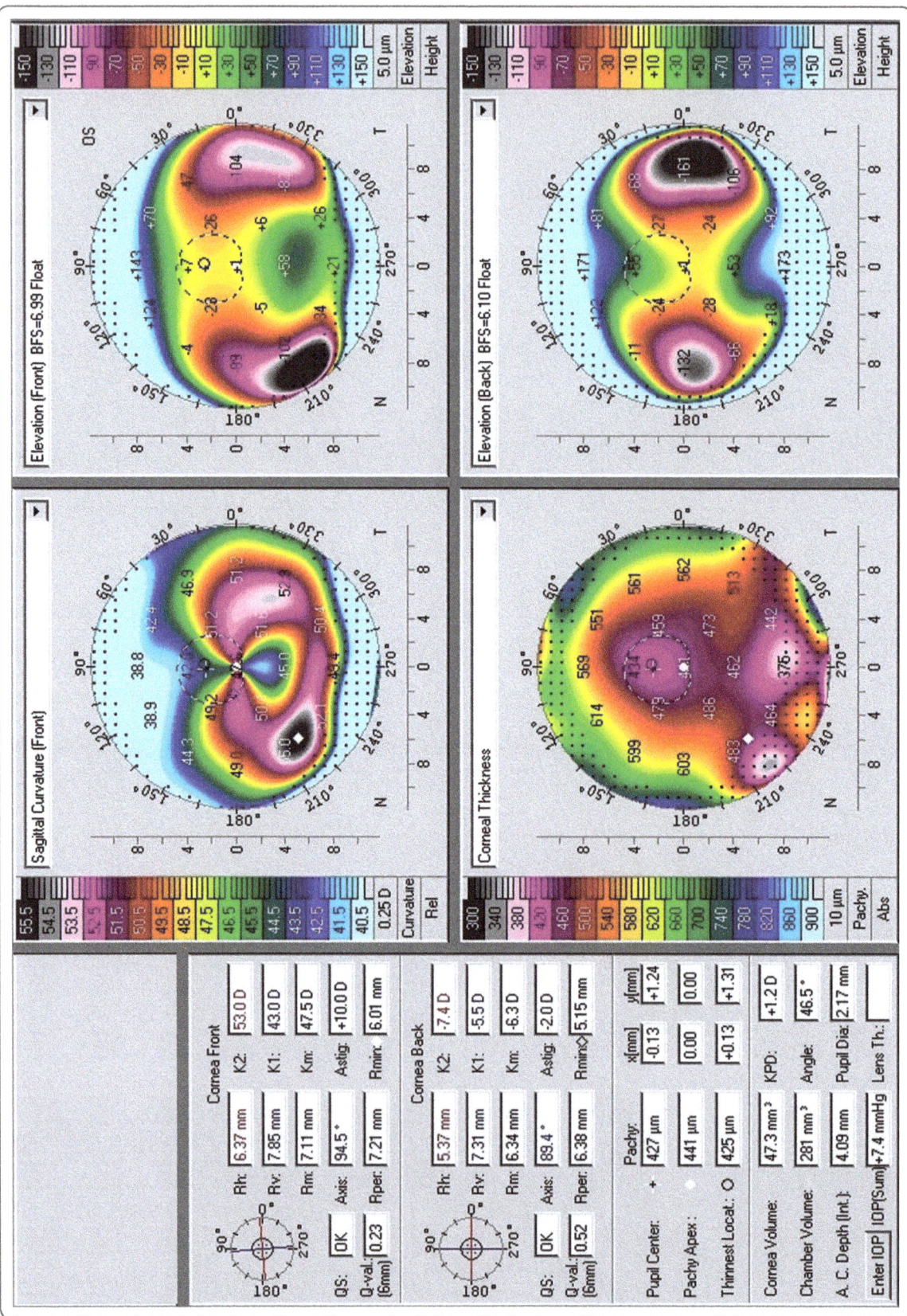

Fig. 19.3: Pellucid marginal degeneration.

Chapter 19: Tomographic Characteristics of Ectatic Corneal Diseases

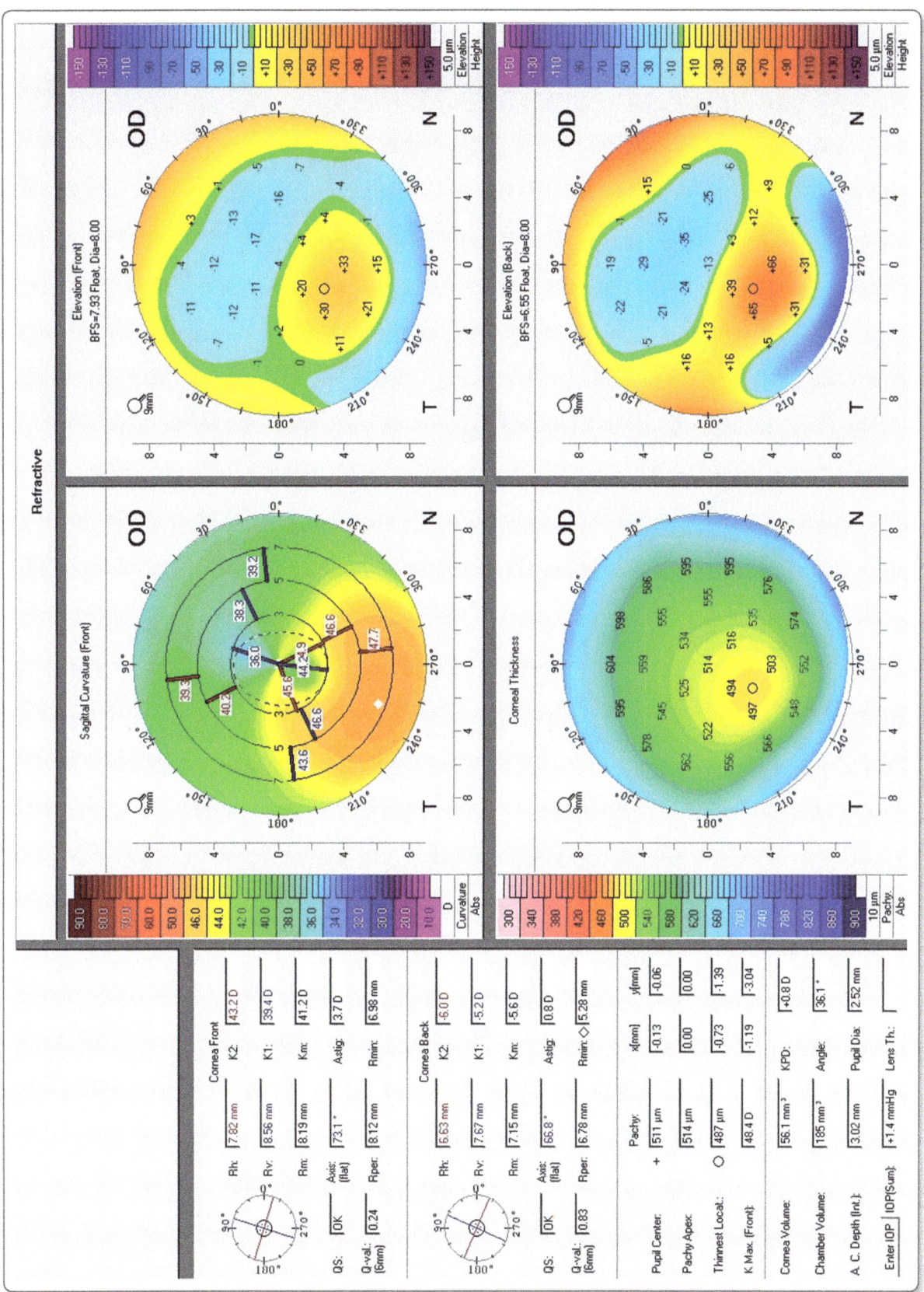

Fig. 19.4: Pellucid-like keratoconus.

172 *Section 6: Corneal Tomography in Ectatic Corneal Diseases*

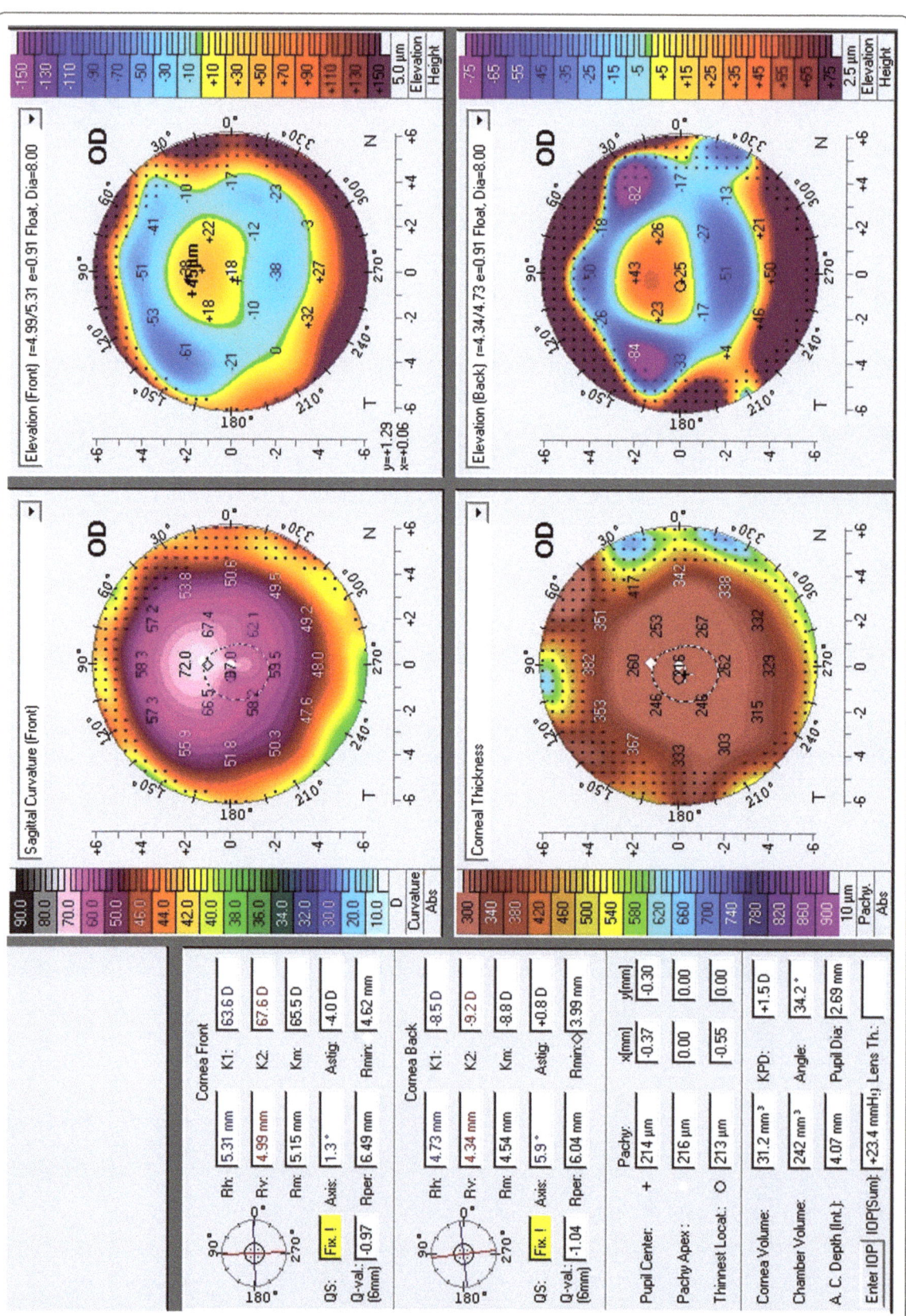

Fig. 19.5: Keratoglobus.

Chapter 19: Tomographic Characteristics of Ectatic Corneal Diseases

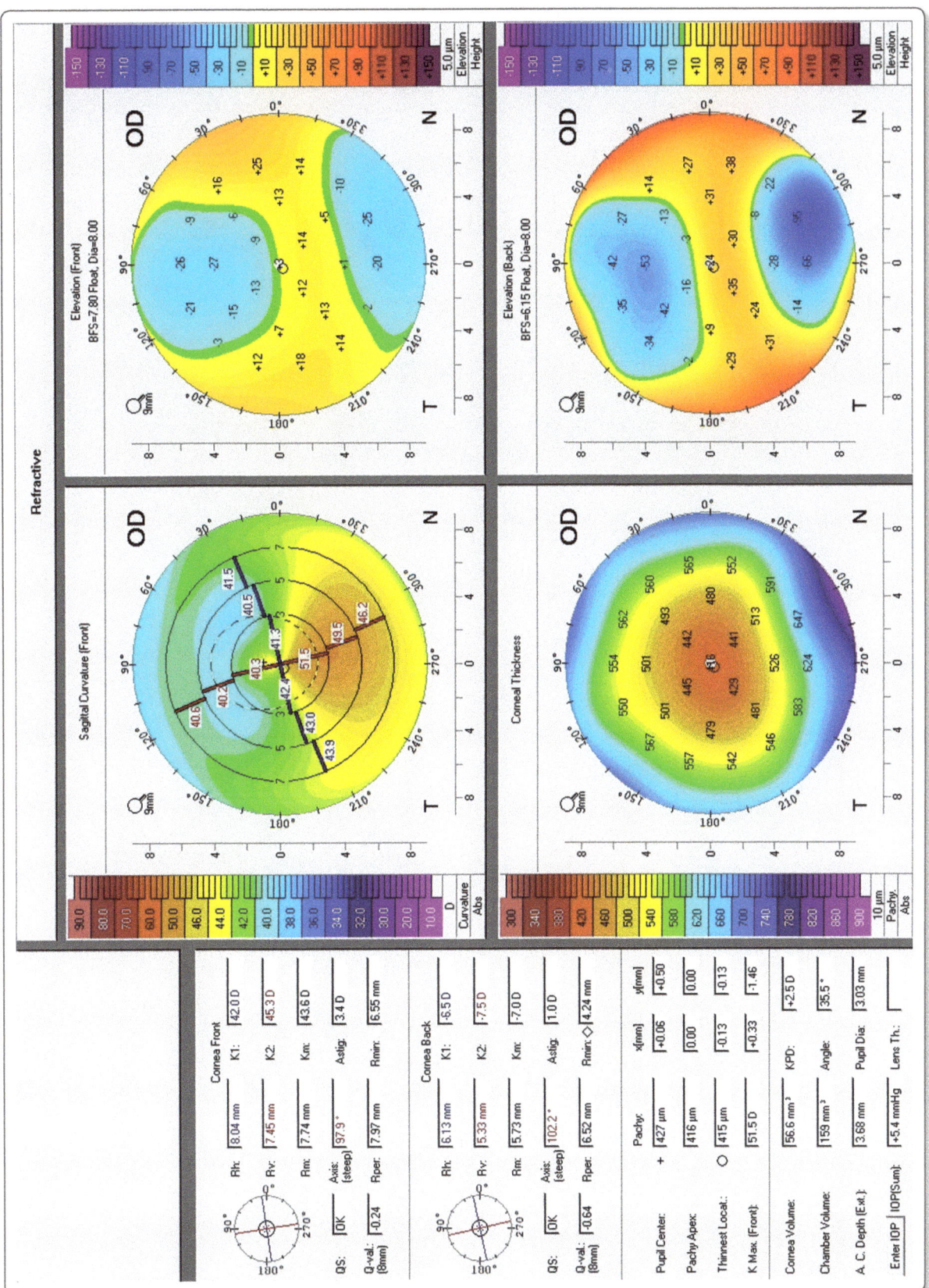

Fig. 19.6: Ectasia after laser vision correction.

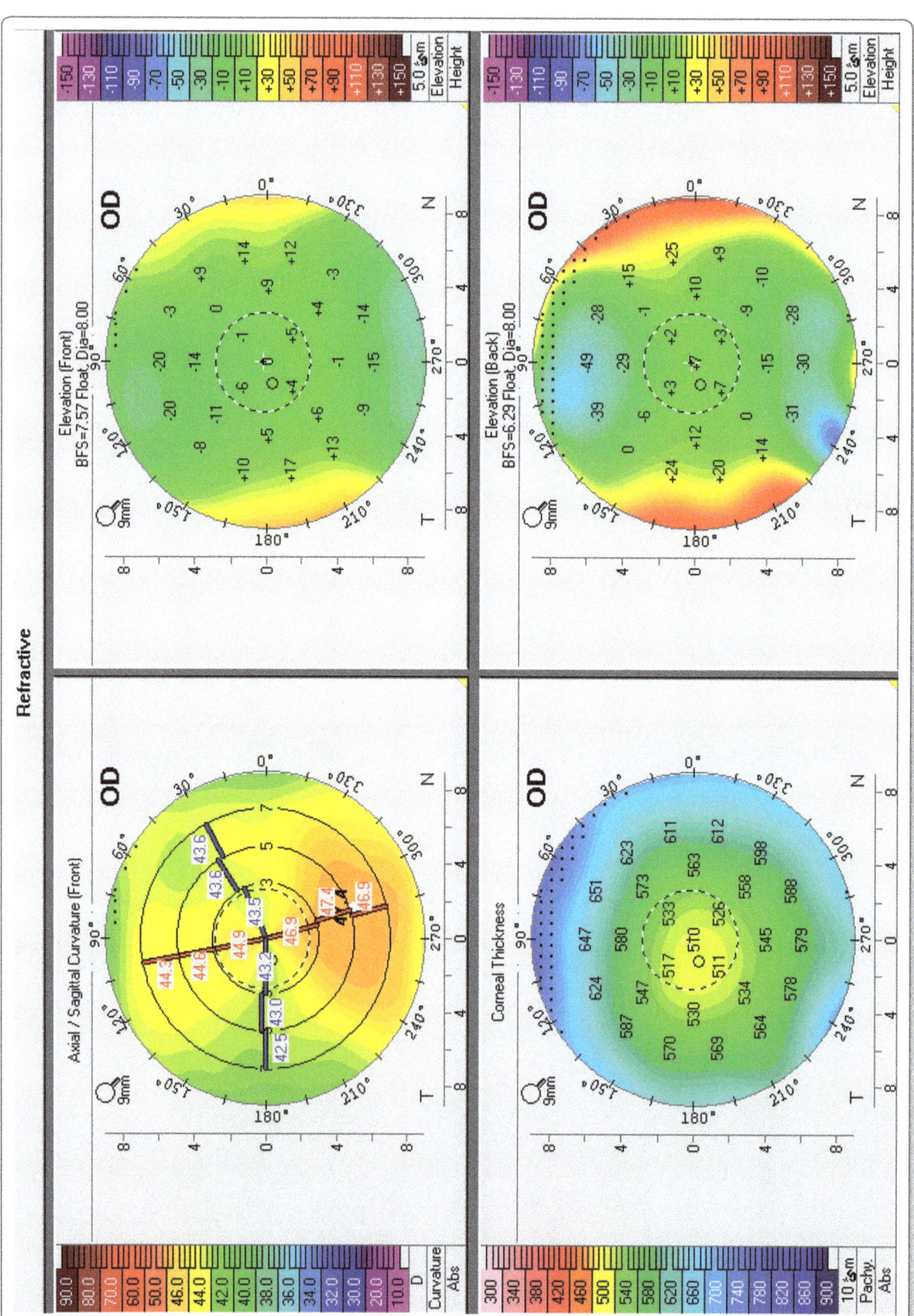

Fig. 19.7: Paraectasia.

Chapter 19: Tomographic Characteristics of Ectatic Corneal Diseases

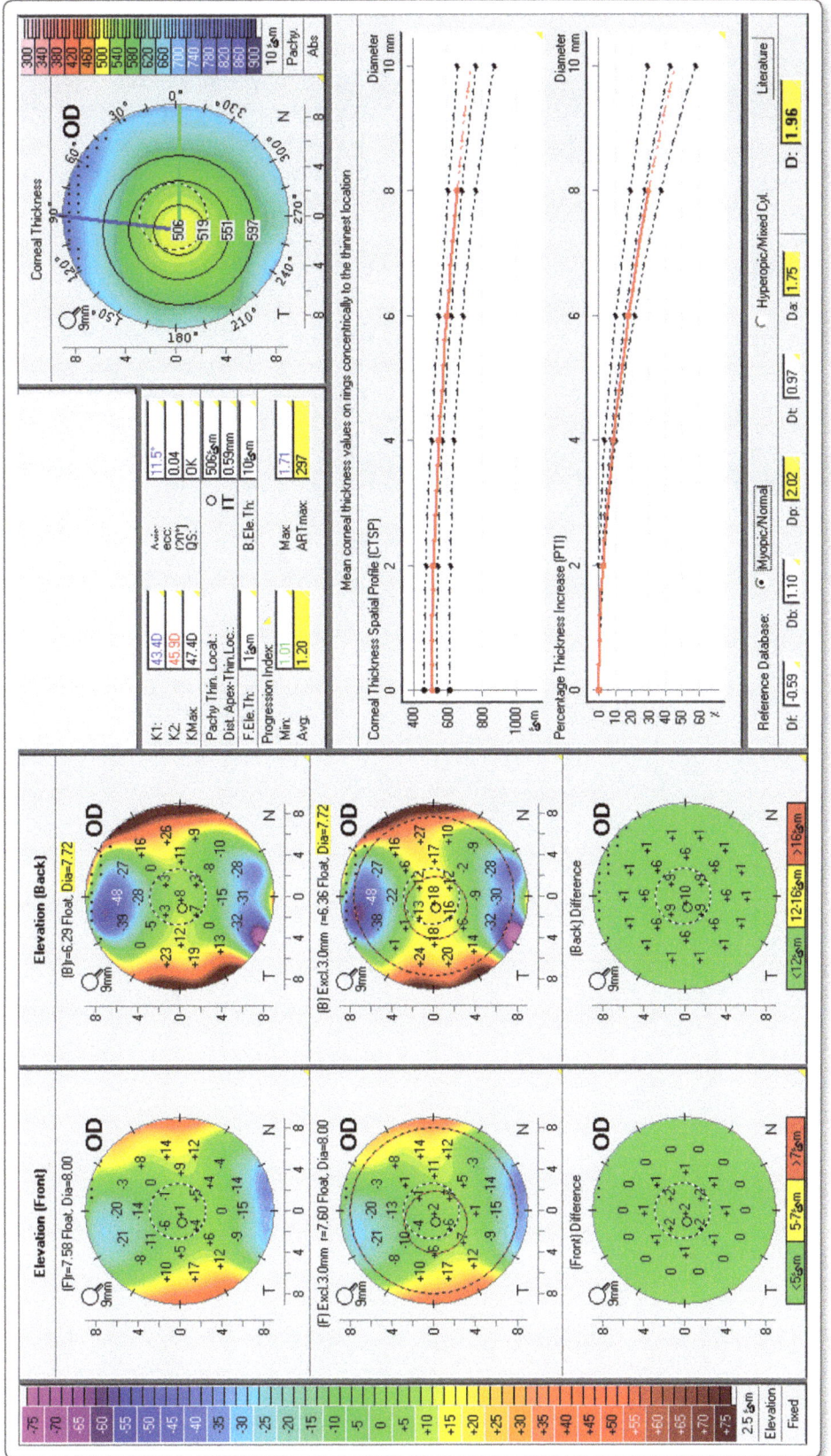

Fig. 19.8: Belin/Ambrósio display for the same eye in Figure 19.7. The display is normal despite paraectasia.

Corneas with High Potential

This entity consists of posterior KC, apparently normal corneas, and unclassified abnormal corneas.

- *Posterior keratoconus*: It is a rare, developmental, and nonprogressive corneal condition first described by T Harrison Butler in 1930 as a "small basin-like depression" in the posterior surface of the cornea. Also known as KC posticus, it is characterized by thinning of the posterior cornea without ectasia of the anterior cornea. It presents as a corneal opacity and is generally considered a developmental anomaly. This anomaly can either be generalized or circumscribed. The former has a uniform corneal steepening. The latter has a localized posterior corneal indentation.

    Posterior KC can be acquired. It may result from corneal trauma, or can be a true ECD known as "subclinical KC". The subclinical KC can be unilateral or asymmetric bilateral and progresses if untreated.

    Tomographically, posterior KC, if not associated with corneal opacity, is characterized by normal anterior curvature with abnormal posterior elevation.

- *Apparently normal corneas*: It is the case of bilateral tomographically normal corneas with a positive family history of an ECD. This category was classified as KCS by Belin and associates; however, I would recommend to use it as an independent term.

- *Unclassified abnormal corneas*: They are corneas that demonstrate abnormalities that are significantly outside the normal range but do not meet the criteria of ECDs. This category was classified as KCS by Belin and associates; however, I would recommend to use it as an independent term to describe corneas *that have* one high risk or two moderate risk factors in the Practical Subjective Scoring System (PS3) *and are not* categorized under any of the previous entities.

Grading Systems of Ectatic Corneal Diseases

INTRODUCTION

A number of grading systems has been developed to classify ectatic corneal diseases (ECDs) into stages. The aim of those systems is to categorize the disease for the purpose of treatment planning and for observation of progression.

AMSLER-KRUMEICH CLASSIFICATION

The first classification of keratoconus (KC) was based on disease evolution and was proposed by Amsler. After that, Krumeich and associates made some modifications to this classification and came up with the Amsler-Krumeich grading system of KC (Table 20.1). This grading system depends on the simulated keratometric readings (Sim-K), central corneal thickness, and clinical examination to grade the severity of KC from 0 (the least) to 4 (the most severe stage). However, this over-20-year-old analysis is limited because it does not reflect much of the more modern diagnostic measurements and depends on clinical signs which are very variable. For example, the cornea may stay transparent even with very advance KC.

ALIO-SHABAYEK MODIFICATION

Alio and Shabayek made some modifications to Amsler-Krumeich grading system, and added corneal higher-order aberrations, especially coma-like aberrations (Table 20.2).

MODIFICATION OF ISHII AND ASSOCIATES

Ishii and associates described a new classification based on Amsler-Krumeich grading system. In their classification, they integrated visual acuity, minimum radius of curvature of the anterior corneal surface, and six indices, namely: (1) ISV, index of surface variance, which describes corneal surface irregularity; (2) IVA, index of vertical asymmetry, which describes curvature symmetry; (3) KI, keratoconus index,

Table 20.1: Amsler-Krumeich classification of keratoconus.

Severity	Mean central K (D)	Thickness (μm)	Spherical equivalent (D)	Cornea
4	> 55	< 200	Not measurable	Central scars
3	53–55	300–400	> –8 Myopia, induced astigmatism, or both	No central scars
2	< 53 D	401–500	(–5, –8) Myopia, induced astigmatism, or both	No central scars
1	< 48 Eccentric steepening	> 500	< –5 Myopia, induced astigmatism, or both	No central scars

which also describes curvature symmetry; (4) CKI, center keratoconus index, which describes the severity of central KC; (5) IHA, index of height asymmetry, which is similar to IVA but based on corneal elevation, and is thus more sensitive; and (6) IHD, index of height decentration, which describes the decentration in elevation data in the vertical direction. Table 20.3 represents the classification.

However, Kanellopoulos and associates showed that the ISV and IHA, both derived from Scheimpflug corneal imaging, may be more sensitive and specific tools than corrected distance visual acuity (CDVA) in evaluating early diagnosis and possible progression in KC patients and corneal ectasia.

BELIN ABCD KERATOCONUS STAGING

This is the most recent system. It depends on four parameters:

1. A for anterior radius of curvature taken from the 3 mm zone cantered on the thinnest point.
2. B for back radius of curvature taken from the 3 mm zone cantered on the thinnest point.
3. C for corneal thickness at the thinnest point.
4. D for best corrected CDVA.

Table 20.4 demonstrates the ABCD classification.

Figures 20.1 and 20.2 are the topometric/keratoconus staging in the Pentacam. The former is for a normal cornea and the latter is for a cornea with KC. Distance visual acuity is not generated by the Pentacam, it should be input manually based on the manifest refraction.

This new classification/grading system has advantages over the older Amsler-Krumeich classification in that it recognizes the importance of the posterior corneal surface and each component (anterior, posterior, thickness, and visual acuity) is individually graded.

Table 20.2: Alio-Shabayek classification of keratoconus.

Stage	Mean central K (D)	Thickness (µm)	Spherical equivalent (D)	Root mean square (RMS) of coma-like aberration (µm)	Cornea
4	> 55	< 200	Not measurable	> 4.5	Central scars
3	> 53–≤ 55	300–400	>–8 Myopia, induced astigmatism, or both	> 3.5–≤ 4.5	No central scars
2	> 48–≤ 53	401–500	(–5, –8) Myopia, induced astigmatism, or both	> 2.5–≤ 3.5	No central scars
1	≤ 48 Eccentric steepening	> 500	<–5 Myopia, induced astigmatism, or both	1.5–2.5	No central scars

Table 20.3: Classification stages of keratoconus adapted from the classical Amsler-Krumeich standards.

	CDVA	ISV	KI	Other indices	Rmin (mm)	Retinoscopy signs	Cornea slit-lamp observation
Prestage (early signs)	20/20–20/15	<30	1.04–1.07	All four indices are "normal"	7.8–6.7	No clear light or shadow movement. Hint of "scissors" reflect	Clear cornea, unobtrusive. Horizontal, oval, or round shades central or slightly decentered, when observed under direct ophthalmoscopy
Level 1	20/25–20/15	30–55	1.07–1.15	Sometimes one value within the "abnormal" range	7.5–6.5	Distorted retinoscopy reflex. Scissors effect	Clear cornea. Fleisher's ring at the apex base. Cone and cone base clearly visible with direct ophthalmoscopy. Decrease in apex thickness not visible, but measurable

Contd...

Contd...

	CDVA	ISV	KI	Other indices	Rmin (mm)	Retinoscopy signs	Cornea slit-lamp observation
Level 2	20/60–20/20	55–90	1.10–1.25	Often one value within the "abnormal" range	6.9–5.3	Clear scissors effect, retinoscopy difficult to perform	Often cornea still clear, apex slightly thinner and eventually decentered. Partial or circular Fleischer's ring. Vogt's striae may be visible
Level 3	20/125–20/30	90–150	1.15–1.45	At least one value within the "abnormal" range	6.6–4.8	Distinct scissors effect, retinoscopy nearly impossible to perform	Apex thinner, decentered, and often slightly cloudy. Clear and mostly circular Fleischer's ring. Vogt's striae clearly visible. Eventually Munson's sign may appear
Level 4	<20/400–20/100	>150	>1.50	At least one value within the "abnormal" range	<5.00	Retinoscopy impossible to perform	Cornea often scarred and opaque in the apex. Munson's sign evident

(CDVA: corrected distance visual acuity; ISV: index of surface variance; KI: keratoconus index; Rmin: minimum radius of curvature)

Source: Bühren J, Kook D, Yoon G, et al. Detection of subclinical keratoconus by using corneal anterior and posterior surface aberrations and thickness spatial proles. Invest Ophthalmol Vis Sci. 2010;51(7):3424-32.

Table 20.4: Belin ABCD keratoconus staging.

Criteria A and ARC (3.0 mm zone)
Anterior radius of curvature—average curvature in the 3.0 mm zone centered on the thinnest location of the cornea
Criteria B and PRC (3.0 mm zone)
Posterior radius of curvature in the 3.0 mm zone—average curvature in the 3.0 mm zone centered on the thinnest location of the cornea
Criteria C and thinnest Pachymetry
Thinnest pachymetry in µm
Criteria D and DCVA
"Distance Best Corrected Visual Acuity"
DCVA is not generated by the Pentacam software. It should be input manually by clicking left mouse into the corresponding field
The input value will be saved to the examination
Whole number stages are rounded down from the numbers with decimal place

ABCD Criteria	A	B	C	D	
	ARC	PRC	Thinnest	BDVA	Scarring
Stage 0	> 7.25 mm (< 46.5 D)	> 5.90 mm	> 490 µm	= 20/20 (= 1.0)	–
Stage I	> 7.05 mm (< 48.0 D)	> 5.70 mm	> 450 µm	< 20/20 (< 1.0)	–, +, ++
Stage II	> 6.35 mm (< 53.0 D)	> 5.15 mm	> 400 µm	< 20/40 (< 0.5)	–, +, ++
Stage III	> 6.15 mm (< 50.0 D)	> 4.95 mm	> 300 µm	< 20/100 (< 0.2)	–, +, ++
Stage IV	> 6.15 mm (< 50.0 D)	< 4.95 mm	= 300 µm	< 20/400 (< 0.05)	–, +, ++

[ARC: anterior radius of curvature; PRC: posterior radius of curvature; Scarring: – (clear), iris details visible (+), iris obscured (++)].

Section 6: Corneal Tomography in Ectatic Corneal Diseases

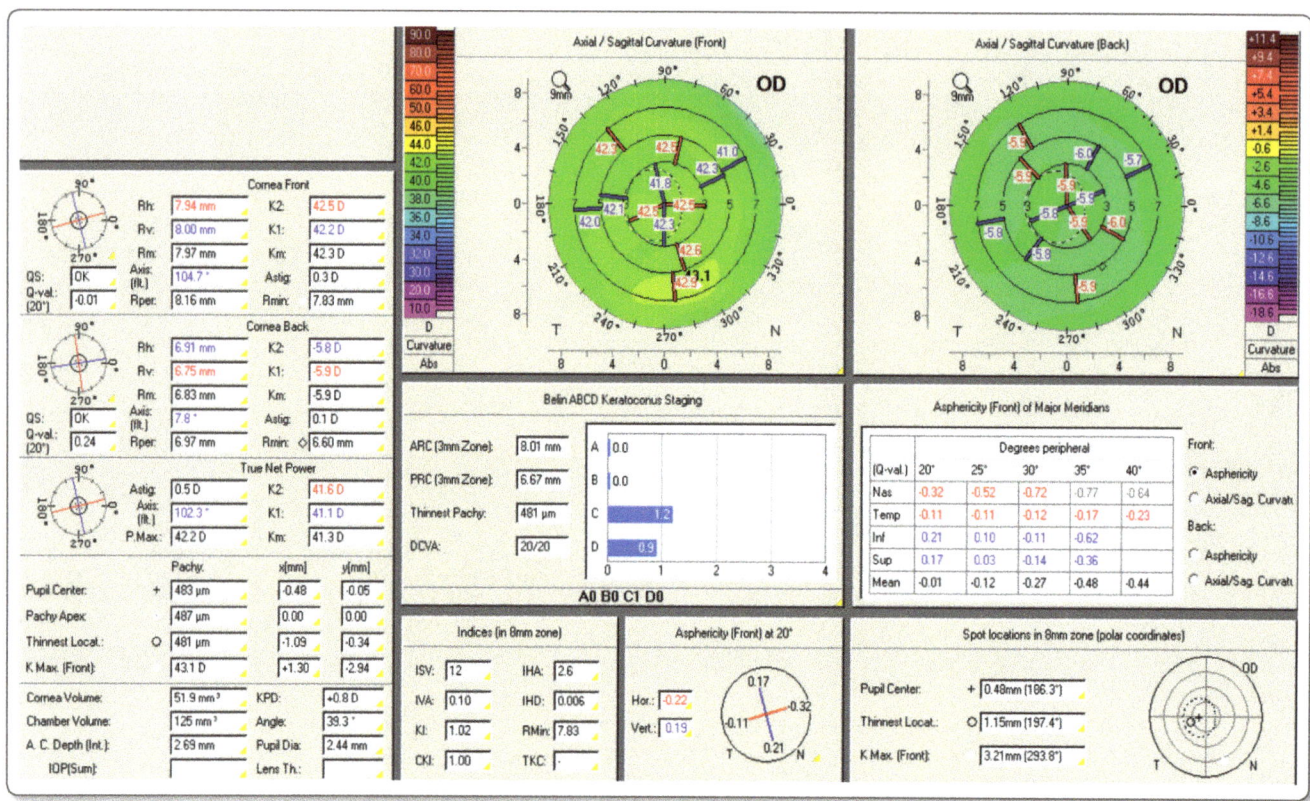

Fig. 20.1: Topometric/Belin ABCD keratoconus staging. Normal cornea.

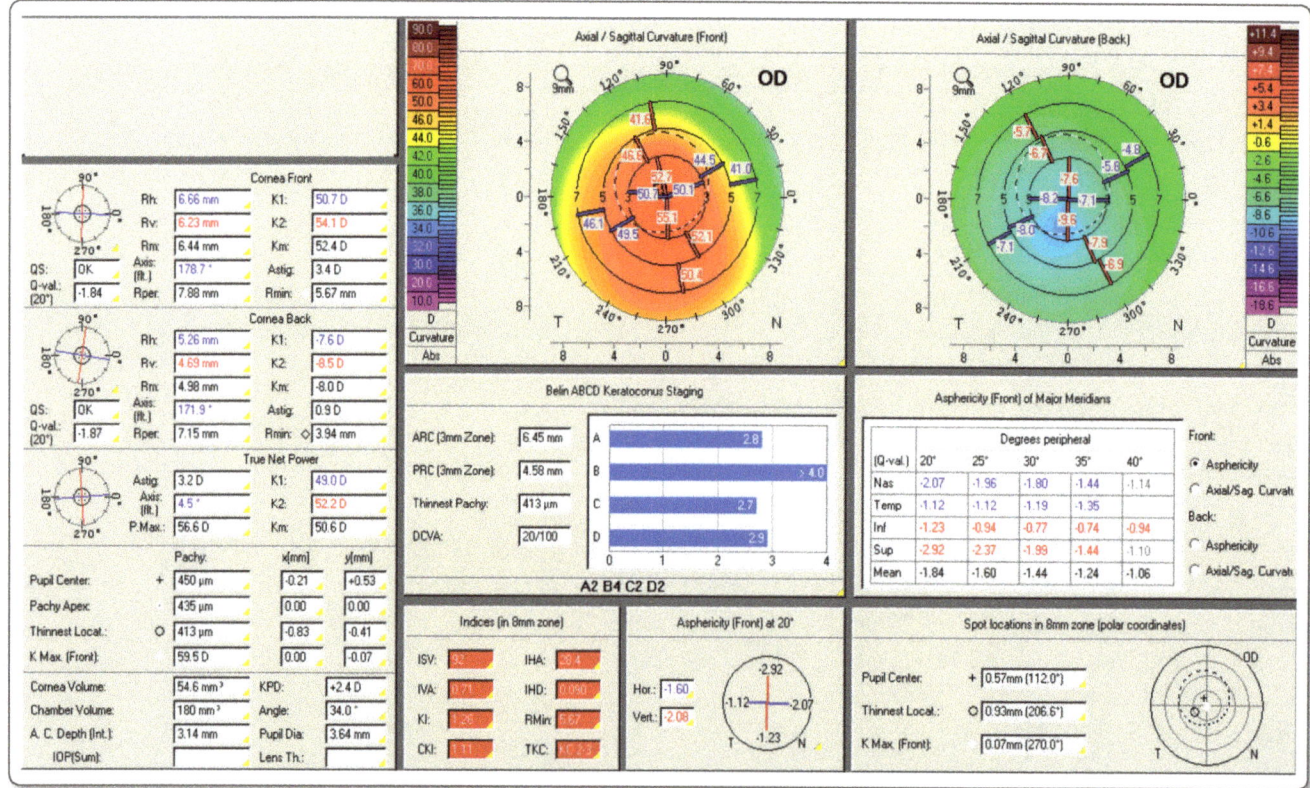

Fig. 20.2: Topometric/Belin ABCD keratoconus staging. Keratoconic cornea.

Progression Criteria

INTRODUCTION

Defining progression of ectatic corneal diseases (ECDs) is a necessity for both indication of treatment, particularly corneal cross-linking (CXL), and follow-up after treatment to observe efficacy and failure. It is also important to differentiate ectasia from entities misdiagnosed as ectasia (Chapter 22).

Definition of progression has been a debate. Different criteria, parameters, and methods were used in different studies throughout the literature. Even when using the same criteria, different cutoff values were used in different studies.

Recently, there is a general consensus on defining progression as a consistent change in at least two of the following parameters where the magnitude of the change is above the "normal noise" of the testing system:

1. Progressive steepening of the anterior corneal surface.
2. Progressive steepening of the posterior corneal surface.
3. Progressive thinning and/or an increase in the rate of corneal thickness change from the periphery to the thinnest point.

On the other hand, this general consensus failed to put clear cutoff values.

The term "normal noise of the testing system" means variability of outcomes. Variability of a test is composed of two terms: (1) repeatability and (2) reproducibility. Repeatability is the variation of outcomes of a test performed in the same conditions and device by the same operator (technician), whereas reproducibility is the variation of outcomes of a test performed in conditions varying within a typical range, by the same device and different operators (technicians) and/or different clinics. Therefore, to neglect the effect of reproducibility, studies are conducted in same clinics to check repeatability.

In normal population, several studies have shown good repeatability of the Pentacam in measuring several parameters such as anterior and posterior corneal curvature, anterior chamber depth, and corneal thickness. However, fewer studies concerning repeatability were conducted on patients with keratoconus (KC), and the results were conflicting.

PARAMETERS OF PROGRESSION

In general, curvature and thickness parameters in addition to visual acuity and manifest refraction are the most commonly used parameters in studies to observe or to define progression. Table 21.1 demonstrates a literature review of studies and the parameters they used. Unfortunately, none of the suggested cutoff values was validated.

Apart from the absence of a general consensus on definite parameters and cutoff values, several factors make depending on many topographic and tomographic progression criteria misleading for the following reasons:

- Different machines generate different values for the same parameters of the same eye. For example, Kmax value on Pentacam is different from that on Sirius for the same captured cornea in the same session.
- Range of variability differs according to number of captures per session. If an eye is captured three times, the range of noise will differ from that when one or five captures are taken.
- Variability increases in distorted corneas. The more distorted the cornea, the larger the noise.
- Patient cooperation during taking the capture. Misalignment during capturing the cornea is a key factor in variability. Other causes of false findings have a large impact as well (Chapter 16).

Table 21.1: Parameters used in the literature to determine progression of ectatic corneal diseases.

Suggested parameters	Value representing progression	Validated
Spherical power, and higher-order irregular astigmatism	Positive rate of change per year	No
Spherical component, regular astigmatism, decentration component, and higher-order irregularity	Positive rate of change per year	No
Kmax (steepest K)	≥ 1 D increase	No
Kmax–Kmin	≥ 1 D increase	No
Kmean (average of Kmax and Kmin)	≥ 0.75 D increase	No
Pachymetry	≥ 2% decrease in central thickness	No
Back optic zone radius of the best fitting contact lens	0.1 mm or more decrease	No
Increase in the central K power	≥ 1.5 D increase from baseline	No
Manifest cylinder	Increase of ≥ 1 D in 24 months	No
Manifest refraction spherical equivalent (MRSE) change	≥ 0.5 D	No
ISV	Specific values for each KC stage	No
IHA	Specific values for each KC stage	No

[IHA: index of height asymmetry; ISV: index of surface variance; Kmax: steepest K reading on anterior corneal surface; Kmin: flattest K reading on anterior corneal surface; Kmean = (Kmax + Kmin)/2; KC: keratoconus].

In the following, the parameters that were used and their pitfalls will be discussed.

Maximum K-reading (Kmax)

- It is the most commonly used parameter to detect or document ectatic progression and is regularly used as an indicator for CXL efficacy or failure.
- Kmax changes were studied by Epstein and associates. In their study "Pentacam HR criteria for curvature change in KC and postoperative LASIK ectasia", they found the change in Kmax between observation visits could be considered as significant with 95% confidence when it exceeded 1.51 D if *single* captures were used. Using an average Kmax of *five* captures in each visit would reduce the real Kmax change to 0.68 D. In other words, if a study is using one capture in each visit, a real Kmax change should be considered as more than 1.51 D over the period of observation. If a study is using five captures in each visit, the significant and real change can be considered as more than 0.68 D. The latter is more reliable and can avoid a lot of factors such as noise, and intra- and interobserver errors. Moreover, they found that Kmax variability was not correlated with measured Kmax magnitude when Kmax was less than 70 D, above which the variability rose sharply.
- On the other hand, the effect of KC grades on variability was studied by Hashemi H et al. In their study "Effect of KC grades on repeatability of keratometry readings: Comparison of five devices", they concluded that when Kmax was more than 55 D, all imaging systems had weak repeatability as a result of measurement error and unreliable K results.
- *Pitfalls*:
  - It is a single point rather than an area, hence it is a poor indicator that is prone to artificats.
  - It fails to reflect the degree of ectasia.
  - It ignores the contribution of the posterior cornea to progression.

Topometric Indices

- There are seven Pentacam-derived topometric indices. The Pentacam software compares the measured values with the means and standard deviations (SDs) of a normal population. Measured values which exceed the SD by more than 2.5 times, are classified as abnormal and highlighted in yellow, and those which exceed the SD by more than 3 times, are classified as pathological and highlighted in red. Namely, these factors are:
  1. *Index of surface variance (ISV)*: The standard deviation of individual corneal sagittal radii from the mean curvature. ISV is, thus, an expression of the corneal surface irregularity. It is elevated in all types of corneal surface irregularity (e.g. scars, astigmatism, deformities caused by contact lenses, and pachymetry). According to the manufacturer's user manual, an ISV larger than 37 is considered as

abnormal (marked with yellow) and larger than 41 is pathological (marked with red).

2. *Index of vertical asymmetry (IVA)*: The measure (expressed in mm) of the mean difference between superior and inferior anterior corneal curvature (similar to the commonly used inferior/superior ratio). IVA is, thus, the value of curvature symmetry, with respect to the horizontal meridian as the axis of reflection. An IVA larger than 0.28 is considered as abnormal and larger than 0.32 is pathological.
3. *Keratoconus index (KI)*: The ratio between mean anterior radius values in the upper and lower segment (r sagittal superior to r sagittal inferior). A KI value larger than 1.07 is considered as abnormal and/or pathological. KI increases with severity of KC.
4. *Center keratoconus index (CKI)*: The ratio between mean anterior radius values in a peripheral ring divided by a central ring: r sag (mean peripheral) to r sag mean center (no units). CKI is elevated especially in central pachymetric, and increases with the severity of central KC. A CKI value larger than 1.03 is considered as abnormal and/or pathological. CKI increases with severity of central KC.
5. *Index of height asymmetry (IHA)*: The mean difference between anterior height values superior minus height values inferior with horizontal meridian as mirror axis (expressed in μm). IHA is calculated by the height data symmetry comparison of the superior and inferior area, and provides the degree of symmetry of height data with respect to the horizontal meridian as the axis of reflection. IHA is similar to the IVA but based on corneal elevation, and is, thus, more sensitive. An IHA value larger than 19 is considered as abnormal and larger than 21 is pathological.
6. *Index of height decentration (IHD)*: The value of the decentration of anterior elevation data in the vertical direction (expressed in μm), and is calculated from a Fourier analysis. This index provides the degree of decentration in the vertical direction, calculated on a ring with radius 3 mm. An IHD value larger than 0.014 is considered as abnormal and larger than 0.016 is pathological.
7. *Rmin expressed in mm*: It is a measurement of the smallest radius of anterior sagittal corneal curvature (i.e. the maximum steepness of the cone). Values of Rmin less than 6.71 mm are considered as abnormal and/or pathological, considering that the average radius of the anterior corneal surface is 7.87 ± 0.27 mm.

- It has been shown that ISV and IHD may be the most sensitive and specific criteria in the diagnosis and progression of KC.
- *Pitfalls*:
    - All of these indices are derived from the anterior corneal surface.
    - They ignore the contribution of the posterior cornea to progression.
    - Changes on the posterior cornea may occur without concurrent anterior changes and there may be posterior progression in spite of a normal anterior surface (posterior KC or subclinical KC).
    - They describe irregularities in general and not specific for ECDs.

Visual Acuity and Manifest Refraction

- *Pitfalls*:
    - Visual acuity methods are very variable.
    - Manifest refraction methods are very variable and observer (optometrist) dependent.
    - Not always accurately measured, especially in advanced cases of ECDs.
    - In some cases, visual acuity remains the same in spite of progression.
    - In some cases, progression may lead to improvement in visual acuity as the cone becomes more peripheral away from the central visual zone, which becomes less irregular.

Corneal Thickness

Three thickness parameters were used to observe progression, namely are: (1) thinnest corneal thickness (TCT), (2) central corneal thickness (CCT), and (3) corneal thickness profiles [cornea thickness spatial profile (CTSP), percentage thickness increase (PTI), and index].

- Alterations in the corneal thickness profiles, such as quick slope and S shape can be seen in early KC even with normal anterior and posterior elevation maps.
- Measuring corneal thickness change at the thinnest point (TCT) should be a more sensitive indicator of progression than apical pachymetry (CCT).
- *Pitfalls*:
    - Central corneal thickness is supposed to be measured at the geometrical center of the cornea. However, the software of the computer considers cornea apex as the geometrical center of the cornea, which is not

true in cases of misalignment or large angle kappa. Therefore, CCT is affected by the previous two factors, while TCT is an absolute point at which the cornea is thinnest, regardless of its location. Therefore, TCT is more reliable than CCT.

- Central corneal thickness often does not adequately reflect the cone, while the TCT usually does. Changes in the decentered cones may occur with insignificant or no changes in the apical cornea.
- Progressive posterior ectasia will be accompanied by further corneal thinning, but this may not be detected by simply taking measurements at corneal apex.
- Corneal thickness measurements are typically altered (thinned) after CXL, thus limiting its value to document progression.

Elevation Maps

Observing changes on the elevation maps are not useful to detect progression. A different reference surface (RS) is used by the computer for every capture. That is because the radius of the RS is automatically determined by the computer based on the mean central radii of the examined corneal surface. The mean central radii changes due to machine variability and causes of false findings as mentioned before. This leads to different radii of the RS in every capture. This variation is usually insignificant in normal corneas, but becomes significant in distorted corneas. Therefore, depending on changes in the elevation maps is not always accurate and yet there are no cutoff values.

Anterior and Posterior Radius of Curvature

Belin ABCD Keratoconus Staging uses the anterior and posterior radius of curvature taken from the 3 mm zone cantered on the thinnest point (Chapter 20).

- Three of the ABCD parameters (A, B, and C) are centered on the thinnest point and limited to the conical region. The three parameters should reflect changes earlier than more global parameters, such as Kmax, IHD, and ISV.
- *Pitfall*: The fourth parameter in the ABCD is visual acuity, which does not always reflect progression.

CONCLUSION

The reader can conclude that there is yet no agreement on the parameters and the cutoff values. In addition, the studies use different methods of inclusion and exclusion criteria, number of captures per studied eye per session, and external validation. Therefore, I recommend the following:
- If the Belin ABCD Keratoconus Staging is available, it is the best to be used to observe progression.
- If the Belin ABCD Keratoconus Staging is not available, Kmax and TCT are to be observed.

In both cases, I recommend the following steps:
- Taking at least three captures for the cornea per visit.
- The three captures are better to be taken by the same technician per visit and in every visit if possible.
- Comparing the averages. The average Kmax of the three captures in a visit is compared with the average Kmax of the three captures in the next visit.
- Along the observation period (usually 3–6 months), an increase in Kmax ≥1.5 D and a thinning in the TCT ≥15 µm is considered as progression.

Figures 21.1 to 21.6 represent an example of KC progression. The Belin ABCD Keratoconus Staging was not available in the device, so the decision was made based on the average change in Kmax and TCT between the two visits. This case shows a very slow progression of KC over 4 years in a female who was 26 years old at the first visit. Figures 21.1 to 21.3 represent the four-composite refractive map in OS in three different dates. Figures 21.4 and 21.5 represent the difference maps between the first visit and the latest visit. Figure 21.6 represents the parametric difference between the first visit and the last visit.

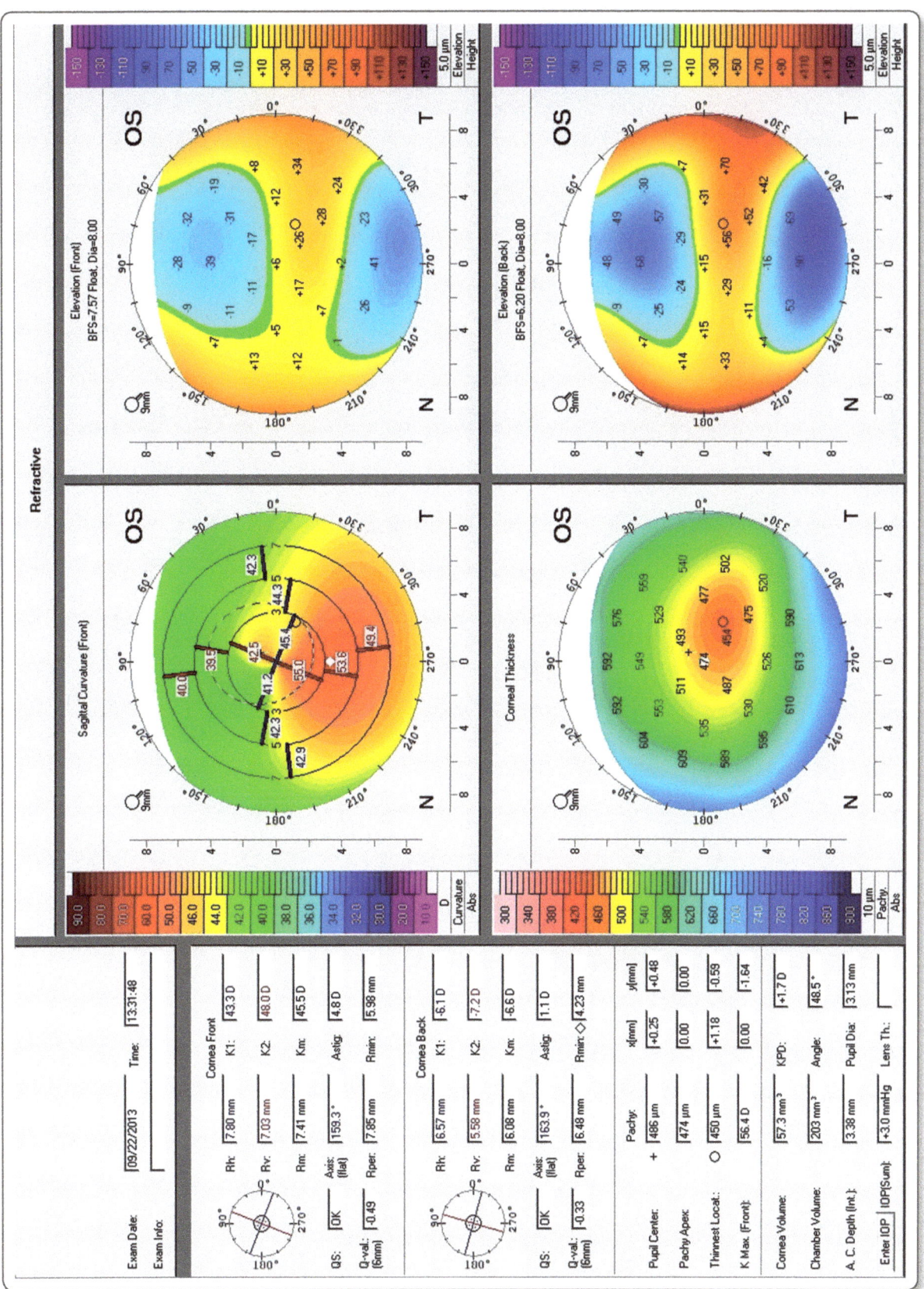

Fig. 21.1: Keratoconus progression. The four-composite refractive map in the first visit.

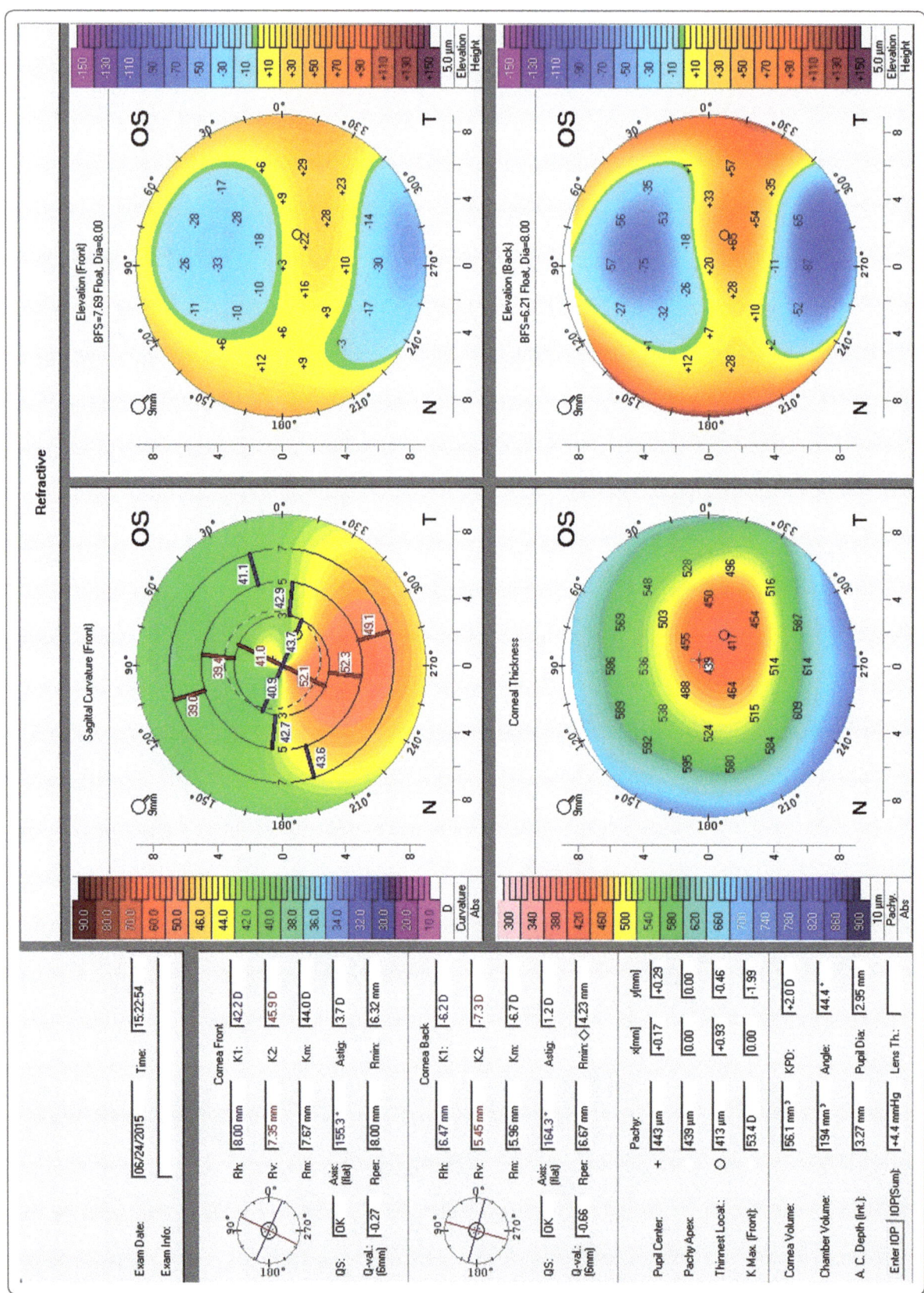

Fig. 21.2: Keratoconus progression. The four-composite refractive map in the second visit.

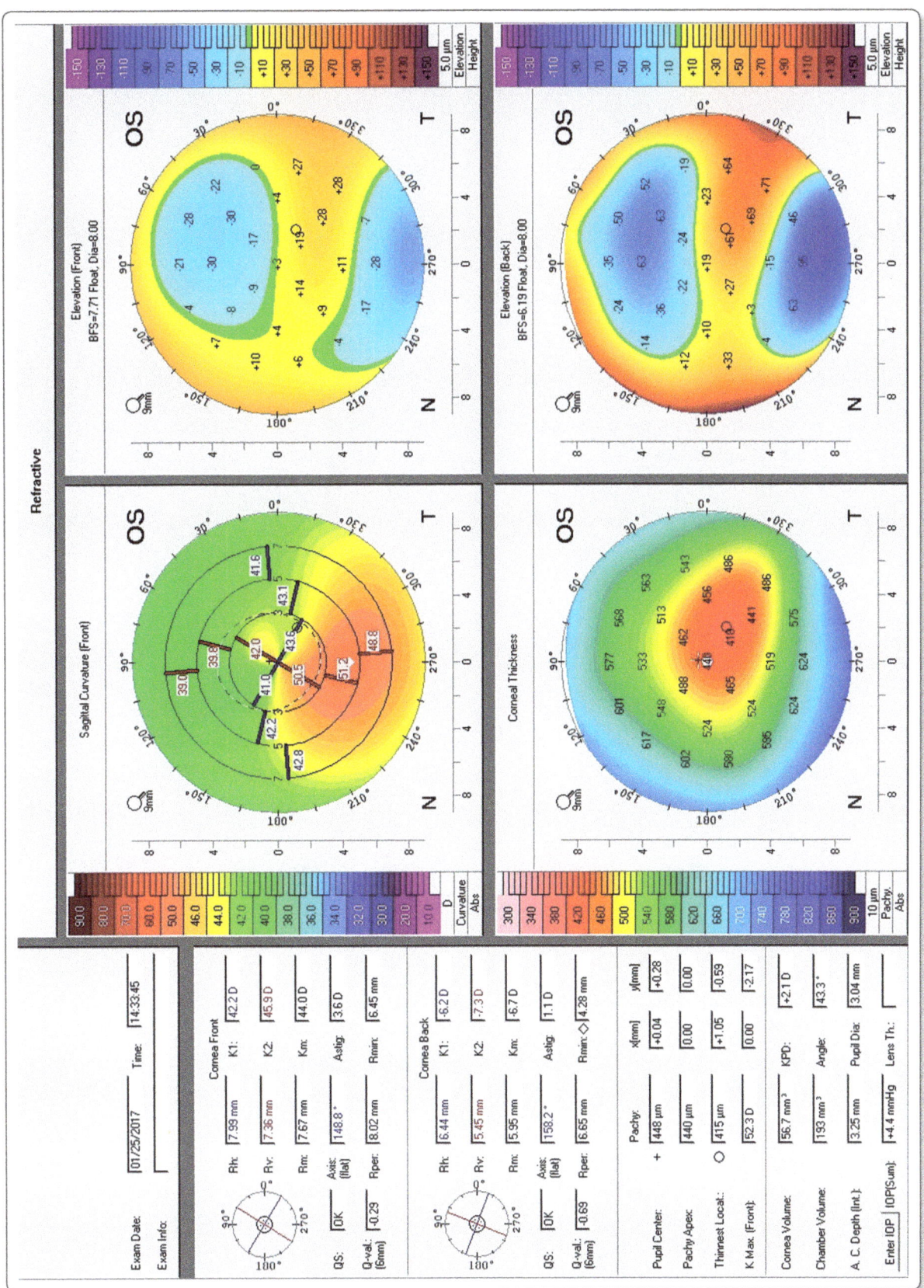

Fig. 21.3: Keratoconus progression: The four-composite refractive map in the third visit.

Section 6: *Corneal Tomography in Ectatic Corneal Diseases*

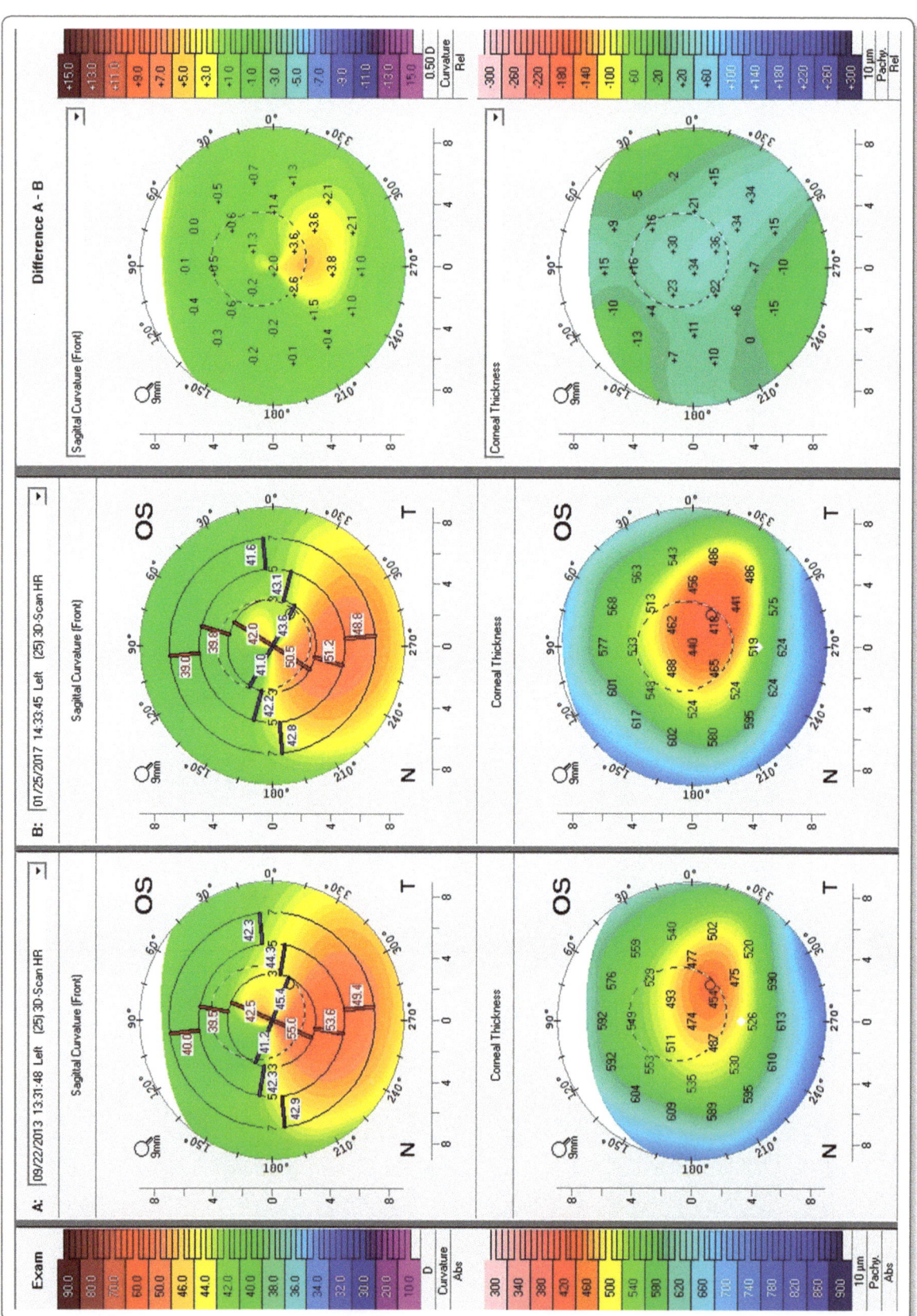

Fig. 21.4: Keratoconus progression. Difference map for the sagittal and the thickness maps between the first and the third visits.

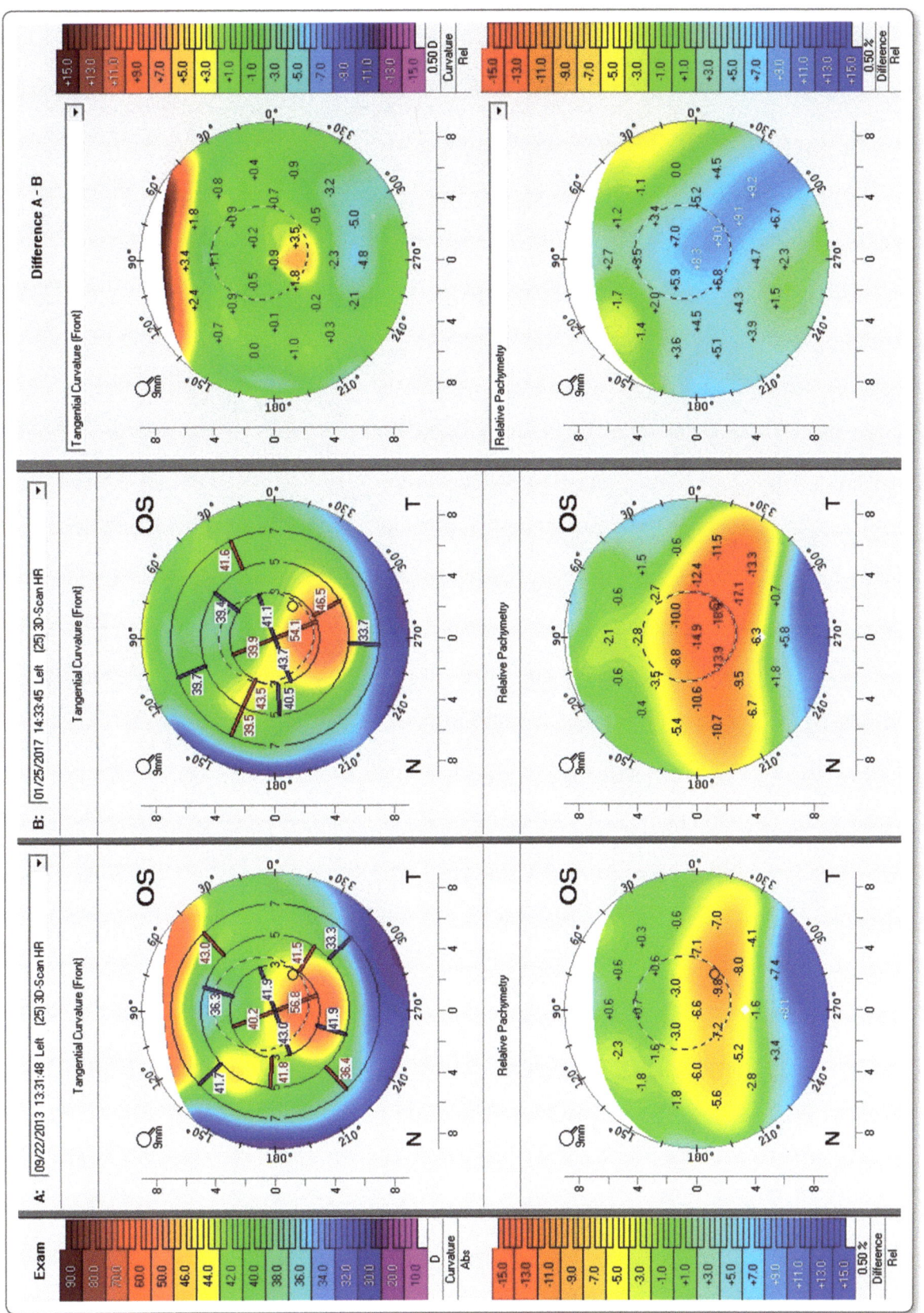

Fig. 21.5: Keratoconus progression. Difference map for the tangential and the relative pachymetry maps between the first and the third visits.

Section 6: Corneal Tomography in Ectatic Corneal Diseases

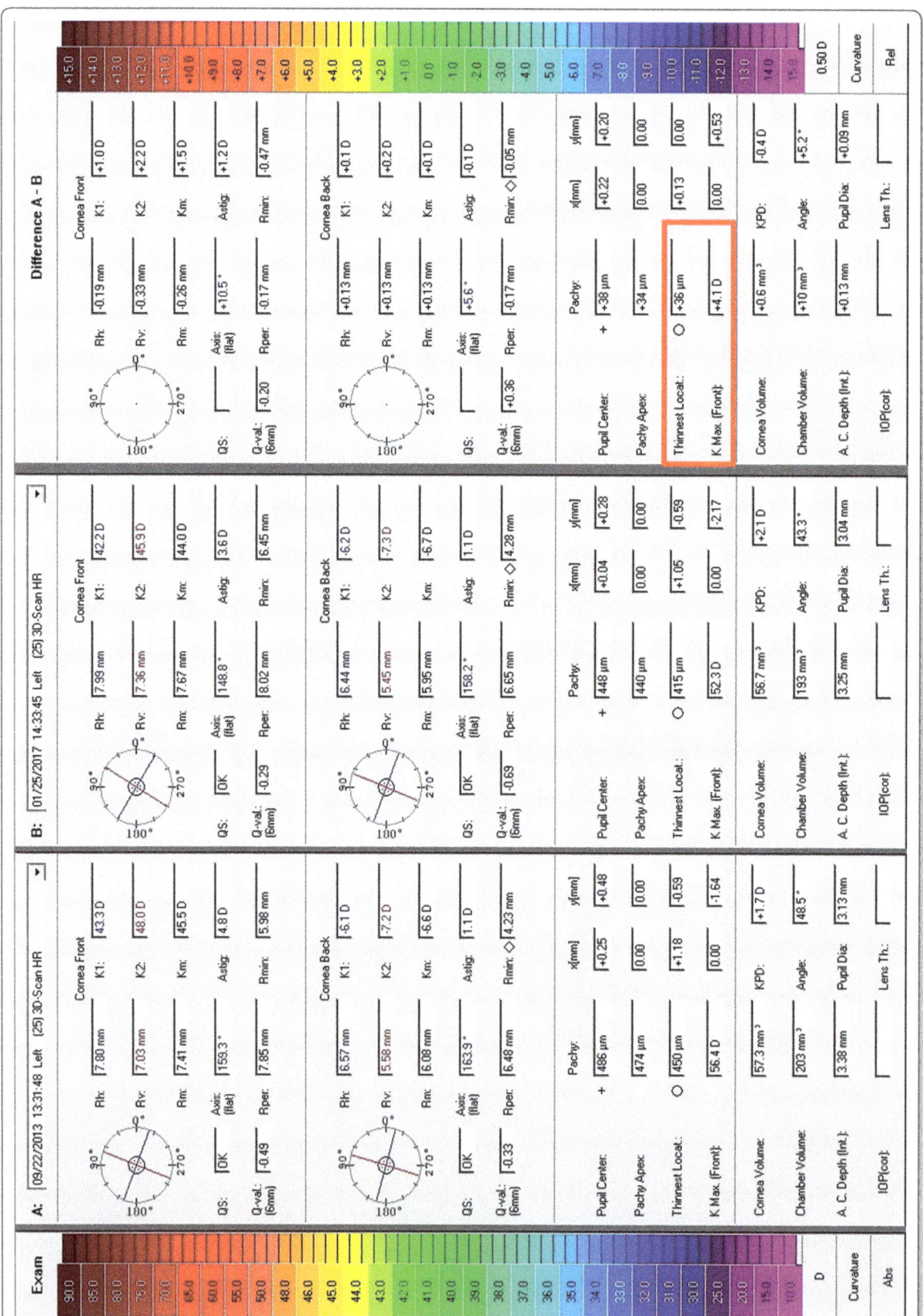

Fig. 21.6: Keratoconus progression. Difference map for the parameters between the first and the third visits.

Entities Misdiagnosed as Ectasia

INTRODUCTION

During daily clinical practice, some irregular corneas may be misdiagnosed as ectatic corneal diseases (ECDs), particularly ECDs per se and para ectasia. This leads to wrong decisions in both management and follow-up. This chapter aims at introducing entities that may be confused and mixed with ECDs. In this chapter, these entities will be classified and discussed in depth to establish a thorough and deep understanding of corneal irregularities.

SOURCE OF ENTITIES MISDIAGNOSED AS ECTASIA

Entities misdiagnosed as ectasia (EMEs) result from factors of false findings, especially corneal surgeries and opacities. Readers are advised to review Chapter 16.

PATTERNS OF ENTITIES MISDIAGNOSED AS ECTASIA

EMEs are classified into three tomographic patterns, namely are: (1) contour, (2) hot spot, and (3) discrete patterns.
The best maps to study the EMEs are:
- *The anterior tangential map*: It is the best curvature map to describe the geography of irregularities and to show the real efficient postoperative optical zone. It is less affected by misalignment, but it exaggerates K-readings.
- *The anterior and posterior elevation maps with best fit sphere (BFS), float, 8 mm reference surface (RS)*: The anterior elevation map is necessary to describe the distribution of the irregularities above and under the RS, while the posterior elevation map is important to rule out ectasia per se and to diagnose posterior keratoconus (KC).
- *The relative pachymetry map*: It shows the ablation zones (AZs), e.g. if the zone of high negative values is circular and central, the ablation was central (myopic treatment); and if it is an oval zone, a myopic-astigmatic correction was done.
- *The Belin Ambrósio Display (BAD)*: It differentiates para ectasia from EMEs, and differentiates ectasia per se from EMEs. In para ectasia, both maps in BAD are normal (green). In EMEs, the anterior BAD map is abnormal, while the posterior map is normal in the vast majority of cases. In ectasia per se, the posterior BAD map is abnormal, while the anterior map may or may not be abnormal.

The best color set is Belin intuitive for the anterior tangential, the American for both elevation maps, and Holladay primary for the relative pachymetry map.

Contour Pattern

The contour pattern usually takes the shape of a ring or a zone, describing the junction between two different corneal zones, the zone of treatment and the untreated corneal zone. These patterns are seen after laser vision correction (LVC), corneal grafts, and after intracorneal rings (ICRs) implantation. In such cases, the contour is seen on the anterior tangential and anterior elevation maps.

Post-Laser Vision Correction Patterns

- Post-myopic LVC pattern (Fig. 22.1). It is characterized by:
  - *Anterior tangential map (Fig. 22.2)*:

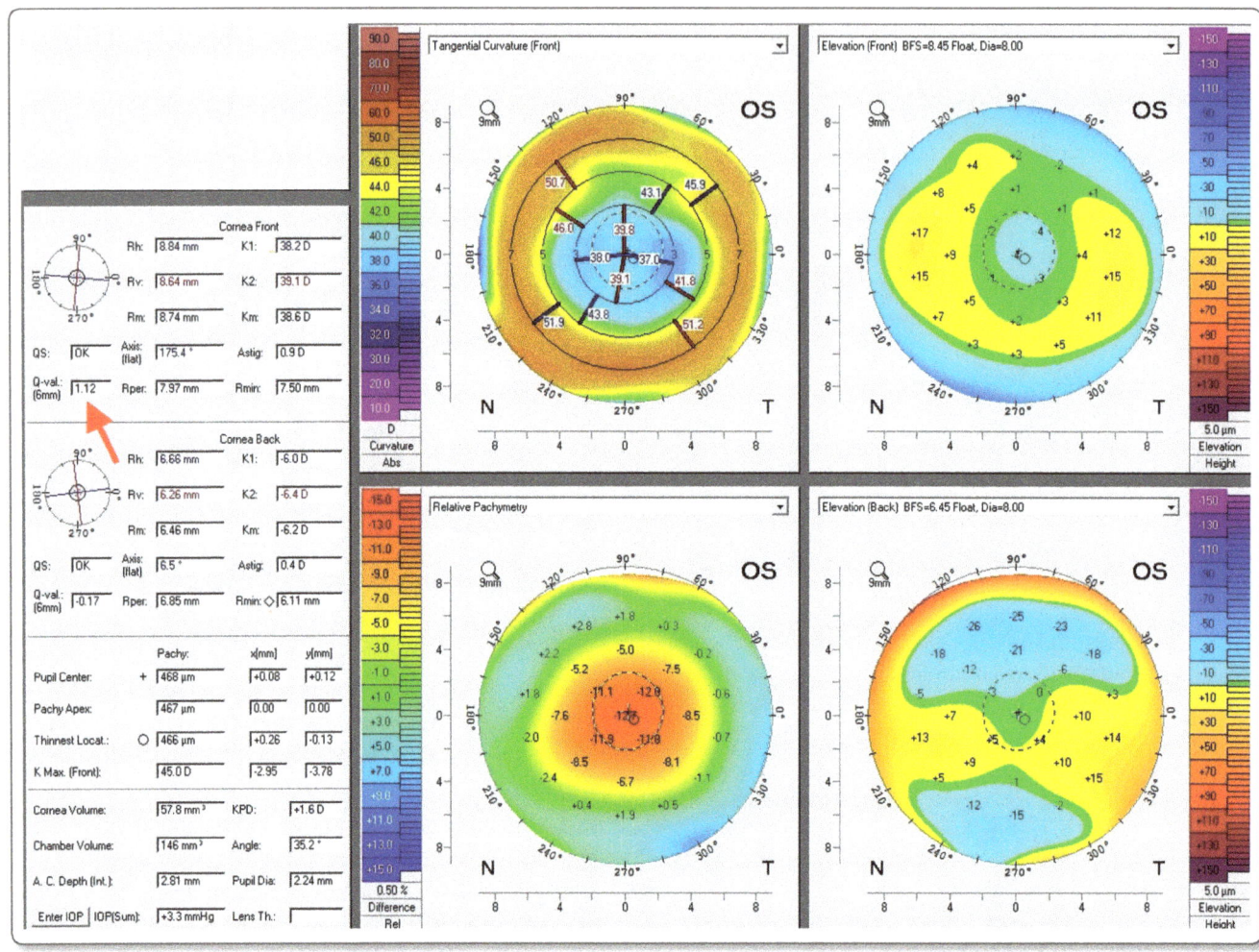

Fig. 22.1: Post-myopic ablation pattern. The four-composite selective map.

- ♦ A flat central zone (cold colors), reflecting an oblate postoperative efficient optical zone (EOZ).
- ♦ A peripheral ring of higher K-readings (hot colors), reflecting the transitional zone (TZ).
- *Anterior elevation map (Fig. 22.3)*:
  - ♦ A very small central island with negative values (cold colors), representing an oblate zone under the RS.
  - ♦ A small ring of neutral values (usually in green) surrounding the central zone, representing the intersection between the anterior corneal surface and the RS.
  - ♦ A peripheral ring with positive values, representing the periphery of the EOZ and the TZ. These positive values do not reflect any ectasia even with high values. That is because the radius of the RS is chosen by the software based on the mean central radii of the examined corneal surface, as mentioned in Chapter 6. This means that the radius of the RS in post-myopic treatment will be large (red arrow in Fig. 22.3) and the RS will be flat so that the periphery of the EOZ and the TZ will appear relatively elevated. This is known as "edge effect". The edge effect explains the tomographical presentation of many of the postsurgical irregularities and differentiates them from true ectasia.
- Posterior elevation map is normal (Fig. 22.1).
- *The relative pachymetry map (Fig. 22.4)*: The central area of the map shows negative values because the ablation was central. This is called "diskiform pattern". The borders of the negative-value zone delineate the area of ablation (black arrows).
- Positive Q-value at 6 mm zone, representing an oblate cornea (Fig. 22.1, red arrow).
- *Anterior corneal topometry at 6 mm*: It is also known as asphericity front at 6 mm (Fig. 22.5). It shows almost equal positive average values of the horizontal and the vertical meridians. This means that a spherical myopic

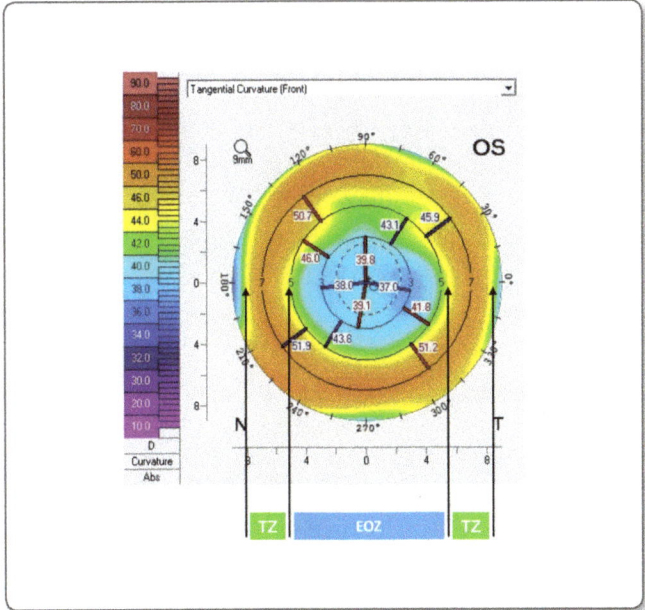

Fig. 22.2: Post-myopic ablation pattern. The anterior tangential map and optical zones. (TZ: transitional zone; EOZ: efficient optical zone)

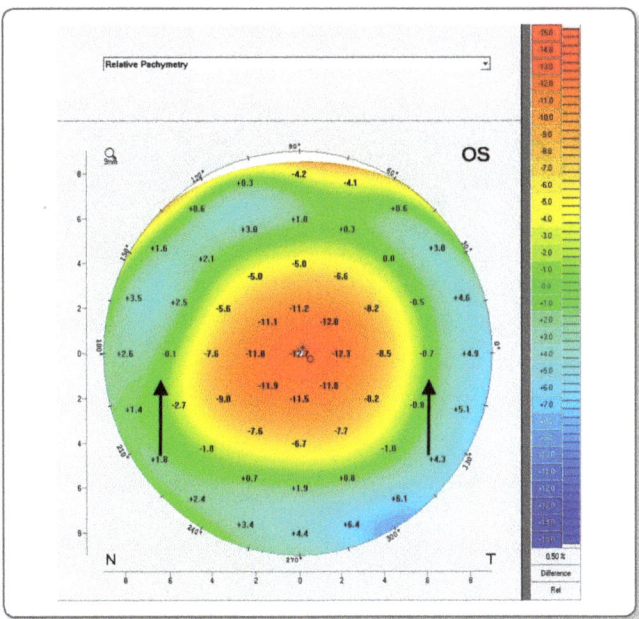

Fig. 22.4: Post-myopic ablation pattern. The relative pachymetry map: the diskiform pattern.

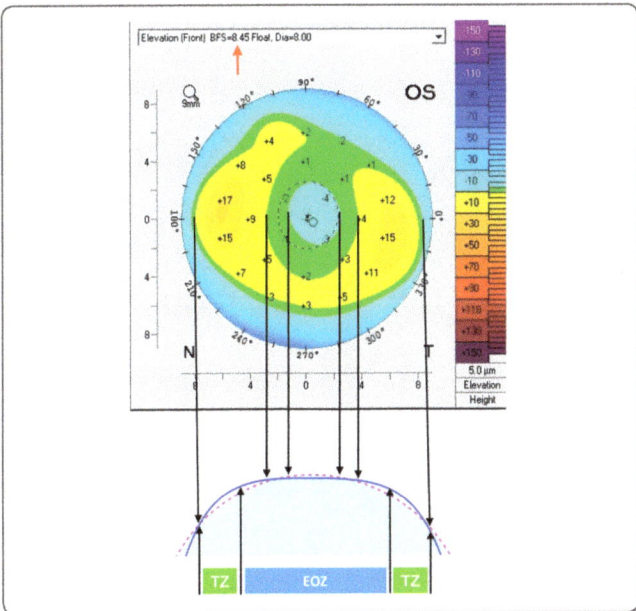

Fig. 22.3: Post-myopic ablation pattern. The anterior elevation map and optical zones. (TZ: transitional zone; EOZ: efficient optical zone)

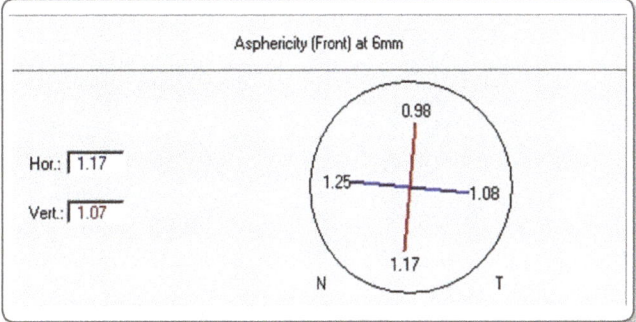

Fig. 22.5: Post-myopic ablation pattern. Anterior corneal topometry at 6 mm.

correction was performed with/without insignificant (<1.0 D) astigmatic correction.

- *Inverse anterior difference Belin Ambrósio Display map (Fig. 22.6):* The center of the anterior difference map is normal (green), surrounded by a yellow ring, followed by a red peripheral ring. This pattern is explained by the edge effect that was previously mentioned. The posterior difference map is usually normal (green) unless it was preoperatively abnormal.
- This pattern is usually confused with ectasia in case of upward decentered AZ. When such a complication occurs, an inferior peripheral hot spot or hot meniscus will be seen on the anterior curvature map, and an inferior "banana" shape of positive values will be encountered on the anterior elevation map. This decentered pattern is differentiated from ectasia by the following:
  ♦ The posterior elevation map is normal.
  ♦ The relative pachymetry map shows an upward displacement of the negative zone. In ectasia, the

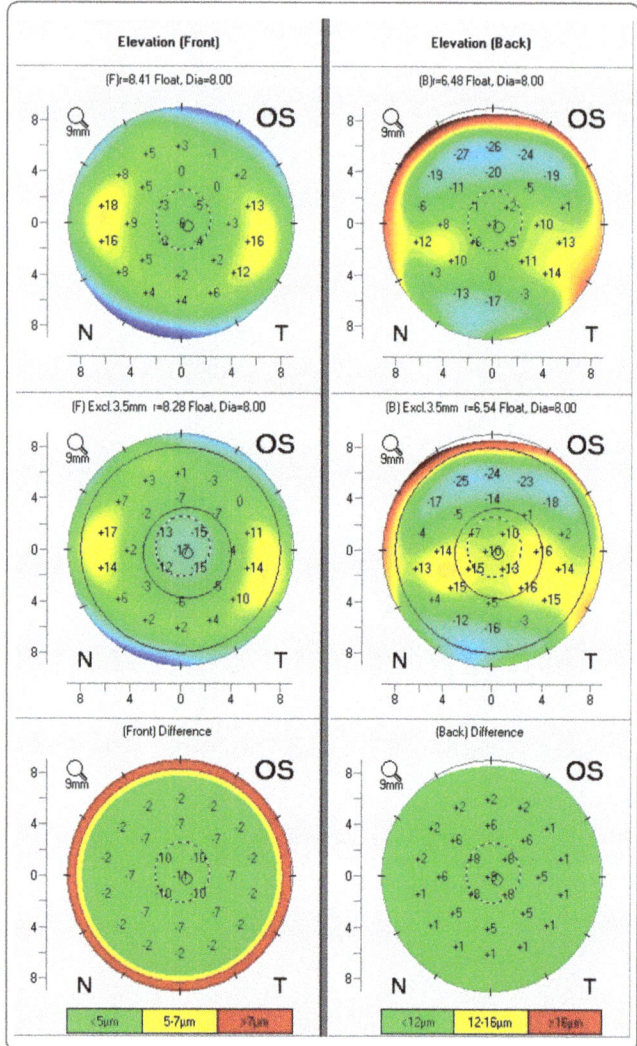

Fig. 22.6: Post-myopic ablation pattern. Belin Ambrósio Display.

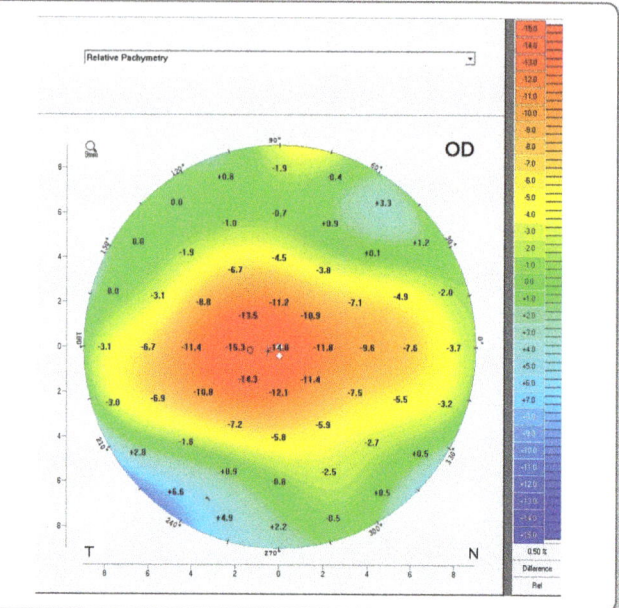

Fig. 22.7: Ectasia. Conic pattern on the relative pachymetry.

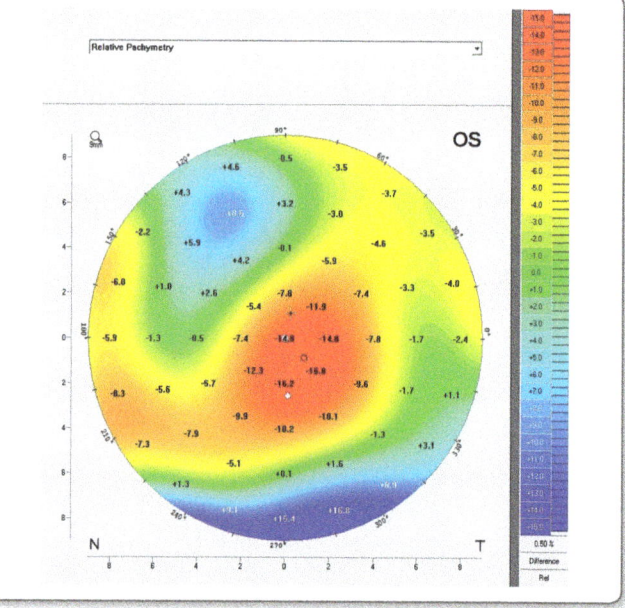

Fig. 22.8: Ectasia. Irregular pattern on the relative pachymetry.

pattern is conic, irregular, and usually inferiorly displaced (Figs. 22.7 and 22.8).
- ♦ The anterior difference BAD map shows the inverse pattern.
- ♦ The posterior difference BAD map is usually normal.
- Post-hypermetropic LVC pattern (Fig. 22.9). It is characterized by:
  - *Anterior curvature map (Fig. 22.10):*
    - ♦ A steep central zone (hot colors), reflecting a prolate or hyperprolate EOZ.
    - ♦ An annular ring at mid-periphery with lower K-readings (cold colors), reflecting the annular AZ or gutter.
    - ♦ Two narrow TZs between the central EOZ and the AZ, and between the AZ and corneal periphery.
  - *Anterior elevation map (Fig. 22.11):*
    - ♦ A small central island with positive values (hot colors), representing the prolate or hyperprolate zone over the RS.
    - ♦ An annular ring at mid-periphery with negative values (cold colors), reflecting the annular AZ.
    - ♦ A peripheral annular ring of positive values surrounding the AZ and representing an untreated corneal periphery (CP).

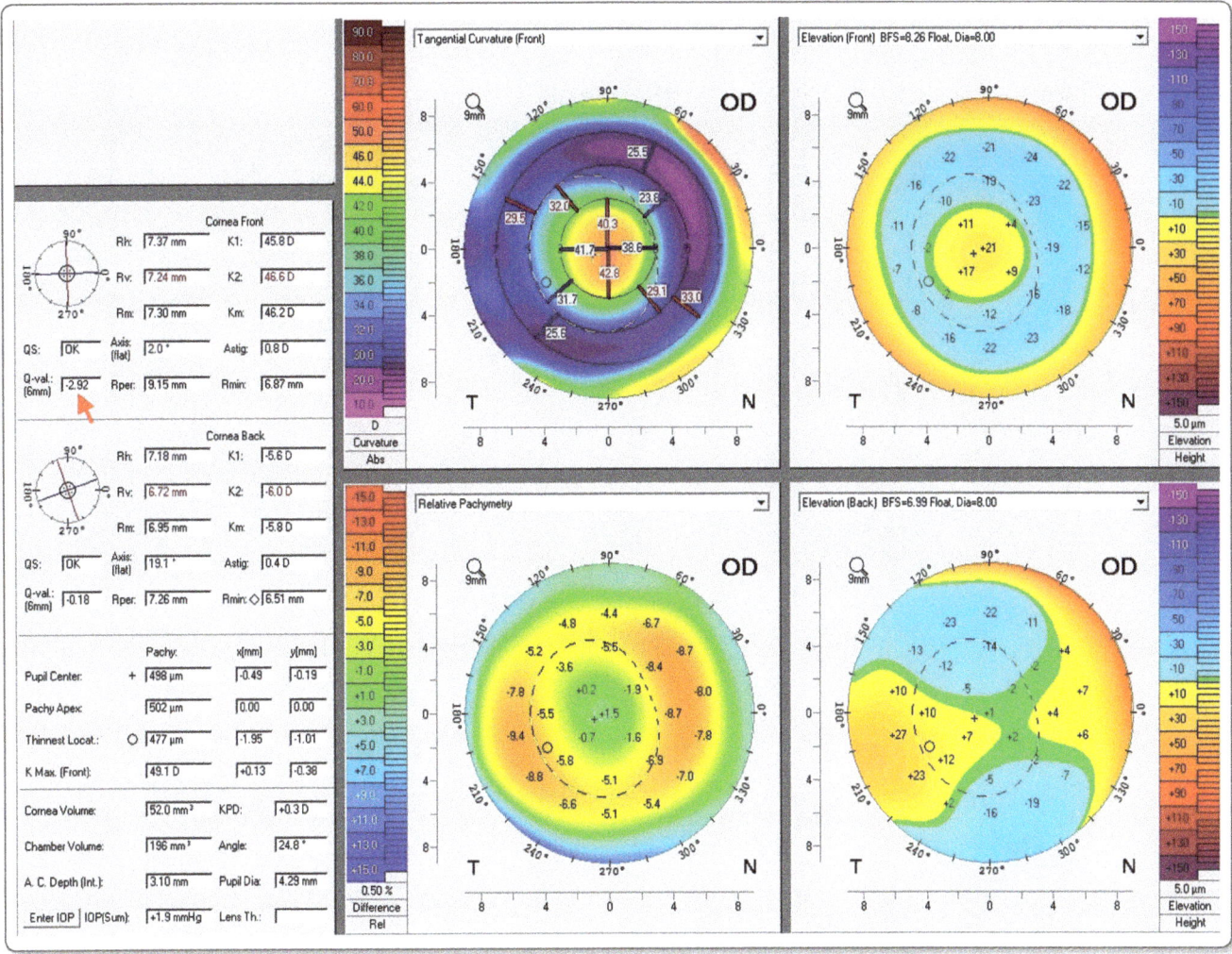

Fig. 22.9: Post-hypermetropic ablation pattern. The four-composite selective map.

- ◆ The central zone and the CP zone are elevated due to edge effect.
- The posterior elevation map is usually normal unless it was preoperatively abnormal (Fig. 22.9).
- *The relative pachymetry map (Fig. 22.12)*: This map is characterized by the "annular pattern". This pattern consists of a central area with normal values, surrounded by a mid-peripheral annular zone with abnormal negative values. This annular zone corresponds to AZ and is surrounded by a peripheral normal zone, representing the untreated CP.
- Negative Q-value at 6 mm zone, representing a prolate or hyperprolate cornea (red arrow in Fig. 22.9).
- Anterior corneal topometry at 6 mm (Fig. 22.13) shows almost equal negative average values of the horizontal and the vertical meridians indicating a pure hypermetropic correction or with insignificant (<1.0 D) astigmatic correction.
- Depending on the amount of hypermetropic correction, the BAD may show a normal anterior difference map in small corrections as in Figure 22.14, or an abnormal anterior difference map in high corrections as in Figure 22.15, but in both cases, the posterior difference map is usually normal unless it was preoperatively abnormal.
- This pattern is frequently confused with ectasia because of the central hot spot on the anterior curvature map, the elevated central island on the anterior elevation map, and the negative abnormal Q-value. The clue of difference is the normal posterior difference BAD map, but the hallmark clue is the annular pattern on the relative pachymetry map.

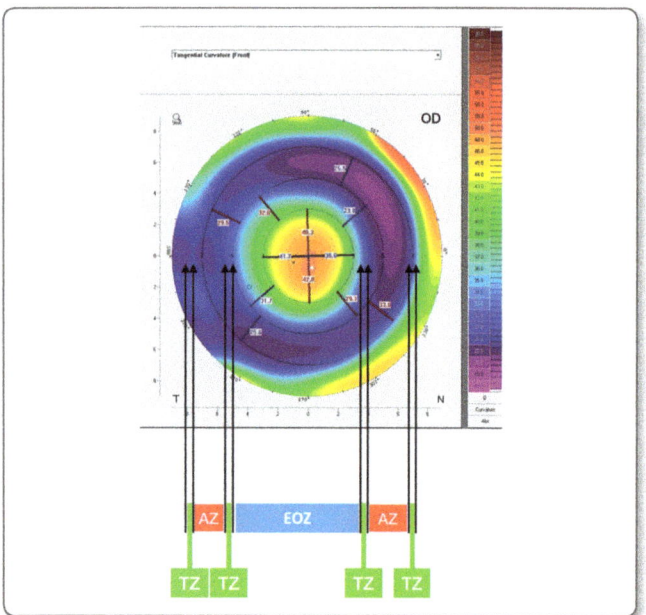

Fig. 22.10: Post-hypermetropic ablation pattern. The anterior tangential map and optical zones. (AZ: ablation zone; EOZ: efficient optical zone; TZ: transitional zone)

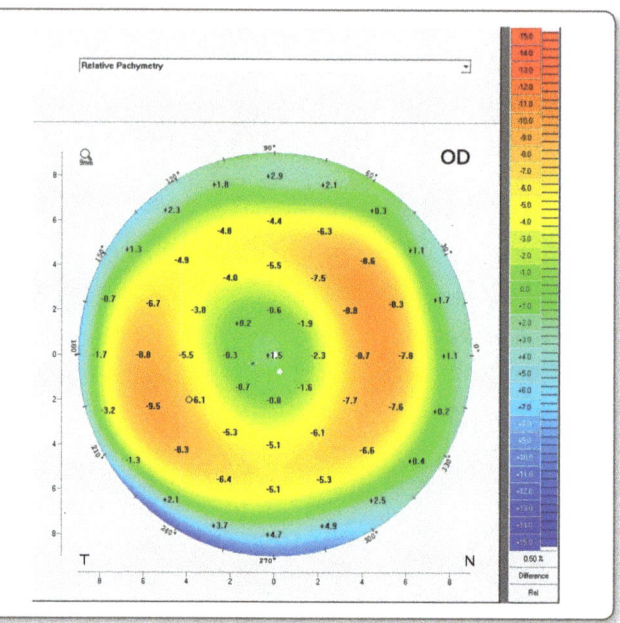

Fig. 22.12: Post-hypermetropic ablation pattern. The relative pachymetry map: the annular pattern.

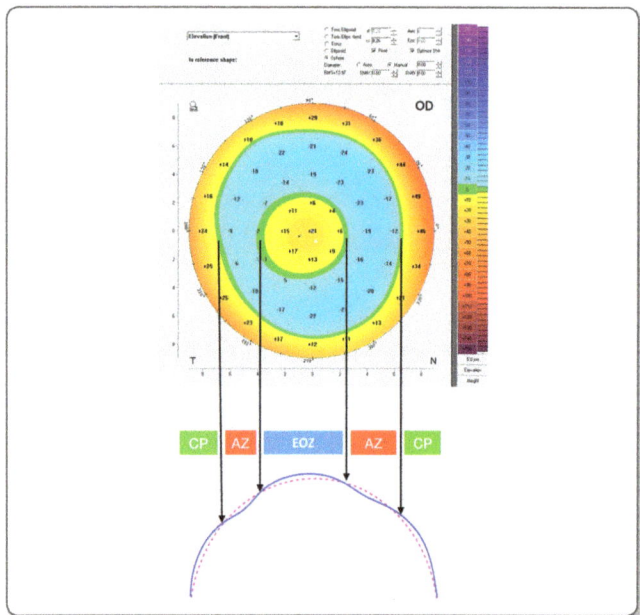

Fig. 22.11: Post-hypermetropic ablation pattern. The anterior elevation map and optical zones. (CP: corneal periphery; AZ: ablation zone; EOZ: efficient optical zone)

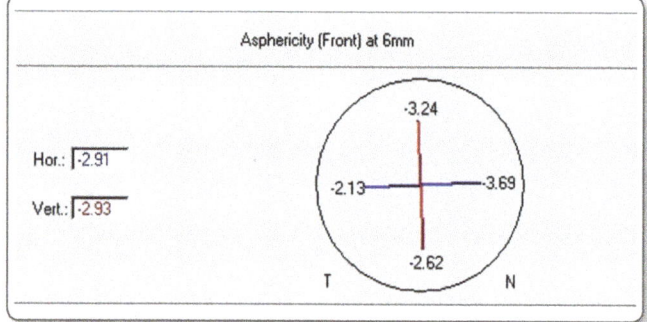

Fig. 22.13: post-hypermetropic ablation pattern. Anterior corneal topometry at 6 mm.

  ♦ *A peripheral surrounding zone with K-readings:*
    ◊ Higher than K-readings of the central zone in post-myopic LVC.
    ◊ Lower than K-readings of the central zone in post-hypermetropic LVC as in Figure 22.16.
  – *Anterior elevation map (Fig. 22.18):*
    ♦ Central island or tongue-like extension with negative values (oblate) in post-myopic-astigmatic correction.
    ♦ Central island or tongue-like extension with positive values (prolate and hyperprolate) in post-hypermetropic-astigmatic correction as in Figure 22.16.
  – The posterior elevation map is usually normal unless it was preoperatively abnormal (Fig. 22.16).

• Post-astigmatic LVC pattern (Fig. 22.16). It is characterized by:
  – *Anterior curvature map (Fig. 22.17):*
    ♦ An elongated central zone, either flat, reflecting a post-myopic-astigmatic ablation, or steep, reflecting a post-hypermetropic-astigmatic ablation.

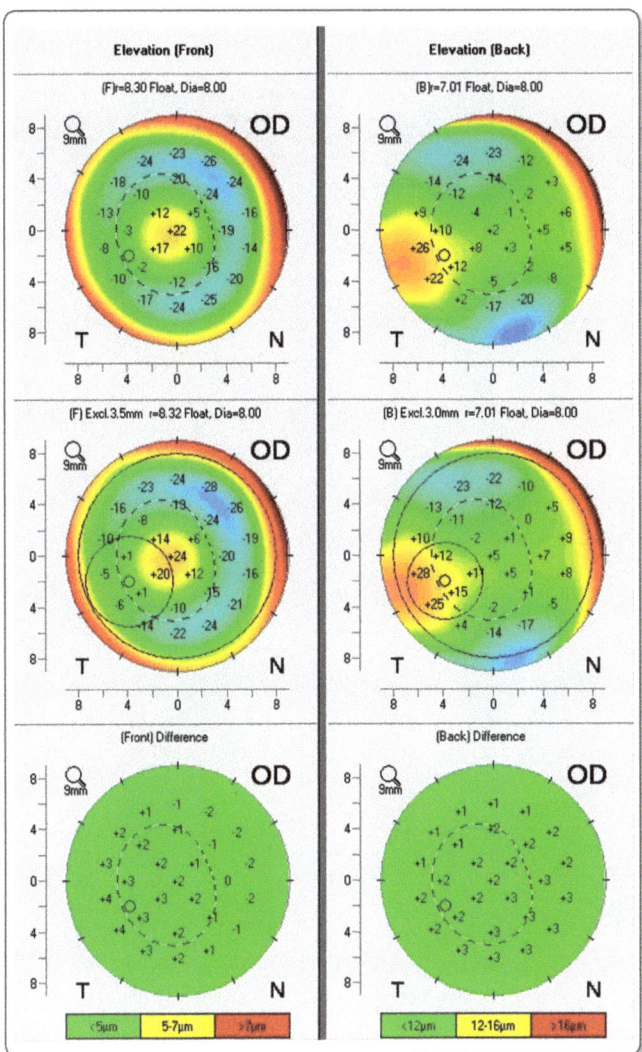

Fig. 22.14: Post-hypermetropic ablation pattern. Belin Ambrósio Display: normal anterior difference map.

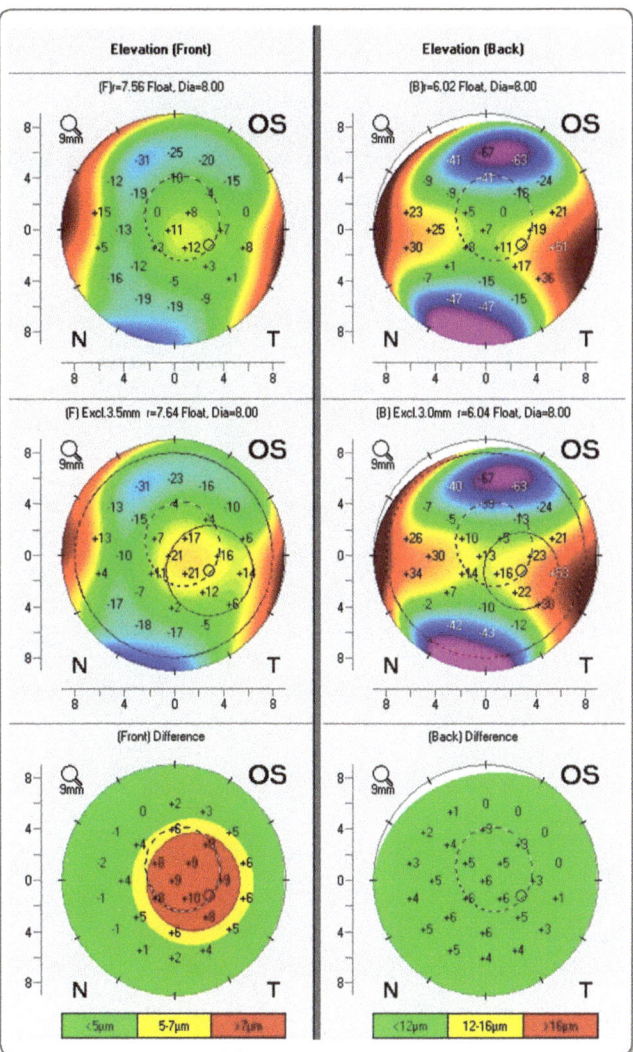

Fig. 22.15: Post-hypermetropic ablation pattern. Belin Ambrósio Display: abnormal anterior difference map.

- *The relative pachymetry map (Fig. 22.19)*: In post-myopic-astigmatic ablation, the map will show an elongated pattern. In post-hypermetropic-astigmatic ablation, the map will show the dual-spot pattern as in Figure 22.19. The black arrows point at the two location of the ablation profile. The case was with-the-rule hypermetropic astigmatism and the ablation was on the horizontal meridian at mid-periphery to steepen it. Since these two locations were ablated, they have negative values. In the post-myopic-astigmatic correction, the central area of the steep meridian will be ablated; therefore, the pattern will be a central oval zone with negative values.
- *Q-value at 6 mm zone is not beneficial in this case while topometry is characteristic*:

- When vertical Q is flatter (more positive) than horizontal Q, it is post-hypermetropic astigmatism treatment on the vertical meridian, or post-myopic astigmatism treatment on the horizontal meridian as in Figure 22.20.
- When vertical Q is steeper (more negative) than horizontal Q, it is post-hypermetropic astigmatism treatment on the vertical meridian or post-myopic astigmatism treatment on the horizontal meridian.
- In oblique astigmatism, treatment is on an oblique meridian, but topometry does not show Q-value on oblique meridians; it shows Q-value on the vertical and horizontal projections of the oblique meridians.

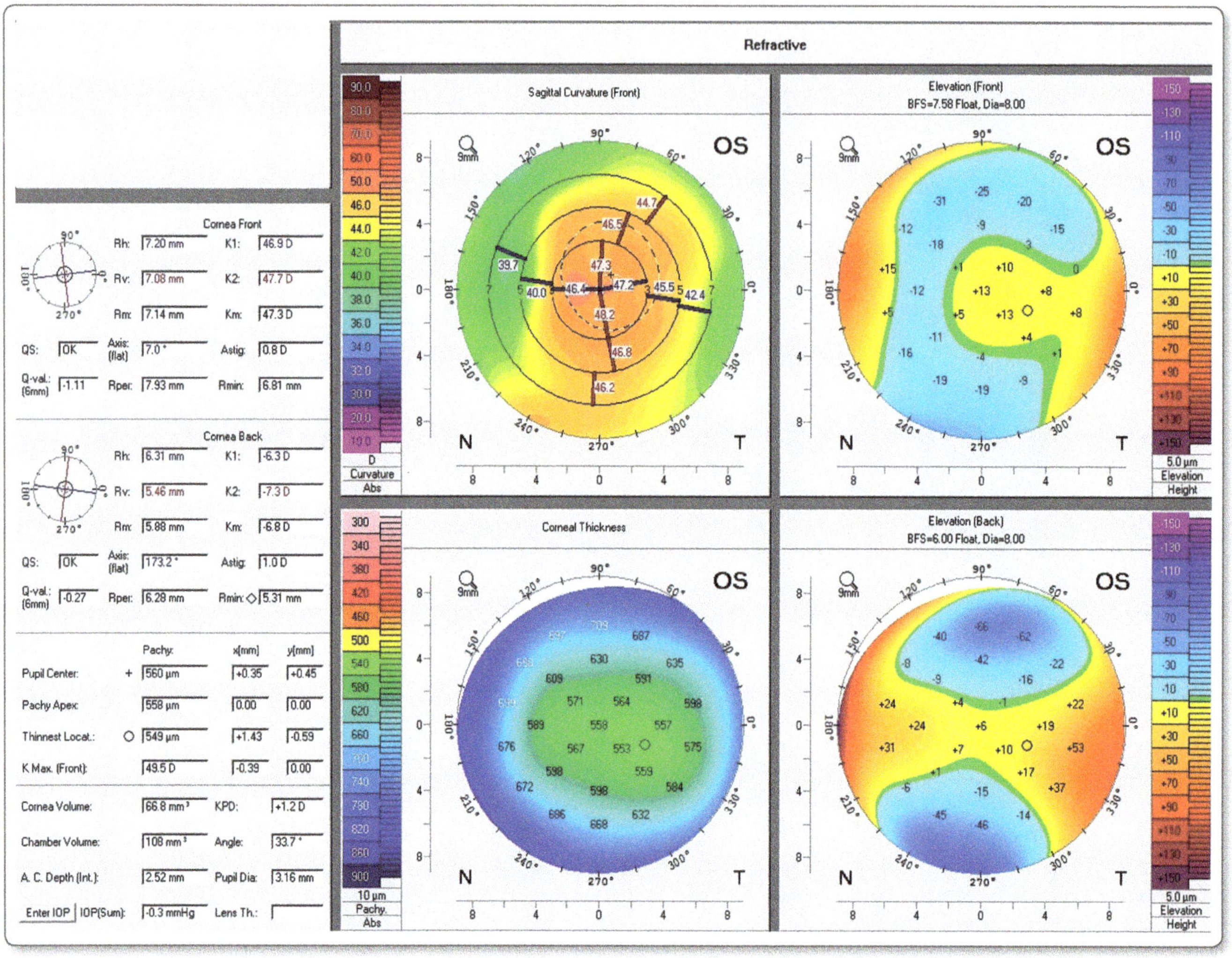

Fig. 22.16: Post-astigmatic ablation pattern. The four-composite selective map.

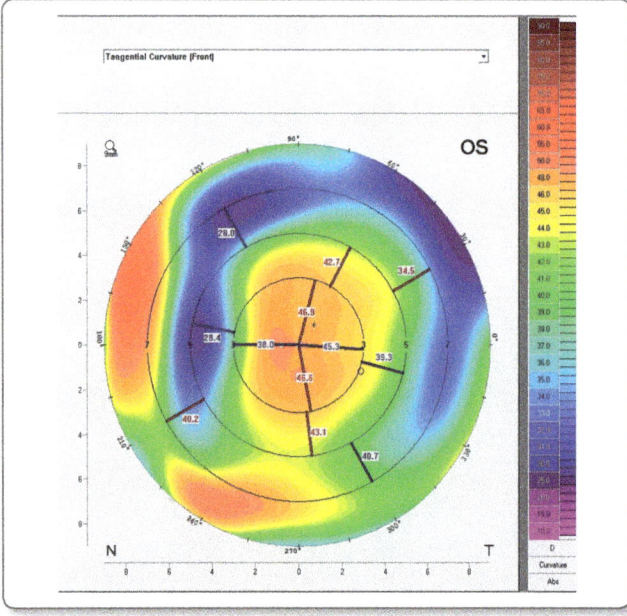

Fig. 22.17: Post-astigmatic ablation pattern. The anterior tangential map; the elongated pattern.

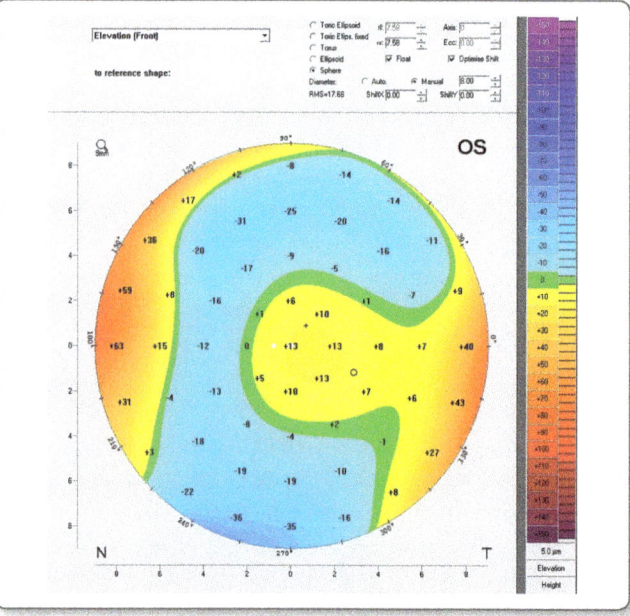

Fig. 22.18: Post-astigmatic ablation pattern. The anterior elevation map.

on the tomography as a ring (although not homogenous and not consistent) in the zone of 6–8 mm depending on the size of the donor graft (Fig. 22.21). In general, the junctional ring shows higher K-readings in the locations of looser sutures and lower K-reading in the locations of tighter sutures.

This pattern is usually associated with other patterns such as the hot spot pattern and/or the discrete pattern in addition to different types of bowtie. Therefore, it is frequently confused with ectasia, especially when only an inferior meniscus is present rather than the whole ring (Fig. 22.22). This usually occurs due to the following reasons:
- Irregular, overlapping and bad suturing technique.
- Inferior dehiscence with bulging out at the junction after early removal of inferior sutures.
- Ignored inferior loose sutures.

In all cases of post-graft, there are no definite patterns on the elevation maps. In addition, the relative pachymetry map may show different patterns based on the thickness of the donor graft. However, apart form slit-lamp examination and history taking, a multiple patterns of irregularity with a ring shape or partial ring shape is the clue of this pattern.

Patterns of Post-Corneal-Rings Implantation

Intracorneal rings implantation is one of the treatment options in ECDs management. Therefore, the pattern after ICR implantation is a combination of ECDs tomographic patterns, such as AB/IS or AB/SRAX, with an arcuate segmental shape pattern (Fig. 22.23). The latter is caused by the hump over the segment, leading to a steep arcuate pattern on the anterior curvature map. In case of a complete ring implantation, such as MyoRing, a circular, rather than segmental, steep shape will be encountered.

Because ICRs are usually inserted in already ectatic corneas, it is nonsense to differentiate the pattern from ectasia. However, the arcuate shape is a clue of an ICR inside the cornea. Moreover, the arcuate shape post-ICR is more regular than that in post-graft pattern.

Hot Spot Pattern

The hot spot is defined as a small (≤3 mm in diameter), circular, or oval area of relatively higher K-readings (≥1.50 D difference) than the K-readings in the surrounding area (Fig. 22.24). It can be located in any sector of the cornea, but is usually encountered in the inferior sector of it.

This pattern results from contact lenses, tear film disturbance, misalignment, *focal* corneal opacities and pathologies, and bad exposure to the camera. These sources are discussed in Chapter 16. The hot spot pattern can also be seen after LVC due to flap complications, such as flap

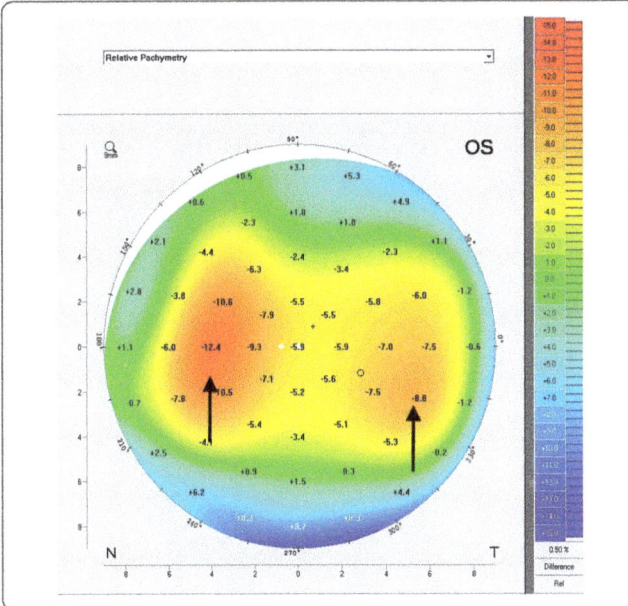

Fig. 22.19: Post-astigmatic ablation pattern. The relative pachymetry map: the dual-spot pattern.

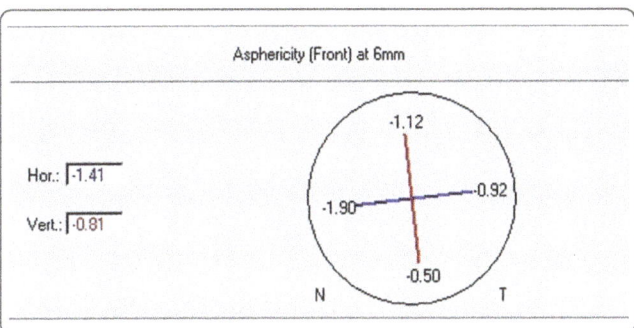

Fig. 22.20: Post-astigmatic ablation pattern. Anterior corneal topometry at 6 mm.

- *The Belin Ambrósio Display* shows the post-myopic pattern after myopic-astigmatic correction (similar to Fig. 22.6), or the post-hypermetropic pattern after hypermetropic-astigmatic correction (similar to Fig. 22.15).
- Post-astigmatic correction may be confused with ectasia in decentered AZs in the same principle that was mentioned earlier with post-myopic and post-hypermetropic corrections.

Post-graft Pattern

The junction between the donor graft and the surrounding recipient cornea is usually abrupt (does not follow the normal corneal slope) and has a high density (due to different degrees of scarring). This junctional ring is shown

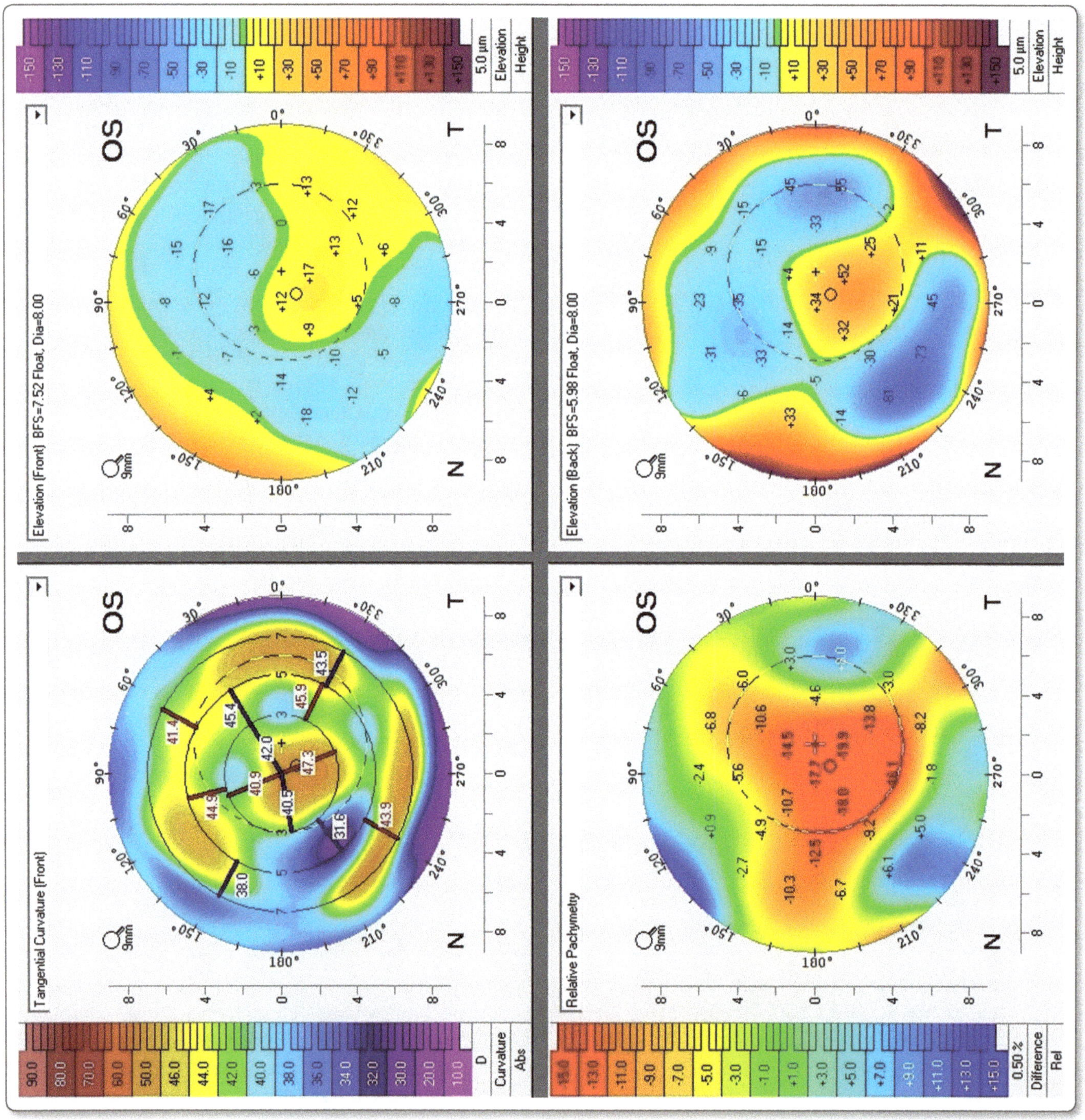

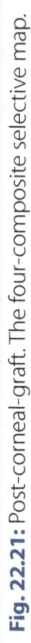

Fig. 22.21: Post-corneal-graft. The four-composite selective map.

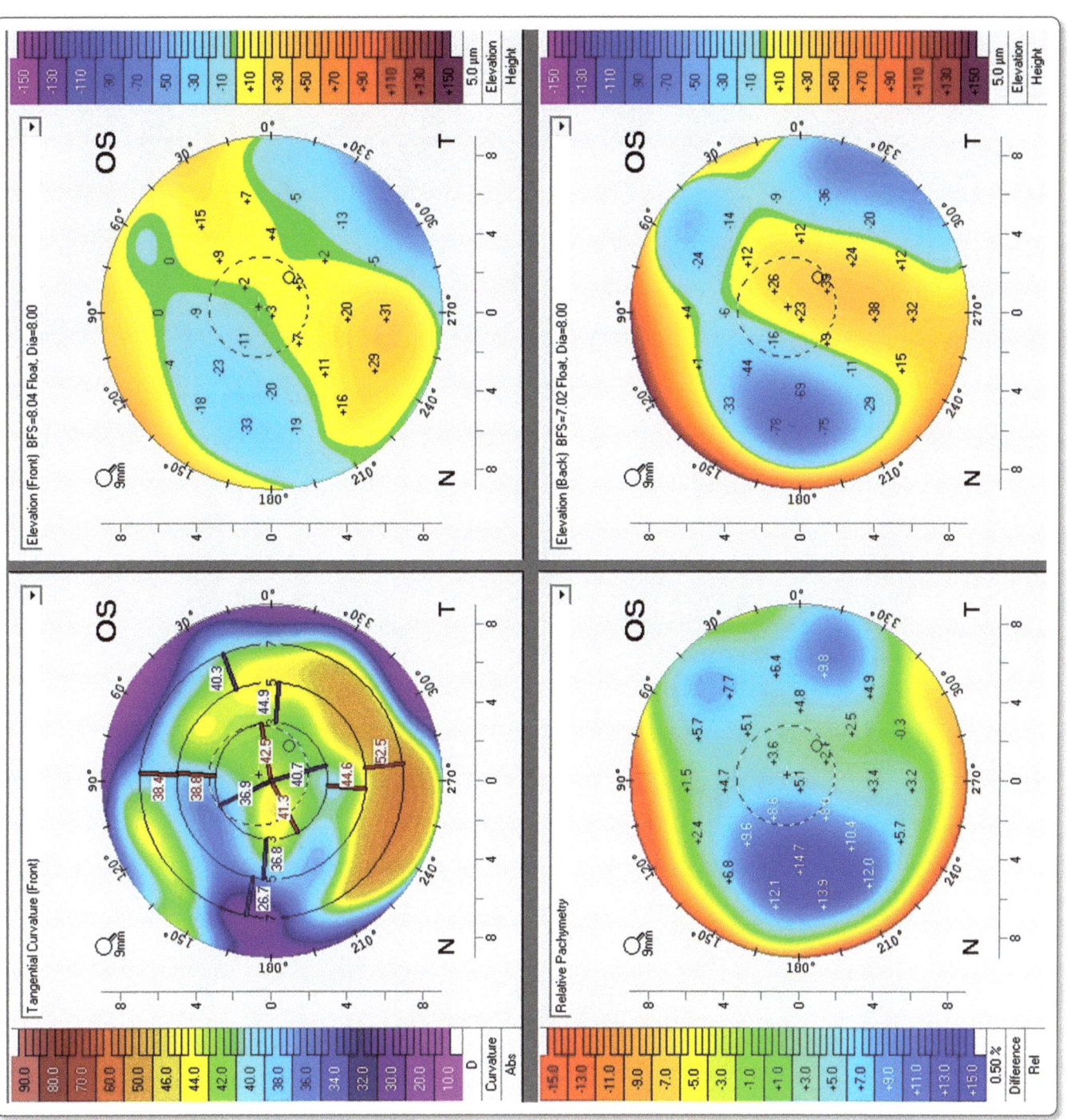

Fig. 22.22: Post-corneal-graft. The four-composite selective map: inferior meniscus pattern.

Section 6: *Corneal Tomography in Ectatic Corneal Diseases*

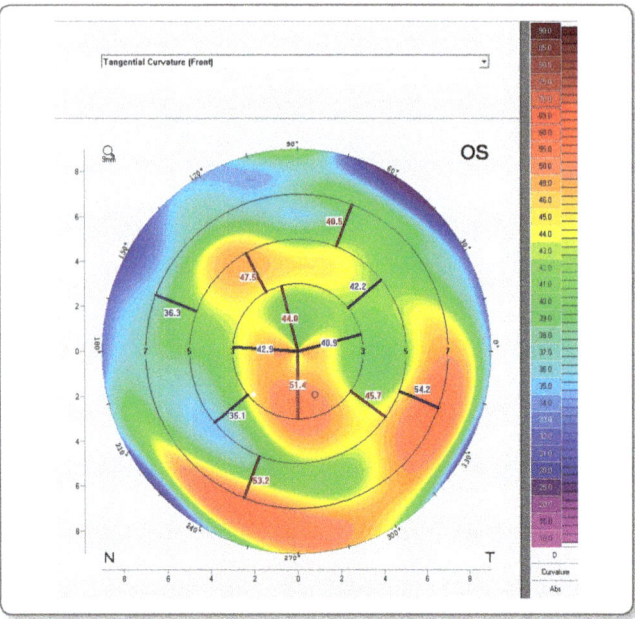

Fig. 22.23: Post-ICR implantation pattern. The anterior tangential map: arcuate segmental shape over the inferior ICR segment.

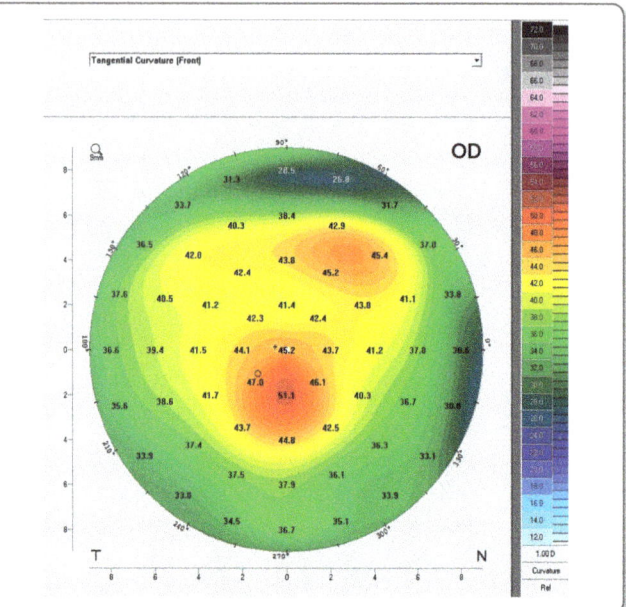

Fig. 22.24: Hot spot pattern.

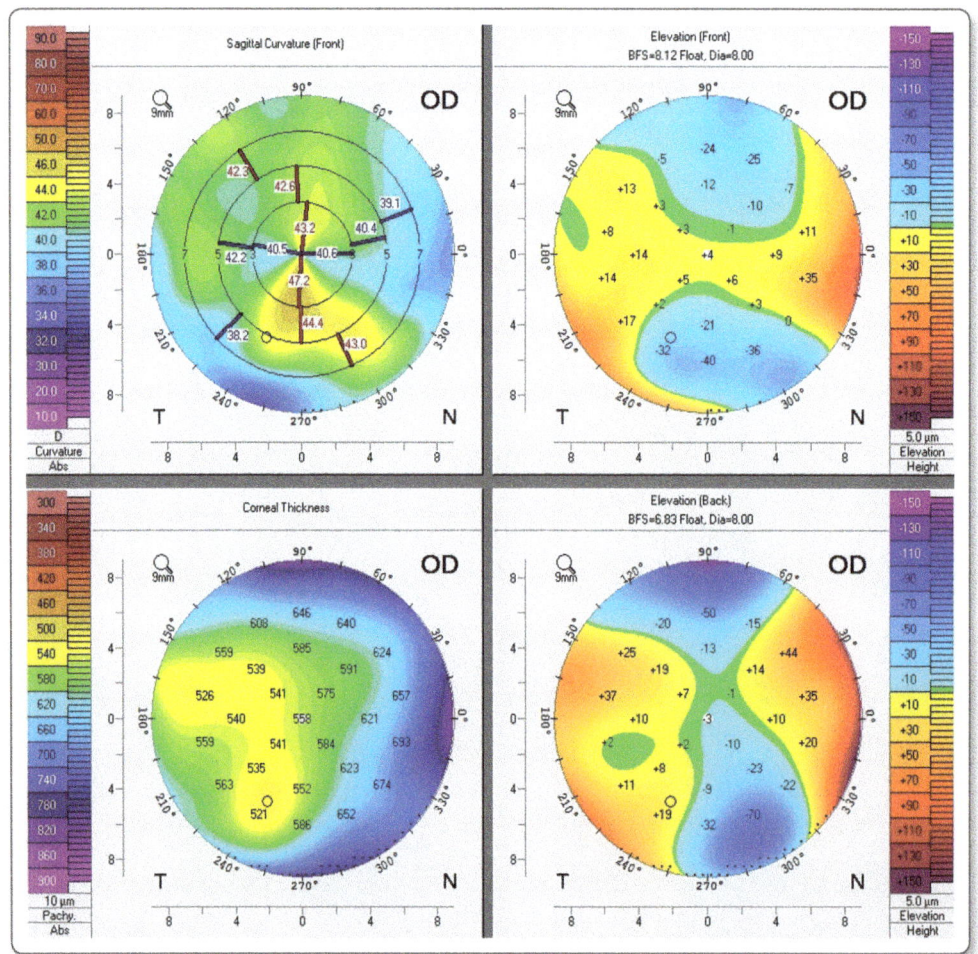

Fig. 22.25: The discrete pattern.

distortion and macrostriae, and interface complications, such as epithelial ingrowth. In addition, it can be seen mixed with other patterns after corneal grafts and post-ICR implantation.

When the hot spot is not associated with posterior elevation abnormality, it is confused with para ectasia. History taking, slit lamp biomicroscopy, and clues of false findings can reveal the cause.

Discrete Pattern

It results from tear film disturbance, *multifocal* corneal opacities and pathologies, corneal grafts, and bad exposure to the camera. Figure 22.25 is an example of this pattern.

This pattern may be confused with ECDs, especially when the elevation maps are abnormal. History taking, slit lamp biomicroscopy, and clues of false findings can reveal the cause.

SECTION 7

Miscellaneous

SECTION OUTLINE

23. Holladay Report
24. Corneal Tomography and Corneal Aberrometry in Cataract Surgery

Holladay Report

INTRODUCTION

The Holladay report is a screening display that was developed by Jack T Holladay and Oculus for diagnosis and treatment purposes.
- It is a general screening display before refractive surgery and cataract surgery.
- It is recommended to diagnose forme fruste keratoconus (FFKC) in terms of Holladay's specific definition of this disease.
- It is used for intraocular lens (IOL) calculations especially in irregular corneas and operated corneas.
- It helps understanding the distribution of corneal power related to corneal zones.

This report is composed of two pages. The first page consists of six maps and some numeric values. It is titled "Holladay Report". The second page consists of a detailed report of corneal power shown as graphs, a table, and numeric values. It is titled "Holladay Detailed Equivalent K-Reading (EKR) Report".

HOLLADAY REPORT

Page 1 of Holladay report consists of numeric values and maps (Fig. 23.1).

Numeric Values

At the top of the page, there are three boxes:
1. *The upper left box*: Patients demographics.
2. *The center upper box*:
    i. EKR65 flat K1, EKR65 steep K2, EKR65 mean, and Astig EKR65. These are the K-readings calculated by the EKR65 method. By default, they are calculated in the 4.5 mm zone around pupil center. The EKR method measures the true K-readings of the cornea taking into consideration the existent back/front ratio in radii of curvature. In other words, it predicts what the K-readings would have been before refractive surgery. It therefore, corrects the error that results from the abnormal back/front ratio, it considers both corneal surfaces and takes into consideration the effect of posterior surface astigmatism, and uses the true refractive index of the cornea (1.376). Holladay found that considering 65% of the EKR (EKR65) in the 4.5 mm zone represents the actual corneal power that the patient uses for distance vision, and it is identical to sagittal keratometric K-readings (Sim-Ks) that are used in IOL calculation formulas. Therefore, the EKR65 can be used for IOL calculation in virgin corneas, and it is more accurate than other methods in measuring the K-readings in post-keratorefractive surgeries, post-keratoplasty, ectatic corneal diseases (ECDs), corneal scars, and any irregular astigmatism. In such cases, the EKR65 together with Astig EKR65 (amount of corneal astigmatism calculated by EKR65 method) are used in the Holladay IOL consultant software, which is useful in toric IOL calculations as well.
    ii. *Q (6 mm)*: Corneal asphericity over a 6-mm zone expressed as Q-value. No spherical aberration (SAs) when Q = –0.53. The average Q in normal population is –0.27.
    iii. *Total SA: Z (4 + 6 + 8, 0)*: Total corneal SA in the 4th, 6th, and 8th Zernike orders in 6-mm zone. The normal average total SA is 0.27 µm. This value is important in choosing the asphericity of the IOL in cataract surgery. A slight negative postoperative Q-value is helpful to increase the depth of field and enhance near vision.

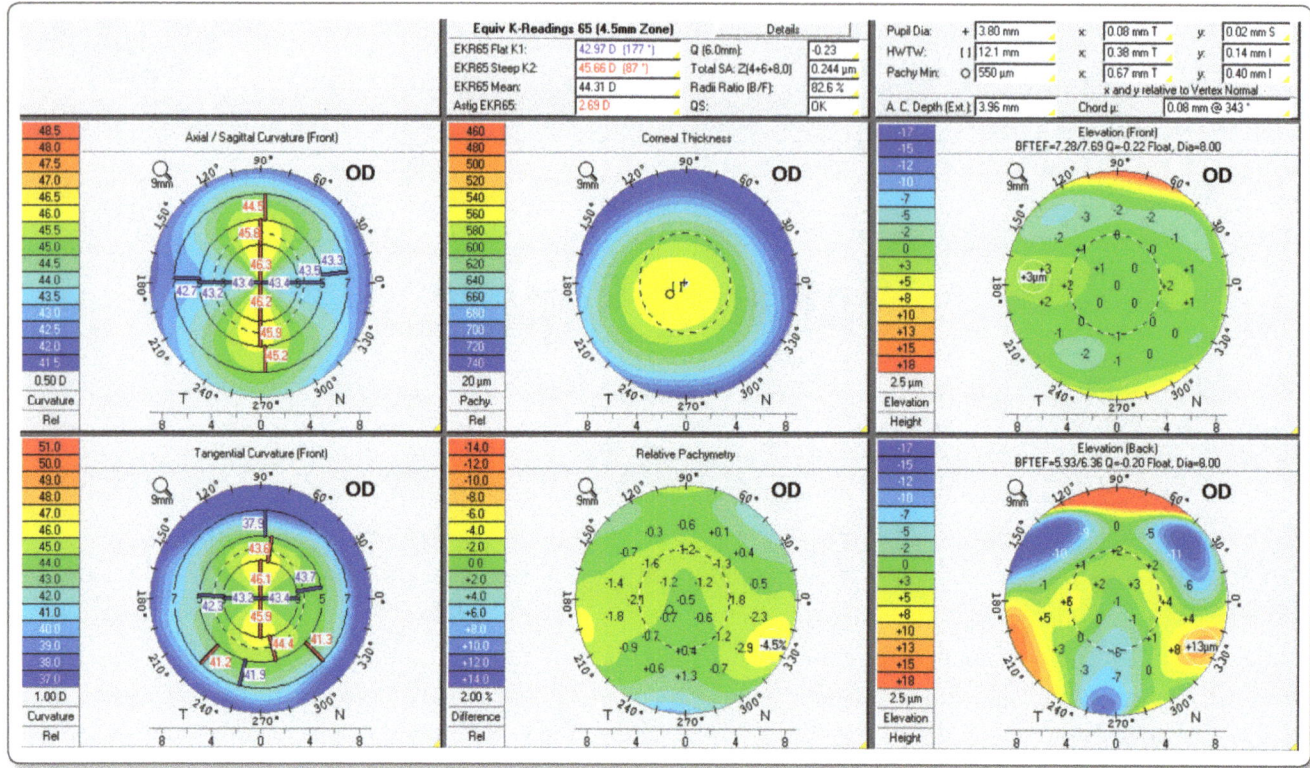

Fig. 23.1: Holladay report. Normal high astigmatic cornea. Page 1.

iv. *Radii ratio (B/F)*: The ratio of back to front radii of curvature. The normal average ratio is 82.2% ± 2.1%. The ratio gets lower after myopic ablation in a proportional relationship.

v. *Qs*: Quality specification.

3. *Upper right box*:
   i. *Pupil diameter*: The mean entrance pupil diameter during the measurements, with X and Y coordinates relative to corneal apex (vertex normal). Pupil diameter depends on the intensity of room illumination when the capture is taken. Even in low intensity light, pupil diameter is smaller than the scotopic diameter when measured by an infrared pupillometry in full darkness. Pupil diameter is important in determining which zone is most suitable for the EKR65 to be used. For example, if the diameter is 3 mm, K-readings of the 3 mm EKR65 are more suitable than the standard 4.5 mm EKR65 for IOL calculations. In general, when the diameter is ≥ 4.5 mm, the 4.5 mm is recommended, when it is ≤ 3 mm, the 3 mm is recommended, and when it is 4 mm, the 4 mm is recommended.
   ii. *HWTW*: Horizontal white-to-white diameter (HWTW). The normal average is 11.77 ± 0.22 mm.
   iii. *The two X and Y boxes next to HWTW*: They are corneal center position coordinates relative to corneal apex (vertex normal). The orientation of decentration relative to vertex normal is indicated by the appendixes T (temporal), N (nasal), I (inferior), or S (superior).
   iv. *Pachy min*: Thinnest corneal thickness with its X and Y coordinates relative to corneal apex (vertex normal). The normal average is 536 μm.
   v. *Anterior chamber (AC) depth (external)*: In Holladay report, AC depth including rather than excluding central corneal thickness is considered.
   vi. *Chord μ*: This is the chord length of angle kappa in polar coordinates relative to the pupil center (average is 0.20 ± 0.11 mm). High toric IOLs, and diffractive and refractive multifocal IOLs perform best when located at the pupillary center and visual axis. If the chord length is more than 0.5 mm, there will be low performance in these premium lenses.
   vii. Position of corneal apex (vertex normal) relative to pupil center in polar coordinates.

Maps

They are six maps as shown in Figure 23.1. They are: (1) the axial (sagittal) curvature front map, (2) the tangential curvature front map, (3) corneal thickness map, (4) relative pachymetry map, and (5 and 6) elevation front and back maps in best fit *toric* ellipsoid (BFTE) float mode and 8 mm diameter.

1. *The anterior sagittal map*: In Holladay report, this map is used to study the pattern (refer to Chapter 5) and the central keratometric reading (front). The latter is suspicious or abnormal if it is more than 48 D or more than 50 D, respectively. The steep (red) and flat (blue) semi-meridians are shown in the 3 mm, the 3-5 mm, and 5-7 mm diameter zones. If these semi-meridians do not form single meridians (one line) and are not orthogonal, irregular astigmatism is present and the axis and magnitude are less accurate.
2. *The anterior tangential map*: In Holladay report, this map is used to highlight irregularities and to study the maximum tangential K (Kmax tangential). Kmax is abnormal if more than 51 D.
3. *Corneal thickness map*: This map is important to study the patterns. Apart from the dashed black circle representing the border of the pupil, there are five landmarks on this map:
   i. The brackets indicate center of limbus, which is considered the *optical center* of the cornea. The center of limbus is always temporal and inferior to vertex normal (average is 0.38 ± 0.22 mm temporal and 0.01 ± 0.14 mm inferior). The IOL will normally center in the bag at the optical center, rather than the pupil center and visual axis.
   ii. The white circle with central black dot indicates *corneal apex* which is known as *vertex normal*.
   iii. Angle alpha is the angle or distance between optical center (shown as brackets [ ] for center of limbus) and apex (considered as visual axis) which has significant vertical and horizontal components.
   iv. The small black circle is the location of thinnest corneal thickness (Pachy thin). It is usually temporal and inferior to the apex.
   v. The black cross is the centroid of the pupil. It is usually less temporal and less inferior to the apex.
4. *Elevation maps*: In Holladay report, the elevation maps are in BFTE float mode. As mentioned in Chapter 6, Holladay believes that BFTE is better to study the shape of the cornea because the cornea is toric ellipsoid. Therefore, matching the cornea with a reference surface that is similar to its shape excludes the effect of corneal astigmatism and highlights corneal irregularities.

   The highest plus value is suspicious or abnormal if it is > +12 µm and > +15 µm on anterior and posterior elevation map, respectively.
5. *Relative pachymetry map*: The minimum relative pachymetry value (%) is suspicious or abnormal if it is < –5% or < –8%, respectively.

Holladay defines FFKC by abnormalities on the anterior tangential map, relative pachymetry map, and posterior elevation map that are correspondent to each others. In other words, in FFKC, a hot spot on the anterior tangential map is located in an area corresponding to the location of areas with abnormal values on the relative pachymetry map and the posterior elevation map.

HOLLADAY DETAILED EQUIVALENT K-READING REPORT

This is page 2 of Holladay report. In this page, EKR values are displayed in more details. The EKR parameters, values, and graphs are relatively sophisticated. To understand these parameters, Figure 23.2 should be understood first. Let us assume that there is a scale of positions ranging from 1 to 12. At each position, there are a number of cubes. For example, at position one, there are three cubes, at position four, there is one cube, and at position 10, there are six cubes. In this graph, the largest number (peak) of cubes is at position 10. The whole range from 1 to 12 is named "global range". The number of cubes in the global range is 40 cubes. Let us look for a range that includes 65% of the cubes (26 out of 40 cubes). There are two ranges, A and B, each of them includes the 65%. Range A extends over nine positions, and range B extends over seven positions. Therefore, the smallest (narrowest) range that includes the 65% is range B. This is the principle of the EKR65.

To understand the EKR report, replace positions by K-readings, and cubes by the frequency of K-readings at each position. Figure 23.3 is an illustration of this concept by using K-readings. Let us assume that a given zone of the cornea measuring 4.5 mm around pupil center is to be studied in terms of the distribution of EKR. The range of EKR found in the 4.5 mm zone is 38–49 D, which is the global EKR. The range of EKR that represents the smallest (narrowest) 65% of the global range is 42–48 D, and that is the EKR65.

The previous example was given as a linear illustration of the EKR. One can imagine a three-dimensional (3D) distribution over the given zone of the cornea, where a flat and a steep axes are present, and therefore, flat EKR65 and steep EKR65 are calculated.

It is important to know that the narrower the range of EKR65, the more reliable the EKR parameters and vice versa. In other words, if the EKR65 range is broad, captures should be repeated, and if they continue to show a broad distribution, errors in IOL calculation should be expected. In general, broad EKR65 range is found in very irregular corneas.

Section 7: *Miscellaneous*

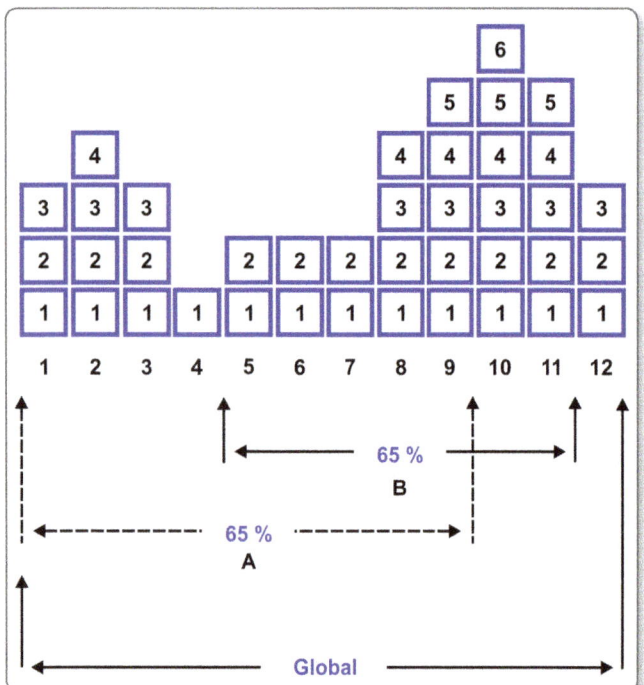

Fig. 23.2: Principle of Holladay equivalent K-reading (EKR) detailed report.

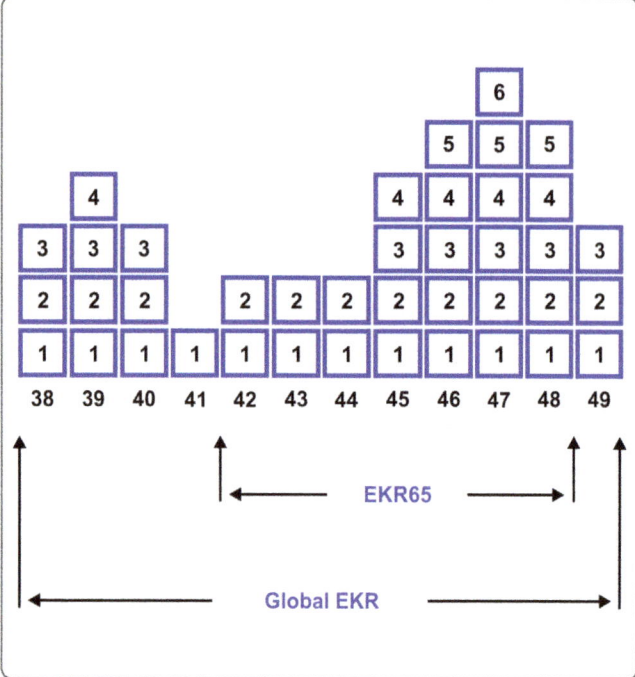

Fig. 23.3: Principle of Holladay equivalent K-reading (EKR) detailed report.

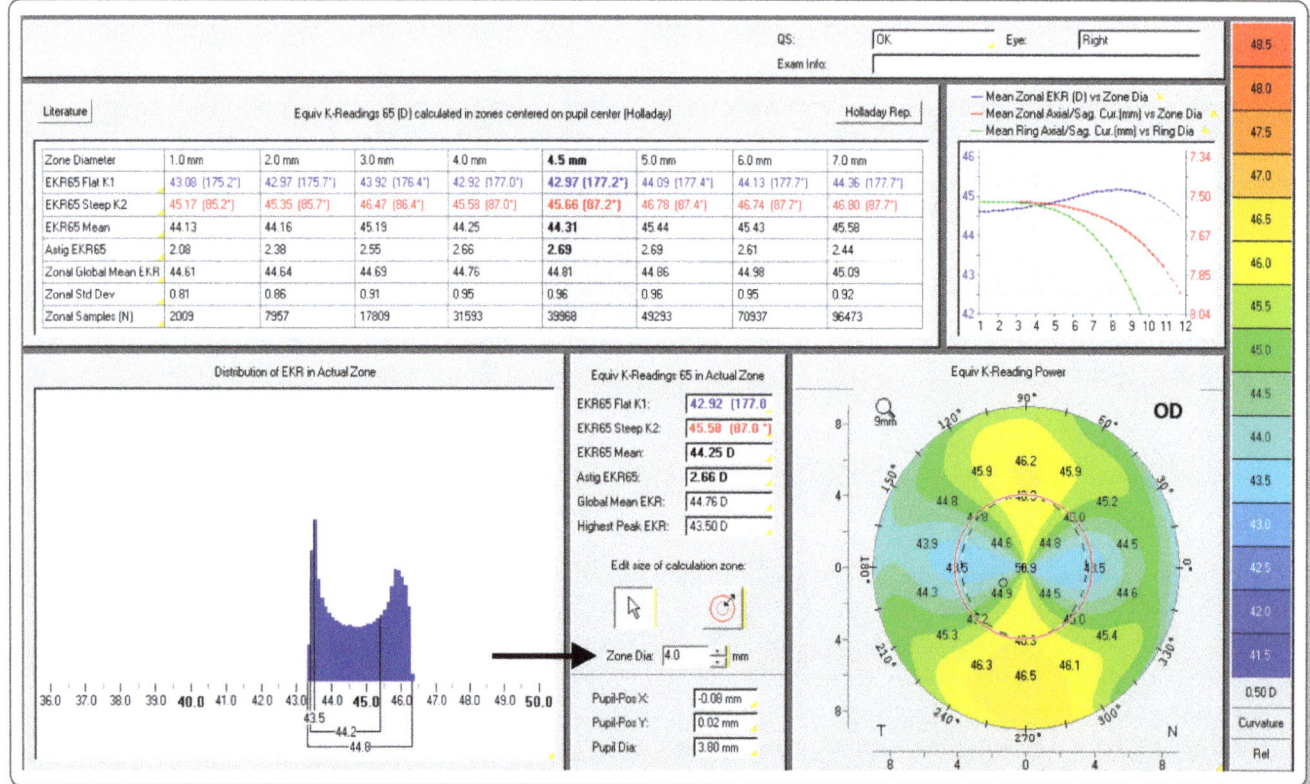

Fig. 23.4: Holladay report. Normal high astigmatic cornea. Page 2.

Figure 23.4 is the EKR detailed report of a normal cornea with regular astigmatism. The report consists of the followings.

Equivalent K-reading Calculated in Zones Centered on Pupil Center

The table at the top left of the page is for EKR65 for various parameters from 1 to 7 mm pupil diameters. By default, the software highlights the 4.5-mm zone because based on the database of Holladay, the EKR65 of this zone is the most accurate for IOL calculations. However, the mesopic pupil of the patient should be considered as was previously mentioned. Moreover, when the EKR65 K-readings are used in an exact toric calculator such as Holladay IOL Consultant Program (www.hicsoap.com), there is no need for additional adjustments because the back surface power and astigmatism have already been implemented.

Power Distribution

The graph at the top right represents the mean zonal EKR (D) versus zone diameter (blue), the mean zonal axial radius of curvature (mm) versus zone diameter (red), and mean ring axial radius of curvature (mm) versus zone diameter (green). The blue values show the refractive power (D) of a *zone* (measured by EKR) as one moves from the center of the pupil. The normal increase in EKR power reflects the normal presence of positive SA in the human cornea (around 2 D from center to 8 mm diameter periphery). The red values illustrate the refractive power (D) of a *zone* (measured by sagittal or keratometric method) as one moves from the center of the pupil. The green values represent the refractive power (D) of a *ring* (measured by sagittal or keratometric method) as one moves from the center of the pupil.

It is important to notice that EKR65 uses Snell's Law, whereas the axial power lines (green and red) do not, and therefore, they do not reflect actual refractive power changes over the cornea.

Equivalent K-reading Parameters

The central lower table displays the main parameters for the selected zone (default is 4.5 mm). In Figure 23.4, the *EKR65 mean* is 44.31 D, the *global mean EKR* is 44.81, and the *highest peak EKR* is 43.5 D. For a normal cornea, these three values vary less than 0.5 D. The EKR65 flat K1 (42.97 D × 177.2°) and steep K2 (45.66 D × 87.2°) are the appropriate values to use. No need for additional adjustment for back surface power, since it is included.

Distribution of Equivalent K-reading in Actual Zone

The lower left graph is a histogram illustrating the relative frequency of EKR power over the selected zone (default is 4.5-mm zone). The graph is rarely symmetrical and often has more than one peak with a normal 2–3 D global range. The shapes of this histogram and the power distribution graph are very important to evaluate the severity of corneal irregularities and the reliability of EKR65 for IOL calculations.

The difference between EKR parameters is a measure of the irregular astigmatism and is a measure of the precision of the EKR65, which is the best value to use. The greater the differences, the broader the range of distribution. Moreover, the greater the number of individual peaks, the lower the reliability of the EKR65, which results in a lower predictability of the IOL power outcome.

Equivalent K-reading Power Map

The lower right map is the EKR map. The dashed black circle shows entrance pupil margin during taking the capture, and the red circle is the study zone (default 4.5 mm). This map allows the clinician to see the power distribution graphically.

CLINICAL EXAMPLES

In the following clinical examples, pages 1 and 2 of Holladay Report will be studied.

Normal High-astigmatic Cornea

Figures 23.1 and 23.4 are pages 1 and 2, respectively, for a normal cornea with high magnitude of astigmatism.
- *Page 1*:
  - *The central upper box*:
    ◆ EKR65 mean value (44.31 D) is slightly steeper than the average K in the normal population (43 D) with a relatively high magnitude of astigmatism (2.69 D).
    ◆ Q-value over a 6-mm zone is –0.23, indicating a prolate cornea approximate to the average in normal population (–0.27). Positive SAs are expected because Q is > –0.53.
    ◆ The total SA (0.244 µm) is approximate to the average of 0.27 µm.
    ◆ Radii ratio (B/F) is 82.6%, which is very approximate to the average.

- *The upper right box*:
    - Pupil diameter is 3.8 mm. In this case, the 4 mm EKR65 is more suitable for IOL calculations as will be shown in Page 2.
    - Horizontal white-to-white is 12.1 mm, which is larger than the average (11.77).
    - Minimal pachymetry (thinnest corneal thickness) is 550 µm, which is slightly thicker than average.
    - ACD is 3.96 mm (>3 mm). It is suitable for phakic intraocular lens (PIOLs).
    - Chord is 0.08 mm which is very appropriate for premium IOLs.
- *The sagittal map*: The pattern is vertically-oriented symmetric bowtie (SB). The semi-meridians are aligned, indicating with-the-rule (WTR) regular astigmatism.
- *The tangential map*: Kmax is less than 51 D.
- *The pachymetry map*: Vertex normal (apex) coincides with pupil centroid. Optical center is very close to them. This is an ideal situation for best performance of premium IOLs. The thinnest location is just inferior and temporal to the optical center, and that is normal.
- *The relative pachymetry map*: The highest minus value is −4.5%, which is normal, but close to the suspicious value (−5%).
- *The elevation maps*: The highest plus values on the anterior elevation map is normal, while the value on the posterior elevation map is suspicious (+13 µm) and corresponds to the location of highest minus value on the relative pachymetry map. However, because there is no corresponding hot spot on the tangential map, this case is not FFKC according to Holladay definition.
- Page 2:
    - The values of the 4.5-mm zone are highlighted in gray by default. However, since the pupil is 3.8 mm, values of the 4-mm zone are recommended for premium IOL calculations, and the diameter of the studied zone should be adjusted to be 4 mm rather than 4.5 mm (black arrow).
    - The blue line shows an increase of power < 1 D over the 8-mm zone. This is usually seen in spherical and slightly prolate corneas.
    - The EKR parameters are mean = 44.25 D, global mean = 44.76 D, and highest peak = 43.5 D. The difference between these parameters is almost 0.5 D, indicating a regular cornea. This is consistent with the histogram.
    - The histogram shows a normal range of distribution (2–3 D), and a bimodal (two peaks) pattern. Each peak corresponds to a major frequency of EKR over the studied zone (4 mm). Although the two peaks are not equal in height and magnitude, they are opposing to each others on the global range, indicating a significant regular corneal astigmatism. One peak corresponds to the flat Ks and the other peak corresponds to the steep Ks. This is consistent with the pattern on the EKR map.
    - *Equivalent K-reading map*: It shows a homogeneous and regular WTR astigmatism.

Normal Low-astigmatic Cornea

Figures 23.5 and 23.6 are pages 1 and 2, respectively, for a normal cornea with low magnitude of astigmatism.
- Page 1:
    - *The central upper box*:
        - EKR65 mean value (42.65 D) is approximate to the average K in the normal population (43 D) with a small magnitude of astigmatism (0.35 D).
        - Q-value over a 6-mm zone is −0.05. This cornea is slightly prolate but positive SA is expected because Q is > −0.53.
        - The total SA (0.312 µm) is much higher than the average of 0.27 µm.
        - Radii ratio (B/F) is 85.7%. This is higher than the average.
    - *The upper right box*:
        - Pupil diameter is 2.44 mm. In this case, the 3-mm EKR65 is more suitable than the 4.5-mm EKR65 for IOL calculations unless the mesopic pupil is measured by a pupillometer.
        - Minimal pachymetry (thinnest corneal thickness) is 481 µm, which is thinner than average.
        - ACD is 3.17 mm (>3 mm). Based on Holladay report, this value is suitable for PIOLs.
        - Chord is 0.48 mm which is border line for premium IOLs.
    - *The sagittal map*: There is no abnormal pattern. Although the semi-meridians are not aligned and do not form one-line meridians, the irregularity is considered as insignificant because of the low magnitude of astigmatism (<1 D).
    - *The tangential map*: Kmax is less than 51 D.
    - *The pachymetry map*: The distribution of vertex normal (apex), pupil centroid, and thinnest location is normal.
    - *The relative pachymetry map*: The highest minus value is −1.1%, which is normal.
    - *The elevation maps*: The highest plus values on both maps are normal.

Chapter 23: Holladay Report

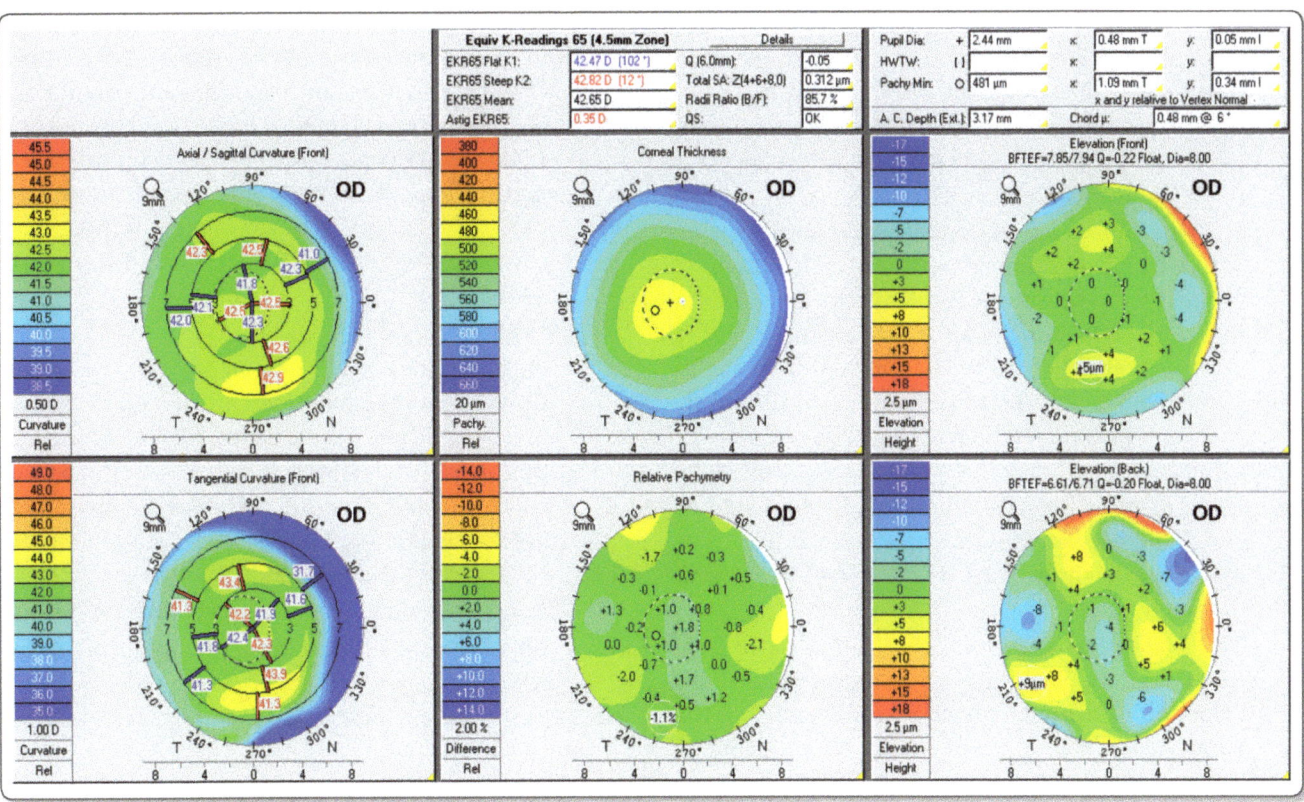

Fig. 23.5: Normal low astigmatic cornea. Holladay report page 1.

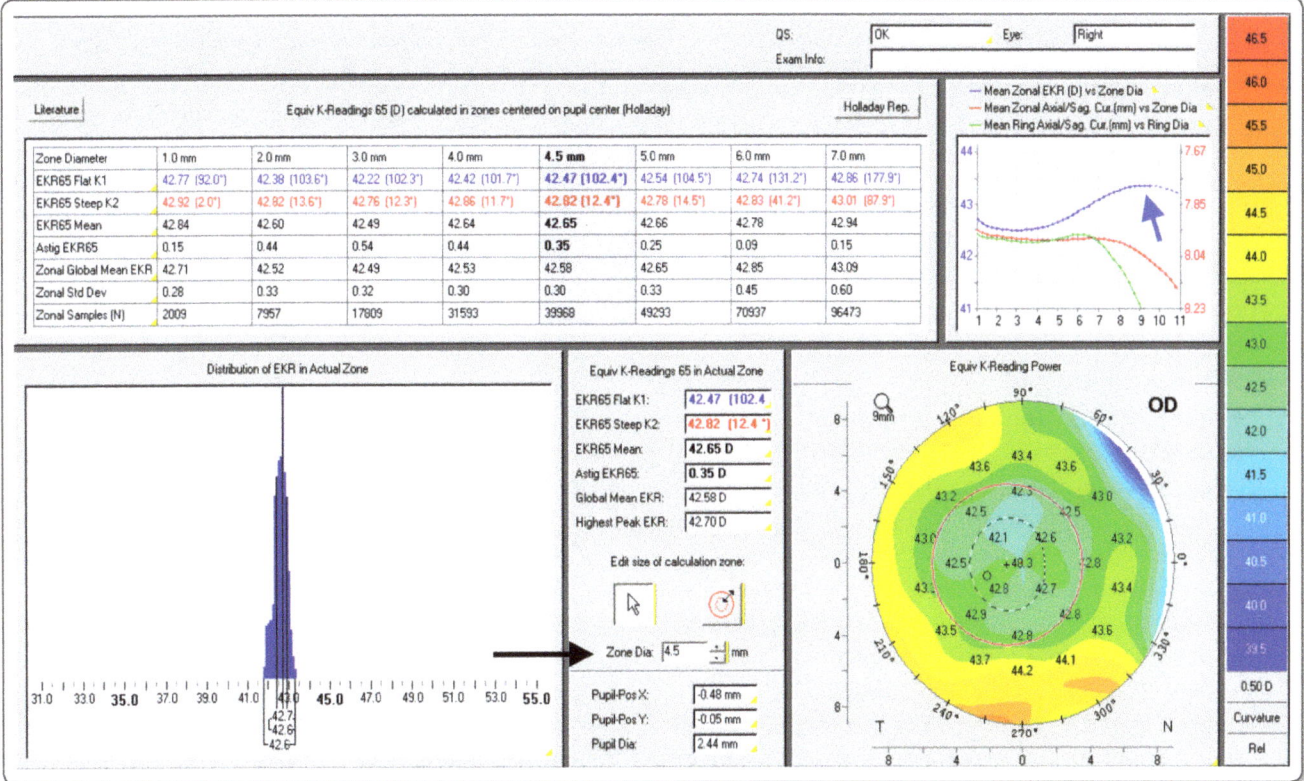

Fig. 23.6: Normal low astigmatic cornea. Holladay report page 2.

- *Page 2*:
  - The values of the 4.5-mm zone are highlighted in gray by default. In this case, infrared pupillometry was performed and the pupil measured 5.3 mm. Therefore, the default zone will be used despite that pupil diameter is showing < 3 mm.
  - The blue curve shows a small increase in EKR power (<1 D) over the 8-mm zone. This is usually seen in spherical and slightly prolate corneas. In addition, the blue curve shows a knee (blue arrow). This is encountered when there is an abrupt increase in corneal curvature toward periphery. This is usually seen after myopic ablation.
  - The EKR parameters are EKR65 mean = 42.65 D, global mean EKR = 42.58 D, and highest peak = 42.7 D. The difference between these parameters is < 0.5 D, indicating a regular cornea. This is consistent with the histogram.
  - The histogram shows a very narrow pattern of distribution (global range = 1.5 D) and a one sharp peak, indicating a very regular studied zone of the cornea.
  - *Equivalent K-reading map*: It shows a homogeneous distribution of power from the center toward the periphery. However, the center is flatter than periphery.

Keratoconus

Figures 23.7 and 23.8 are pages 1 and 2, respectively, for a keratoconic cornea.

Patterns of keratoconus (KC) differ according to cone pattern and cone location in addition to the difference between ECDs. The following case is a moderate KC with an oval cone pattern and central cone location.

- *Page 1*:
  - *The central upper box*:
    - EKR65 mean value (50.51 D) is much higher than the normal average K, indicating a high myopia generated by the cornea. The magnitude of astigmatism is moderate (1.9 D). In KC, the dissociation between the EKR and the standard keratometry measurements (Sim-Ks) is proportional to the severity of KC. In other words, the more advanced the disease, the larger the dissociation. The standard keratometry usually overestimates the power leading to a hypermetropic shift after treatments. In advanced cases, this dissociation may be up to 3 to 4 D.
    - Q-value over a 6-mm zone is –1.66, indicating a hyperprolate cornea and a high negative SA. This is consistent with the very high value of total SA (1.113 µm), which is much higher than the normal average (0.27 µm).
    - Radii ratio (B/F) is 77.5%. This is much lower than the average. This indicates a steeper posterior corneal surface in comparison with the anterior surface.
  - *The upper right box*:
    - Pupil diameter is 3.64 mm. In this case, the 4-mm EKR65 is more suitable for IOL calculations unless the mesopic pupil is measured by a pupillometer.
    - Minimal pachymetry (thinnest corneal thickness) is 413 µm, which is much thinner than the normal average and is borderline if the standard epi-off corneal cross-linking is indicated.
    - ACD is 3.57 mm (>3 mm). It is suitable for PIOLs.
    - Chord is 0.57 mm which is not suitable for premium IOLs.
  - *The sagittal map*: It shows asymmetric bowtie/inferior steep (AB/IS).
  - *The tangential map*: It shows an oval cone pattern.
  - *The pachymetry map*: It shows a dome pattern with temporal and inferior displacement of the thinnest location.
  - *The relative pachymetry map*: The highest minus value is –18.4% which is very abnormal.
  - *The elevation maps*: The highest plus values on both maps are abnormal with the posterior value being much higher, which is usual in KC. In all corneal irregularities and because of the remodeling effect of the epithelium, the anterior corneal surface is usually smoothened by the thinned epithelium over the steep areas.
- *Page 2*:
  - The values of the 4.5-mm zone are highlighted in gray by default. However, since the pupil is 3.64 mm, values of the 4-mm zone are recommended for premium IOL calculations, and the diameter of the studied zone should be adjusted to be 4 mm rather than 4.5 mm (black arrow).
  - The power distribution graph shows a sharp decline in the three curves. This is characteristic to the central pattern of KC. The reader can see the difference when looking at Figures 23.9 and 23.10 for a KC with eccentric cone (pellucid-like KC), and Figures 23.11 and 23.12 for a case with peripheral cone (pellucid marginal degeneration).

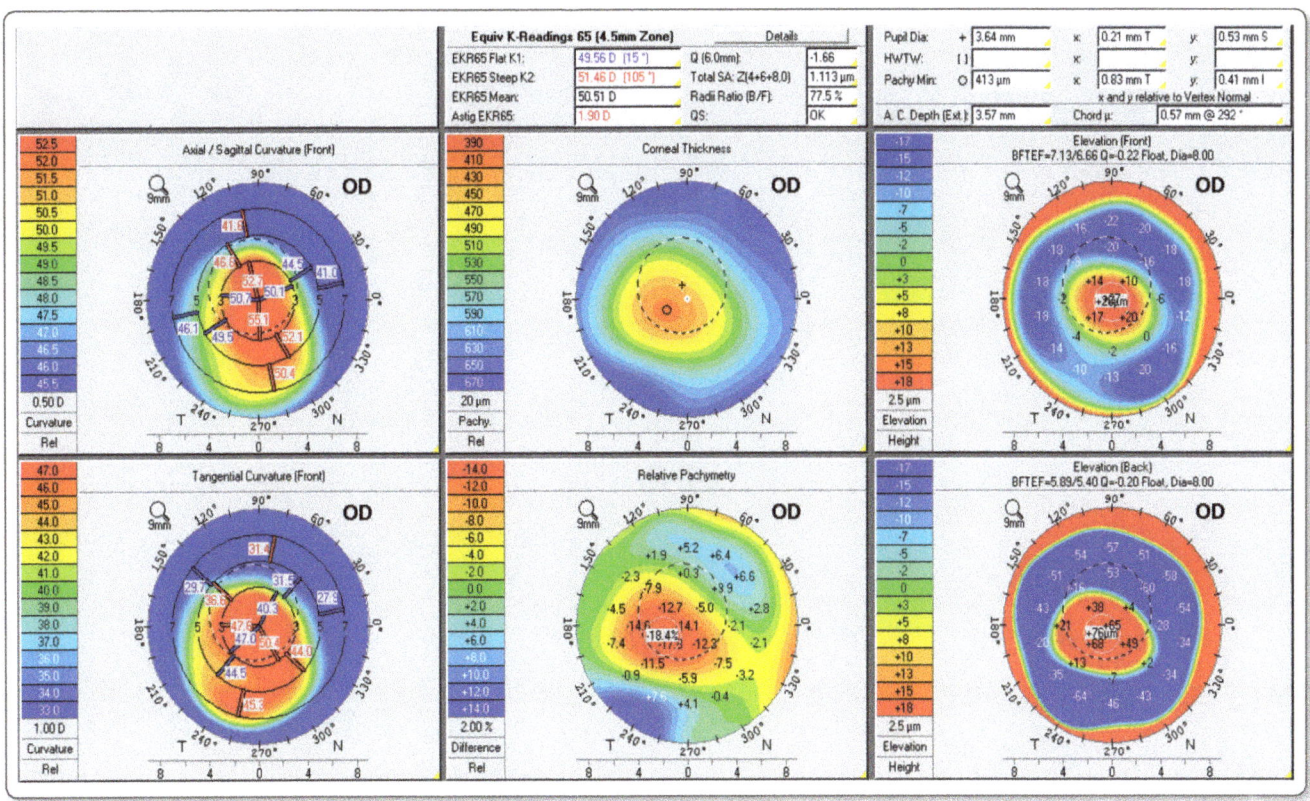

Fig. 23.7: Keratoconus. Holladay report page 1.

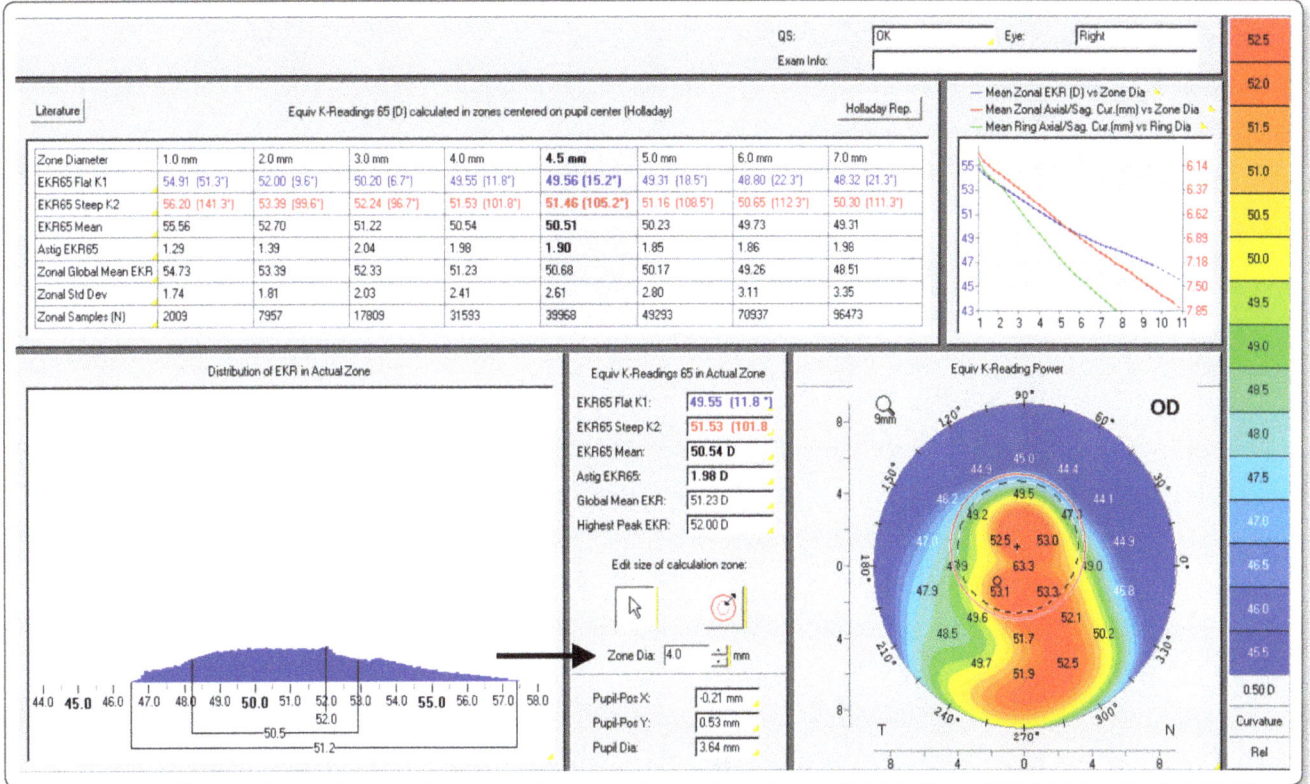

Fig. 23.8: Keratoconus. Holladay report page 2.

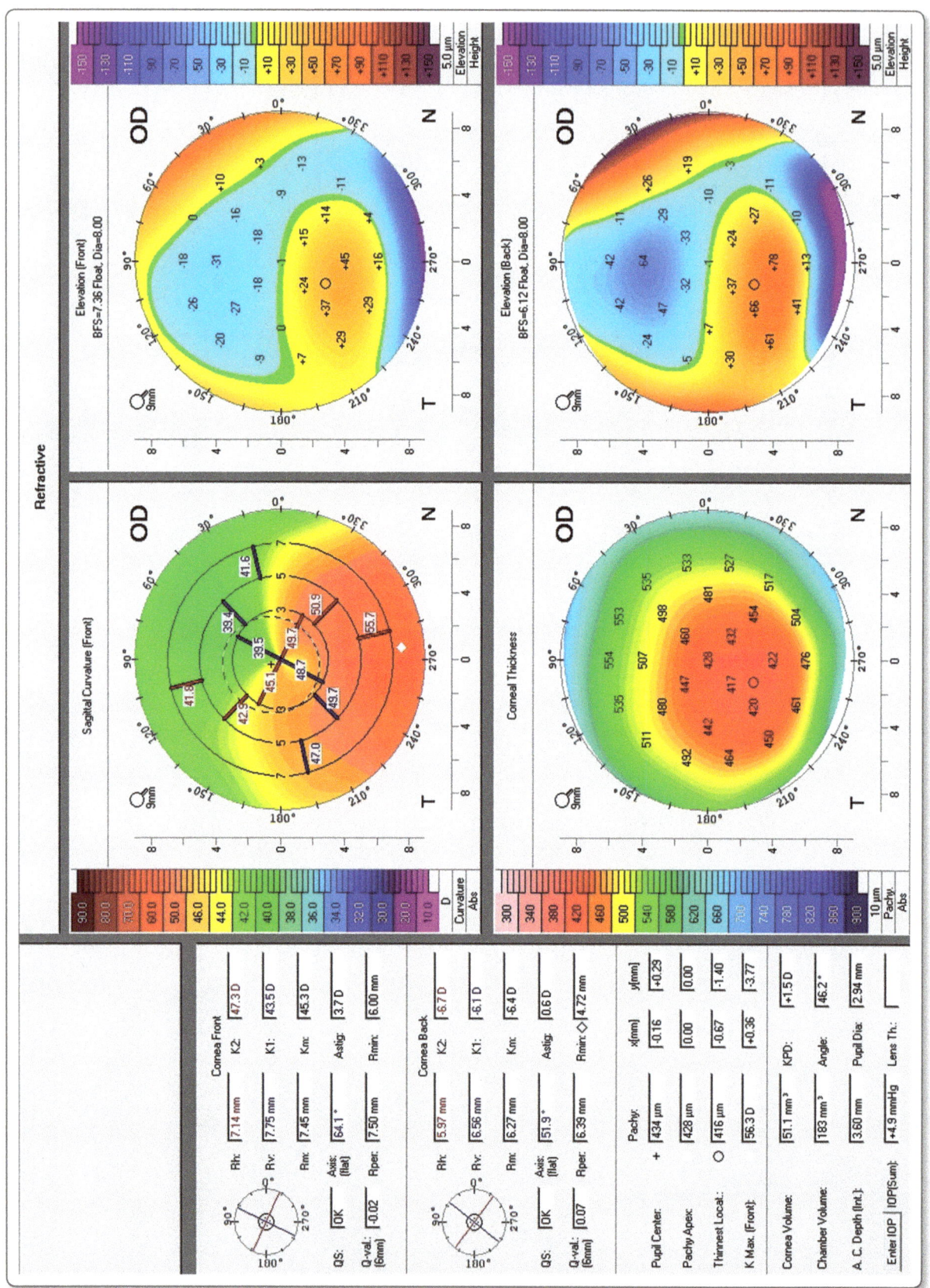

Fig. 23.9: Pellucid-like keratoconus. Holladay report page 1.

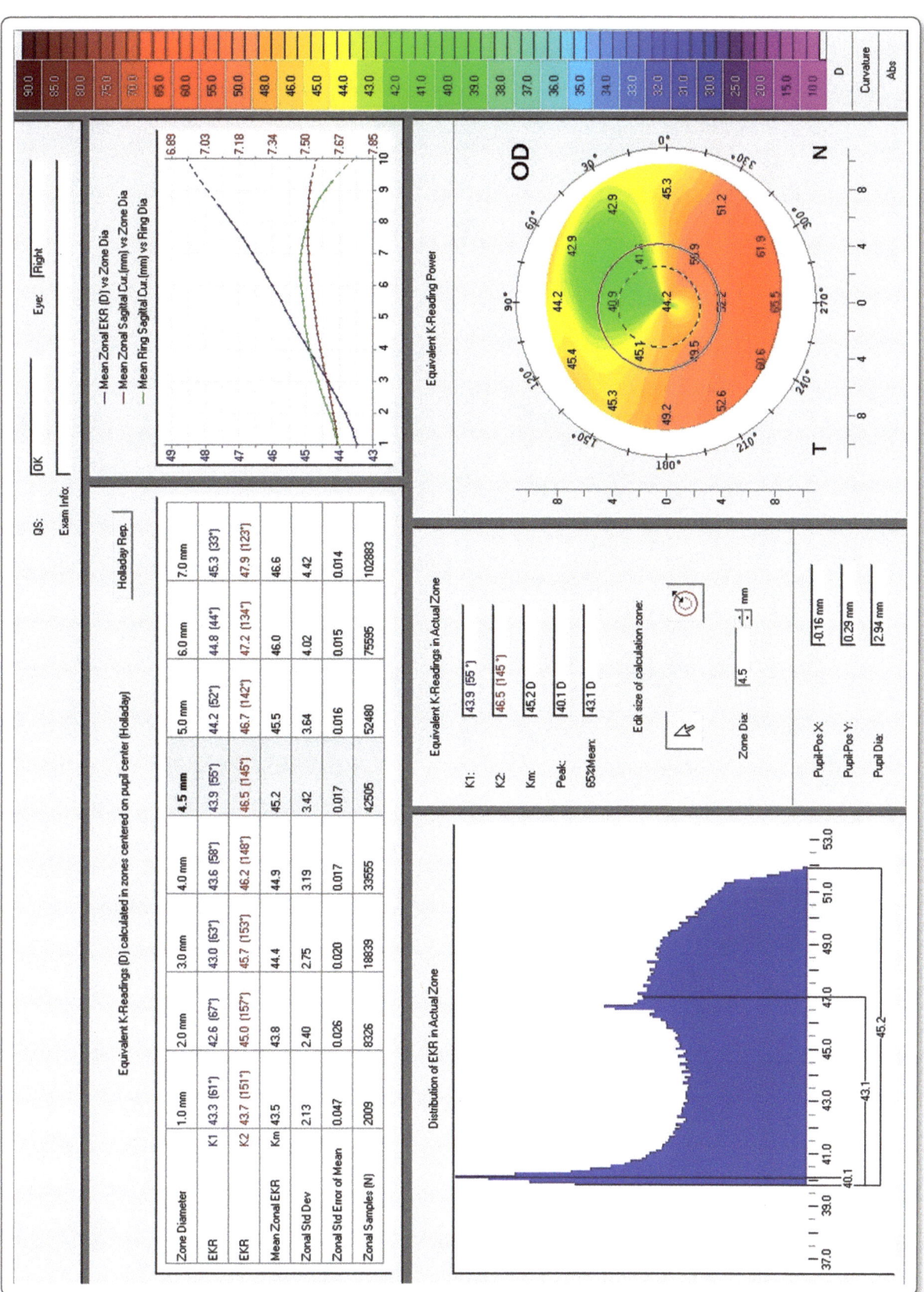

Fig. 23.10: Pellucid-like keratoconus. Holladay report page 2.

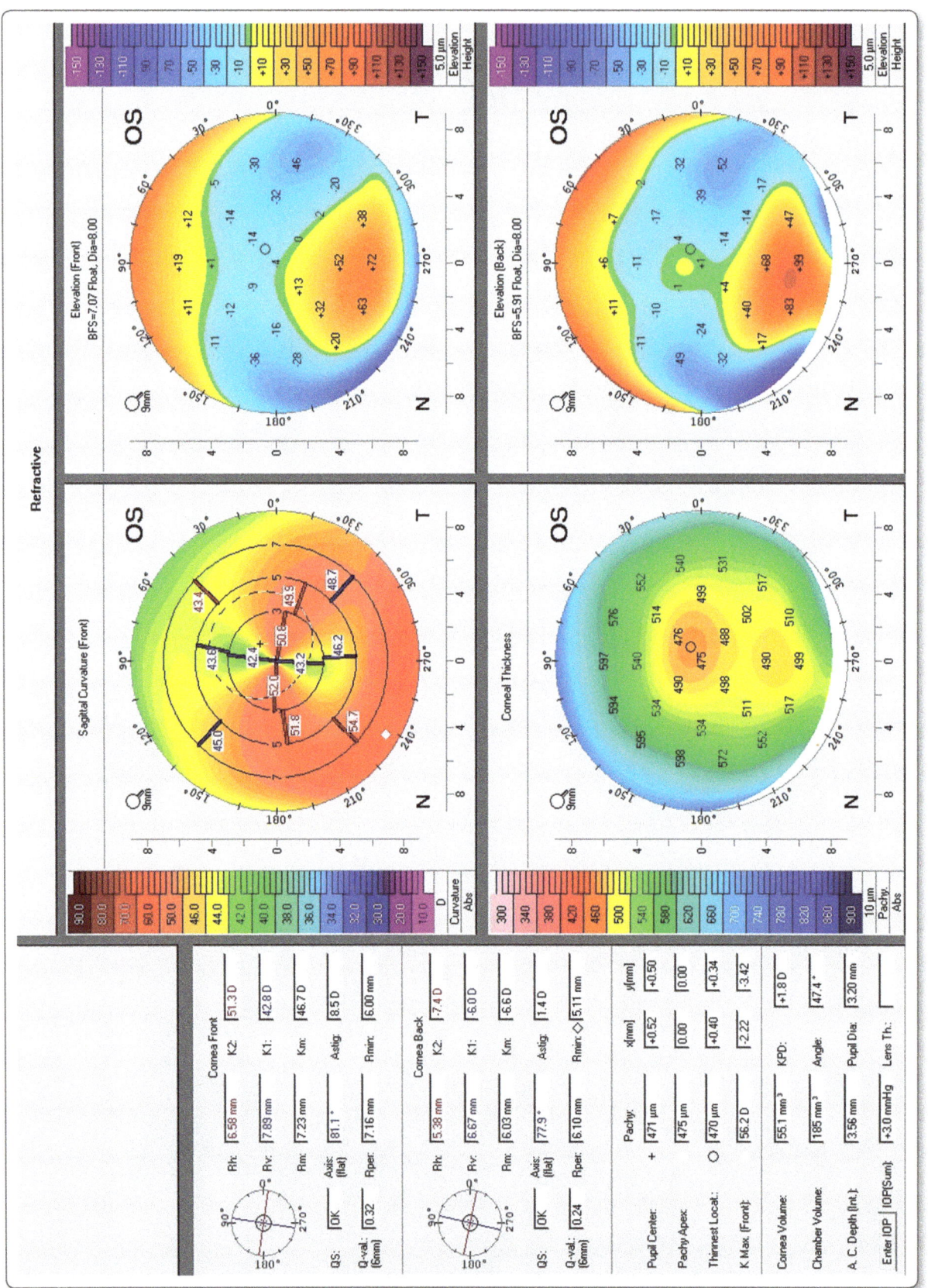

Fig. 23.11: Pellucid marginal degeneration. Holladay report page 1.

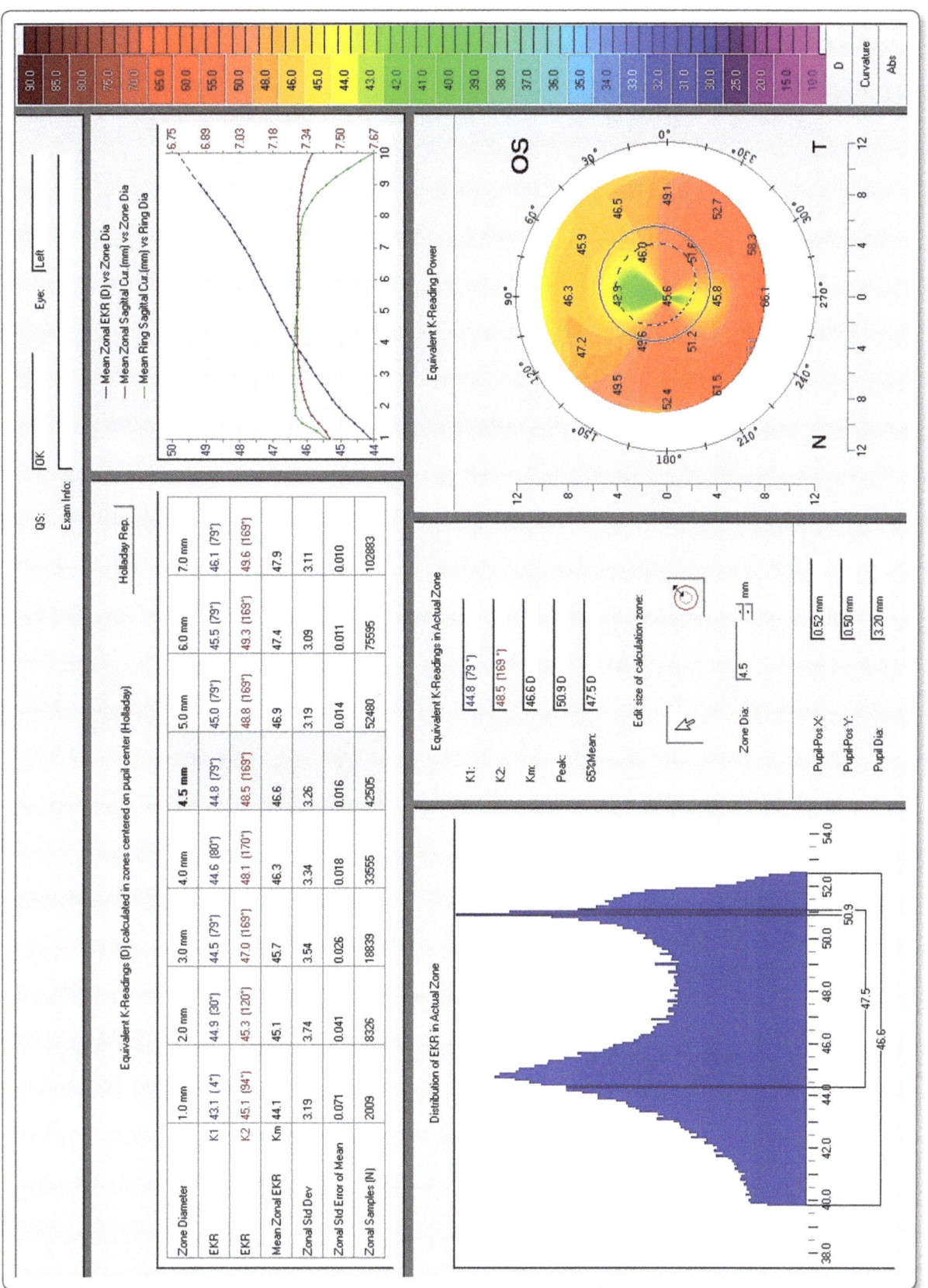

Fig. 23.12: Pellucid marginal degeneration. Holladay report page 2.

- The EKR parameters are mean = 50.54 D, global mean = 51.23 D, and highest peak = 52 D. The difference between these parameters is > 0.5 D, indicating an irregular cornea.
- The histogram shows a very wide pattern of distribution (global EKR range = 11 D and EKR65 range = 4.5 D), indicating a very irregular cornea. This point is very important in differentiating post-hypermetropic treated cornea from central KC as will be shown in the next case.
- *Equivalent K-reading map*: It is consistent with KC.

Post-Hypermetropic Laser Vision Correction

Figures 23.13 and 23.14 are pages 1 and 2, respectively, for a cornea after hypermetropic laser vision correction (LVC).

- *Page 1*: Patterns of the tangential map, elevation maps, and relative pachymetry map were studied in Chapter 22.
- *Page 2*:
  - The graph on the top right shows an S-shape in both blue and red curves (blue arrow). This shape correlates to the high K-readings in the center of the cornea and the sudden flatness of corneal surface toward the untreated peripheral cornea.
  - The histogram on the bottom left shows a one-peak pattern, indicating a regular cornea. In spite of a broad global range (9 D), the EKR65 is relatively narrow (3.5 D), which differentiates this case from a case of central KC as mentioned before.
  - The EKR map on the bottom right shows the steep central area.

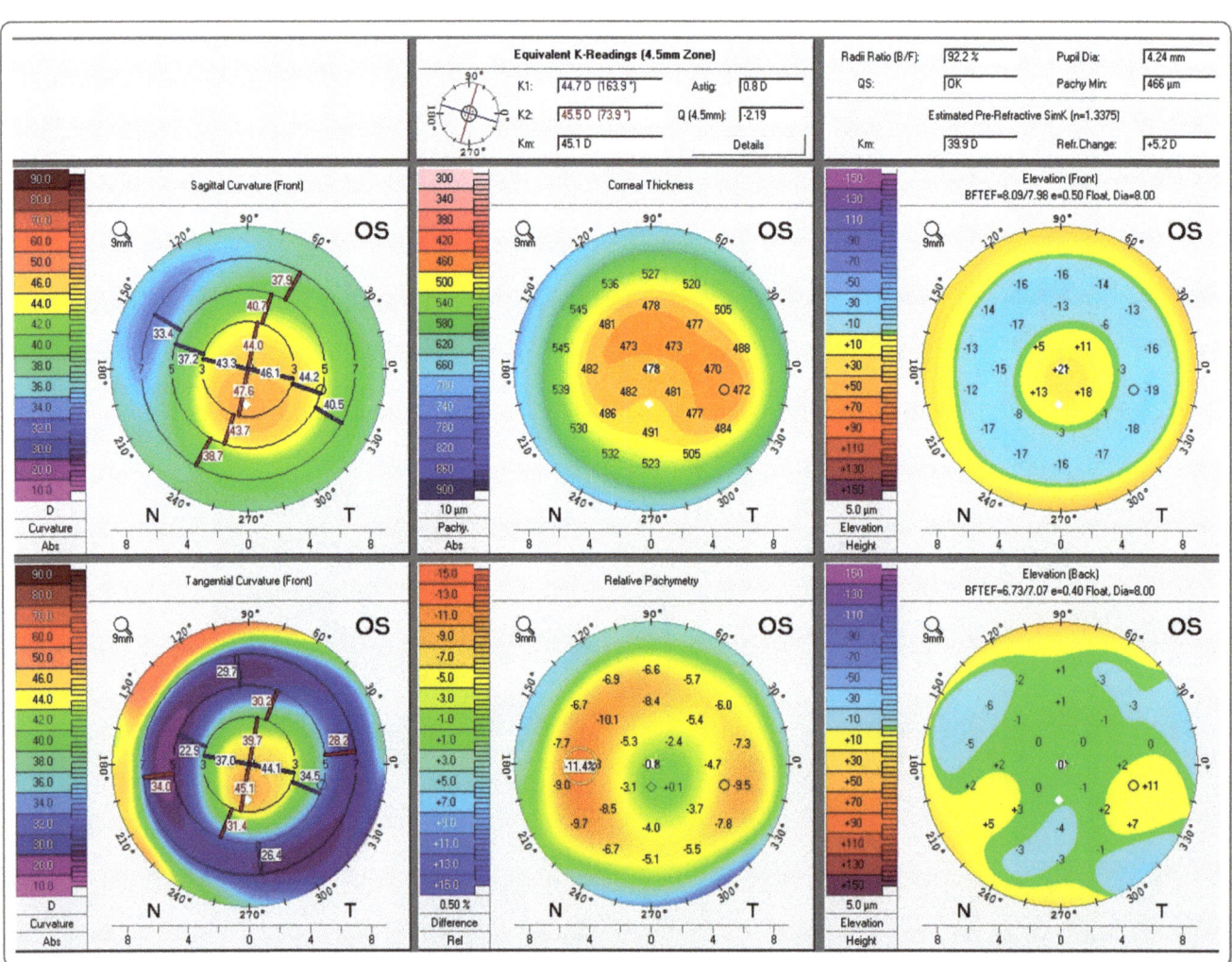

Fig. 23.13: Post-hypermetropic laser vision correction (LVC). Holladay report page 1.

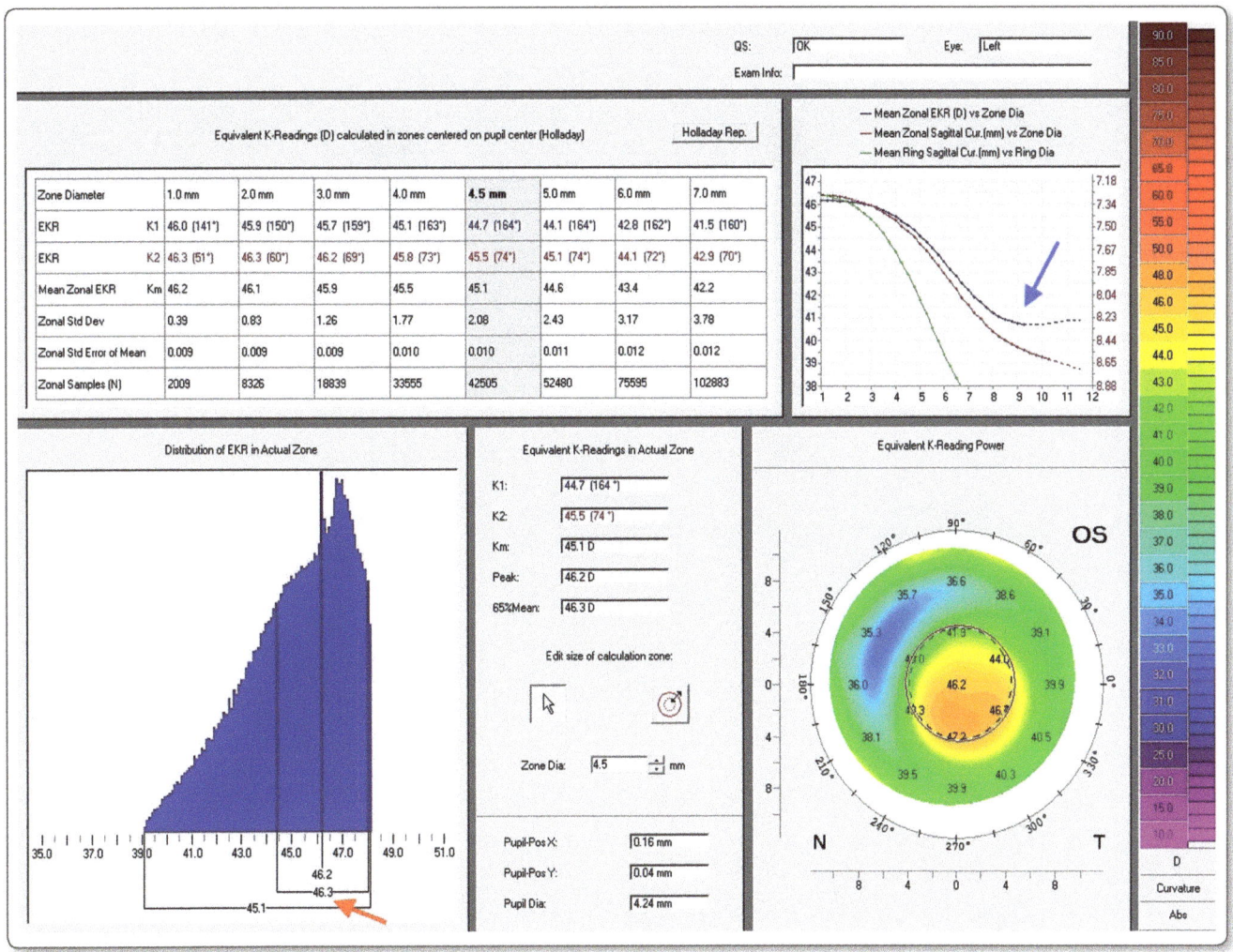

Fig. 23.14: Post-hypermetropic laser vision correction (LVC). Holladay report page 2.

Post-Myopic Laser Vision Correction

Figures 23.15 and 23.16 are pages 1 and 2, respectively, for a cornea after myopic LVC.
- *Page 1*: Patterns of the tangential map, elevation maps, and relative pachymetry map were studied in Chapter 22. However, in this case, the semi-meridians are broken in the sagittal map indicating an irregular ablated zone, which is better seen on the tangential map.
- *Page 2*:
  - The graph on the top right shows a knee in all curves (black arrow). This shape correlates to the transitional zone.
  - The histogram on the bottom left shows a global EKR range with flat K-readings which is consistent with the oblate shape of this operated cornea. The EKR65 is narrow (1.75 D) but shows a multipeak pattern, indicating an irregular cornea.
  - The EKR map on the bottom right shows an oblate cornea with an irregular ablated zone.

Section 7: Miscellaneous

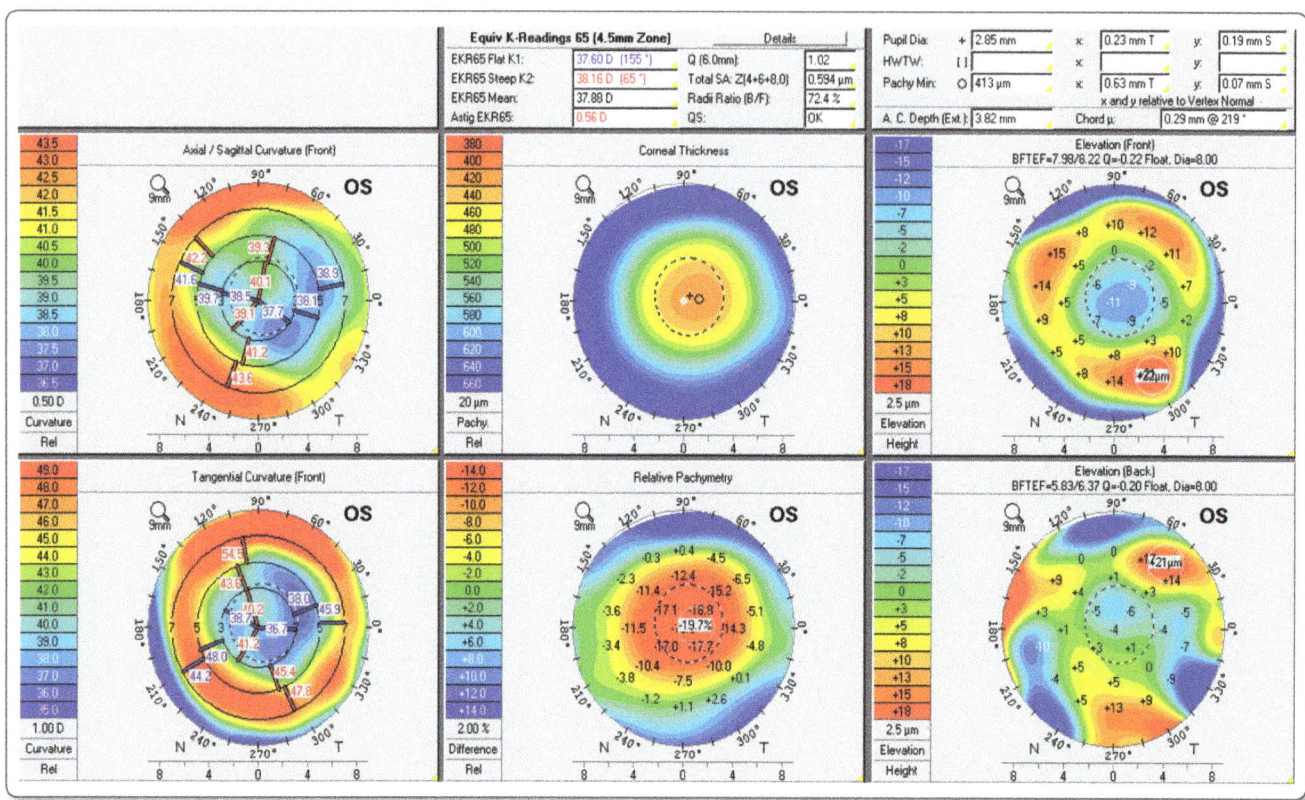

Fig. 23.15: Post-myopic laser vision correction (LVC). Holladay report page 1.

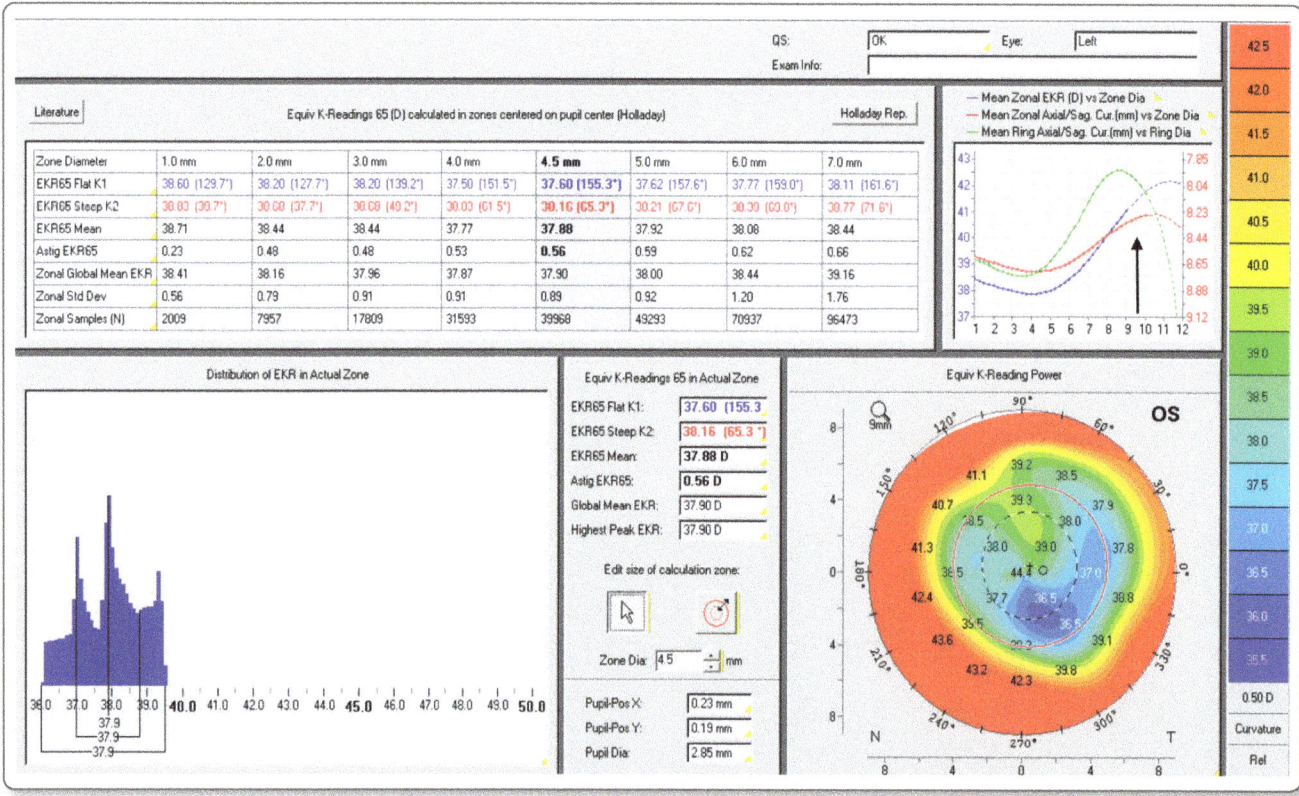

Fig. 23.16: Post-myopic laser vision correction (LVC). Holladay report page 2.

Corneal Tomography and Corneal Aberrometry in Cataract Surgery

INTRODUCTION

The role of corneal tomography and aberrometry in cataract surgery is becoming more important in the screening and planning processes, both pre- and postoperatively.

PREOPERATIVE SCREENING PROCESS

It is not uncommon to see patients after cataract surgery suffering from reduced quality and quantity of vision due to higher-order aberrations (HOAs) resulting from unrecognized preoperative corneal irregularities, ectatic corneal diseases (ECDs), or abnormal corneal asphericity. Such patients may or may not have preoperative significant astigmatism. The problem increases by folds in case of significant astigmatism and the use of premium intraocular lens (IOLs), where HOAs will definitely affect the final outcomes. Recognizing such disorders during the preoperative assessment process are necessary not only from a medical viewpoint but also from a legal viewpoint in regard with the consent form.

Corneal tomography and aberrometry can be used as a screening process to look for:
- Irregular astigmatism and ECDs because:
  - May be they are the limiting factor of patient's vision, not the cataract.
  - They increase the risk of postoperative glare and halos.
  - They reduce the quality of vision.
  - They are contraindicated for multifocal lenses.
  - They reduce the efficacy and safety of astigmatic keratotomy (AK) and limbal relaxing incisions (LRIs).
  - They affect the accuracy of IOL calculations.
  - A two-step plan of treatment can be discussed with the patient before the operation. For example: a 17-year-old patient with mild keratoconus (KC) and presenile cataract. His cataract is due to prolong abuse of topical steroids because of vernal keratoconjunctivitis. His KC should be considered as progressive and treated with corneal cross-linking at least 6 months before the cataract surgery. Should the cornea has become stable and the K-readings have stopped changing, IOL calculations are more accurate.
- Corneal surface irregularities, such as epithelial basement membrane dystrophy (EBMD) or Salzmann's nodular degeneration. These disorders are usually treated in a three-step approach:
  1. *Step 1*: Epithelial debridement or peeling of Salzmann's nodules.
  2. *Step 2*: A healing period of 2–3 months.
  3. *Step 3*: If visual acuity has improved to an efficient level, the cataract surgery can be delayed, otherwise the surgery can be performed but with more regular cornea and more accurate IOL measurements.
- *Previous refractive surgery*: Some patients may have refractive surgery when they were in the 30s and came back in the 50s with cataract. It may be very difficult to recognize the previous refractive surgery on the regular slit lamp biomicroscopy; therefore, when the K-readings are taken, it cannot be known whether the 40 D K is the patient's native K or an iatrogenic K. Corneal tomography will give the answer (Chapter 22).
- *Dry eye*: It is one of the causes of distorted tomography. Sometimes, dry eye can more easily be seen on

tomography because at the slit lamp, the surgeon probably will primarily be looking at the cataract rather than at ocular surface.

PREOPERATIVE PLANNING PROCESS

- *Intraocular lens calculation*: Corneal tomography is essential in case of: irregular astigmatism, ECDs, post-laser vision correction (LVC) and post-RK, and EBMD. In such cases, keratometry cannot be simply taken from the Sim-Ks. Equivalent K-readings (EKRs) from Holladay report, or K-readings measured by the total corneal refractive power (TCRP) are more accurate. EKR can directly be input into the IOL formulas, while the TCRP K-readings may need to be modified by a factor for some formulas. Therefore, the guidelines of the manufacturer should strictly be followed.
- *Intraocular lens types*:
  - Aspheric IOLs are used to enhance contrast sensitivity and reduce spherical aberrations in cataract patients either by compensating for corneal spherical aberration or by not affecting it at all. Corneal tomography and aberrometry measure corneal asphericity.
  - Toric IOLs are used to neutralize corneal astigmatism in cataract patients. Corneal tomography, and not the keratometry (Sim-Ks), help to know the type, magnitude, and axis of corneal astigmatism, and to check the regularity of astigmatism. It also measures posterior surface astigmatism, which has an effect on the accuracy of IOL calculations.
- *Shape, type, size, and location of cataract incision*: Several factors affect the impact of cataract incision on corneal astigmatism and regularity. Location, shape, and length of the incisions, wound construction, and the manner of wound closure are the key factors. Any incision has a flattening effect on the meridian of the incision. This effect is known as surgically-induced astigmatism (SIA). There are general rules:
  - The farther the incision from visual axis, the less the flattening effect it induces.
  - The more symmetric the incision, the less the flattening effect it induces (Fig. 24.1).
  - Scleral incisions have less flattening effect than limbal and clear corneal incisions.
  - Scleral bent frown incision has less flattening effect than scleral arcuate incision (Fig. 24.2).
  - Limbal (vascular, near-clear corneal) incisions have less flattening effect than avascular, truly clear corneal incisions.
  - Temporal incisions and oblique-meridian incisions have less flattening effect than superior incisions because they have less influence from the eyelid and extraocular muscle and are farther from the center of the cornea. In elderly patients with against-the-rule (ATR) astigmatism, the flattening effect of the temporal incision is an advantage.
  - The narrower and the longer the tunnel of incision, the less flattening effect it induces (Figs. 24.3 and 24.4).
  - Arcuate corneal incisions have more flattening effect than straight linear corneal incisions. If arcuate incisions were made on the steep axis in cases with a small preoperative astigmatism, the astigmatism would be overcorrected.
- *Pterygium and corneal scars*: They affect the accuracy of IOL calculations and the visual outcome by terms of

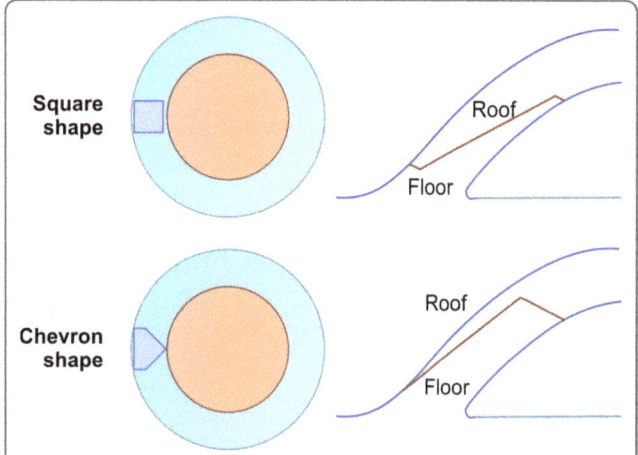

Fig. 24.1: Incision symmetry. In the square shape, roof equals floor in terms of thickness. In the chevron shape, shallow roof, and thick floor.

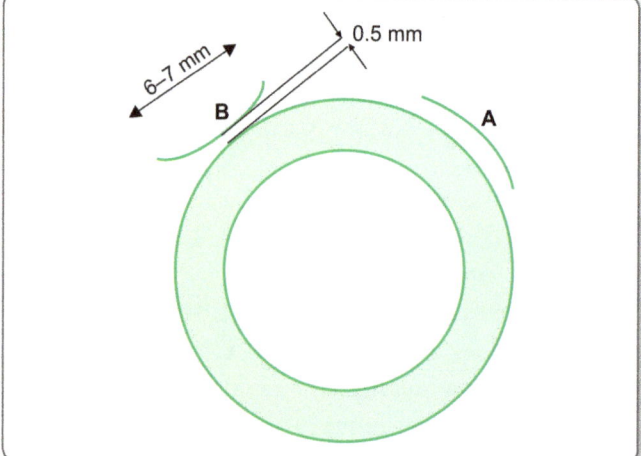

Fig. 24.2: Scleral incisions. A, The bent frown incision; and B, The arcuate incision.

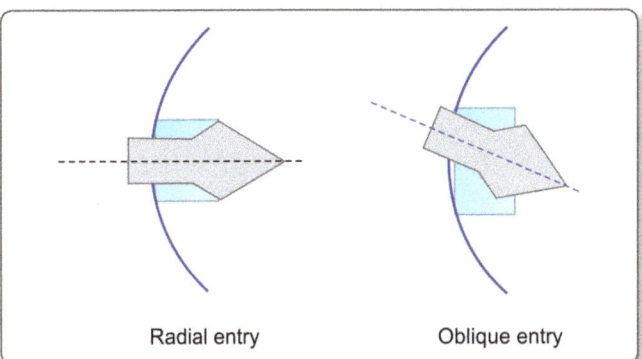

Fig. 24.3: Dimensions of the incision. Good form: radial entry, straight in-straight out, proper incision width, and less astigmatic effect. Poor form: oblique entry, different in and outpaths, incision is too wide, and more astigmatic effect.

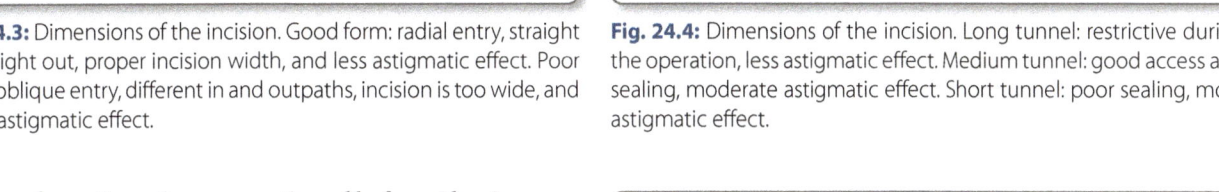

Fig. 24.4: Dimensions of the incision. Long tunnel: restrictive during the operation, less astigmatic effect. Medium tunnel: good access and sealing, moderate astigmatic effect. Short tunnel: poor sealing, more astigmatic effect.

irregular astigmatism as mentioned before. Also, in a case of pterygium, tomography will help in deciding whether to remove the cataract first or to remove the pterygium first, in terms of which would give the patient better vision. If there is a significant irregular astigmatism on the tomography due to the pterygium, it will be wise to address the pterygium first.

- *Astigmatic keratotomy and limbal relaxing incisions*: Corneal tomography is essential here for the following reasons:
  - Number, length, depth, and location of the incisions are determined by the magnitude and type of astigmatism [with-the-rule (WTR), ATR, or oblique] in addition to patient's age.
  - In astigmatism with skewed radial axis (SRAX), the cornea does not respond normally to AK and LRIs, and they may produce more irregularity.
  - *Customizing the incisions*: It is not uncommon to have an asymmetric bowtie (AB). Keratometry cannot recognize this irregularity. In AB pattern, the incision on the steeper side can be made a little longer than on the other side. In symmetric bowtie with SRAX (SB/SRAX) and AB/SRAX patterns, incisions should not be done on opposite sides, but should be placed at the tips of the astigmatism to round it out and make it more symmetrical. This can be planned by tomography and topography rather than keratometry.
  - Tomography can give regional pachymetry values in the areas where the relaxing incisions are planned; therefore, the depth of incisions can be precisely calculated.
  - Prohibiting AK and LRIs when the sagittal curvature map shows an unspecific irregular pattern such as in Figure 24.5.

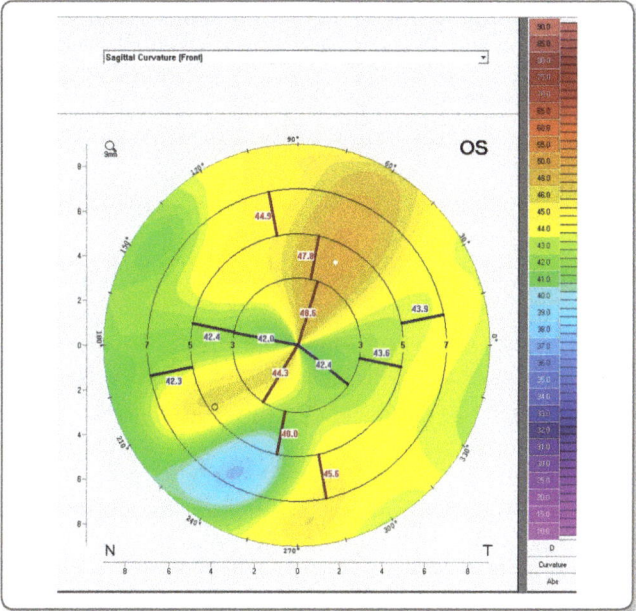

Fig. 24.5: Unspecific irregular pattern. Not suitable for AK and LRIs. (AK: astigmatic keratotomy; LRIs: limbal relaxing incisions)

- *Cornea guttata and Fuchs' dystrophy*: Corneal tomography can reveal these two important entities by corneal thickness spatial profile (CTSP) and percentage thickness increase (PTI) (Chapter 8).

POSTOPERATIVE PLANNING PROCESS

Corneal tomography and aberrometry should be performed after cataract surgery when the postoperative corrected distance visual acuity (CDVA) is not optimal with no clear reason, where corneal irregularities and HOAs are the first accusers.

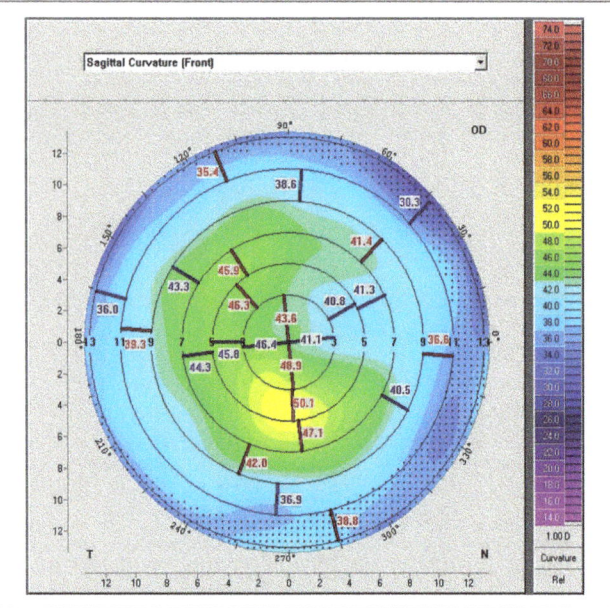

Fig. 24.6: Incision-related corneal steepening due to tight superior sutures.

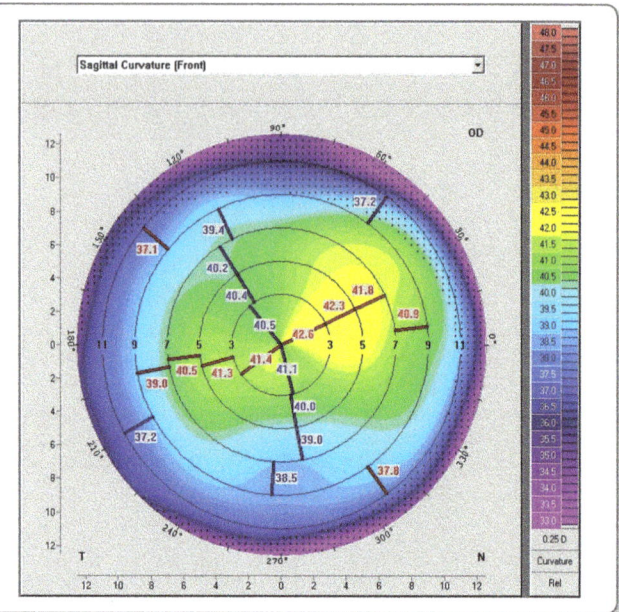

Fig. 24.7: Incision-related corneal flattening due to loose superior sutures.

In general, postoperative corneal tomography is useful in detecting tight sutures, torsion of the wound, internal wound gap, and irregular astigmatism, as well as to guide suture removal. In wounds closed by nonabsorbable sutures, selective suture manipulation at 8–12 weeks postoperatively is an effective way for reducing wound-related corneal astigmatism. For interrupted sutures, this involves removal of the tight suture(s) on the steep axis/axes. Continuous sutures may partly or entirely be removed, or alternatively, the tension in the suture may be redistributed by easing it loop by loop from flat areas to steep areas. Corneal tomography is superior to keratometry for suture adjustment; it can identify more accurately the location of the tight sutures, particularly if more than one is tight and if the K-readings cannot be read by the keratometer.

Postoperative Corneal Steepening

Wound-related corneal steepening (WTR astigmatism for a superior incision) occurs secondary to compression of tissue at the wound site. This is commonly a result of the overtightening of sutures or edema of the wound margins. It may also be due to vertical wound misalignment in which the central edge under rides the peripheral edge, or due to cautery causing tissue contraction. The compression of tissue at the limbus depresses the limbal cornea toward the center of the globe, thereby increasing the curvature of the infracentral cornea (that is a reduction in the radius of curvature). There is a small area of flattening immediately within the area of the suture and a secondary flattening in the meridian perpendicular to the suture, as a result of the coupling effect (Fig. 24.6).

Postoperative Corneal Flattening

Wound-related corneal flattening (ATR astigmatism for a superior incision) occurs as a result of wound gap. This is sometimes seen to a small extent in unsutured wounds, but more commonly if sutures are too loose, either at the time of surgery or if there is subsequent cheese-wiring, knot slippage, suture-related inflammation, degradation, or early removal. Sutures which are placed too superficially may result in posterior wound gap, which has a similar tomographic appearance. Vertical misalignment of the wound with the central edge of the incision flattens the incision meridian (Fig. 24.7).

Irregular Astigmatism

If wound-related flattening or steepening is due to a single or a uniform structural defect, regular astigmatism is most likely and is relatively easy to correct optically or surgically. However, more complex anatomical changes can result in irregular astigmatism, which produces greater visual dysfunction and is more difficult to correct. Bioblique astigmatism (nonperpendicular axes) may occur if nonadjacent sutures are overtightened. A torsional effect results from a horizontal misalignment of the wound, which may result from mismatching of its edges or nonradial suture bites.

Bibliography

1. Abad JC, Rubinfeld RS, Valle MD, et al. Vertical D: A novel topographic in some keratoconus suspects. Ophthalmology. 2007;114(5):1020-6.
2. Alio JL, Shabayek MH. Corneal high order aberrations: A method to grade keratoconus. J Refract Surg. 2006;22:539-45.
3. Alio JL. Corneal irregularity. In: Alio J, Azar D (Eds). Management of Complications in Refractive Surgery. Berlin, Heidelberg: Springer-Verlag; 2008. pp. 143-6.
4. Alpins N, Ong JKY, Stamatelatos G. Corneal topographic astigmatism (CorT) to quantify total corneal astigmatism. J Refract Surg. 2015;31(3):182-6.
5. Ambrósio R Jr, Alonso RS, Luz A, et al. Corneal-thickness spatial profile and corneal-volume distribution: tomographic indices to detect keratoconus. J Cataract Refract Surg. 2006;32(11):1851-9.
6. Ambrósio R Jr, Belin MW. Imaging of the cornea: topography vs tomography. J Refract Surg. 2010;26(11):847-9.
7. Ambrósio R Jr, Caiado AL, Guerra FP, et al. Novel pachymetric parameters based on corneal tomography for diagnosing keratoconus. J Refract Surg. 2011;27(10):753-8.
8. Ambrósio R Jr, de Oliveira Ramos IC, Luz A, et al. Comprehensive pachymetric evaluation. In: Belin MW, Khachikian SS, Ambrósio R Jr (Eds). Elevation Based Corneal Tomography, 2nd edition. Panama: Jaypee-Highlights Medical Publisher, Inc; 2012. pp. 25-45.
9. Ambrósio R Jr, Klyce SD, Wilson SE. Corneal topographic and pachymetric screening of keratorefractive patients. J Refract Surg. 2003;19(1):24-9.
10. American Academy of Ophthalmology. (2018). Zones of the Cornea. [online] Available from https://www.aao.org/bcscsnippetdetail.aspx?id=65c7bff9-4f1e-4717-8585-40318390fc7c [Accessed August 2018].
11. Amsler M. Keratocone classique et keratocone fruste, arguments unitaires. Ophthalmologica. 1946;111:96-101.
12. Amsler M. Le keratocone fruste au javal. Ophthalmologica. 1938;96:77-83.
13. Amsler M. The "forme fruste" of keratoconus. Wien Klin Wochenschr. 1961;73:842-3.
14. Arbelaez MC, Versaci F, Vestri G, et al. Use of a support vector machine for keratoconus and subclinical keratoconus detection by topographic and tomographic data. Ophthalmology. 2012;119(11):2231-8.
15. Armitage JA, Bruce AS, Philips AJ, et al. Morphological variants in keratoconus: Anatomical observation or aetiologically significant? Aust N Z J Ophthalmol. 1998;26 (Suppl 1):S68-70.
16. Baillif S, Garweg JG, Grange JD, et al. Keratoglobus: review of the literature. J Fr Ophthalmol. 2005;28:1145-9.
17. Barbara R, Castillo JH, Hanna R, et al. Keratoconus expert meeting, London, 2014. J Kerat Ect Cor Dis. 2014;3(3):141-58.
18. Basmak H, Sahin A, Yildirim N, et al. Measurement of angle kappa with synoptophore and Orbscan II in a normal population. J Refract Surg. 2007;23:456-60.
19. Basmak H, Sahin A, Yildirim N, et al. The angle kappa in strabismic individuals. Strabismus. 2007;15:193-6.
20. Beiko GH, Haigis W, Steinmueller A, et al. Distribution of corneal spherical aberration in a comprehensive ophthalmology practice and whether keratometry can predict aberration values. J Cataract Refract Surg. 2007;33(5):848-58.
21. Belin MW, Asota IM, Ambrósio R Jr, et al. What's in a name of: Keratoconus, pellucid marginal degeneration, and related thinning disorders. Am J Ophthalmol. 2011;152:157-62.
22. Belin MW, Khachikian SS, Ambrósio R Jr. Suggested set-up and screening guidelines. Elevation Based Corneal Tomography, 2nd edition. Panama: Jaypee Highlights Medical Publisher, Inc; 2012. pp. 57-69.
23. Belin MW, Khachikian SS, Ambrósio R Jr. Understanding elevation based topography: How elevation data is displayed. Elevation Based Corneal Tomography, 2nd edition. Panama: Jaypee Highlights Medical Publisher, Inc. 2012. pp. 25-45.
24. Belin MW, Khachikian SS. An introduction to understanding elevation based topography: How elevation data are displayed—a review. Clin Experiment Ophthalmol. 2009;37(1):14-29.

25. Belin MW, Khachikian SS. Introduction and overview. In: Belin MW, Khachikian SS, Ambrósio R Jr (Eds). Elevation Based Corneal Tomography, 2nd edition. Panama: Jaypee Highlights Medical Publisher, Inc; 2012. p. 2.
26. Belin MW, Khachikian SS. Keratoconus: It's hard to define, but. Am J Ophthalmol. 2007;43(3):500-3.
27. Belin MW, Kim JT, Zloty P, et al. Simplified nomenclature for describing keratoconus. Int J Kerat Ect Cor Dis. 2012;1(1):31-5.
28. Belin MW, Litoff D, Strods SJ, et al. The PAR technology corneal topography system. Refrac Corneal Surg. 1992;8:88-96.
29. Benes P, Synek S, Petrova S. Corneal shape and eccentricity in population. Coll Antropol. 2013;37(Suppl 1):117-20.
30. Berti T, Ghanem V, Ghanem R, et al. Moderate keratoconus with thick corneas. J Refract Surg. 2013;29:430-5.
31. Binder PS, Trattler WB. Evaluation of a risk factor scoring system for corneal ectasia after LASIK in eyes with normal topography. J Refract Surg. 2010;26(4):241-50.
32. Bogan SJ, Waring GO III, Ibrahim O, et al. Classification of normal corneal topography based on computer-assisted videokeratography. Arch Ophthalmol. 1990;108(7):945-9.
33. Boxer W, Huynh VN, El-Shiaty AF, et al. Evaluation of corneal functional optical zone after laser in situ keratomileusis. J Cataract Refract Surg. 2002;28:948-53.
34. Bühren J, Kook D, Yoon G, et al. Detection of subclinical keratoconus by using corneal anterior and posterior surface aberrations and thickness spatial proles. Invest Ophthalmol Vis Sci. 2010;51(7):3424-32.
35. Bühren J, Kuhne C, Kohnen T. Defining subclinical keratoconus using corneal first-surface higher-order aberrations. Am J Ophthalmol. 2007;143:381-9.
36. Bühren J, Kuhne C, Kohnen T. Wavefront analysis for the diagnosis of subclinical keratoconus. Ophthalmologe. 2006;103:783-90.
37. Butler TH. Two rare corneal conditions: I acute conical cornea II keratoconus posticus circumscriptus. Br J Ophthalmol. 1932;16(1):30-5.
38. Cameron JA, Al-Rajhi AA, Badr IA. Corneal ectasia in vernal keratoconjunctivitis. Ophthalmology. 1989;96(11):1615-23.
39. Cameron JA. Keratoglobus. Cornea. 1993;12(2):124-30.
40. Cavara V. Keratoglobus and keratoconus: A contribution to the nosological interpretation of keratoglobus. Br J Ophthalmol. 1950;34:621-6.
41. Chan JS, Mandell RB, Burger DS, et al. Accuracy of videokeratography for instantaneous radius in keratoconus. Optom Vis Sci. 1995;72:793-9.
42. Chang DH, Waring GO 4th. The subject-fixated coaxially sighted corneal light reflex: a clinical marker for centration of refractive treatments and devices. Am J Ophthalmol. 2014;158(5):863-74.
43. Chatzis N, Hafezi F. Progression of keratoconus and efficacy of pediatric corneal collagen cross-linking in children and adolescents. J Refract Surg. 2012;28(11):753-8.
44. Chen D, Lam AK. Intrasession and intersession repeatability of the Pentacam system on posterior corneal assessment in the normal human eye. J Cataract Refract Surg. 2007;33:448-54.
45. Choi JA, Kim MS. Progression of keratoconus by longitudinal assessment with corneal topography. Invest Ophthalmol Vis Sci. 2012;53(2):927-35.
46. Choi SR, Kim US. The correlation between Angle Kappa and ocular biometry in Koreans. Korean J Ophthalmol. 2013;27(6):421-4.
47. Correia FF, Ramos I, Lopes B, et al. Topometric and tomographic indices for the diagnosis of keratoconus. Int J Kerat Ect Cor Dis. 2012;1(2):92-9.
48. Dai G-M. Zernike aberration coefficients transformed to and from Fourier series coefficients for wavefront representation. Opt Lett. 2006;31:501-3.
49. De sanctis U, Loiacono C, Richiardi L, et al. Sensitivity and specificity of posterior corneal elevation measured by Pentacam in discriminating keratoconus/subclinical keratoconus. Ophthalmology. 2008;115(9):1534-9.
50. De Sanctis U, Missolungi A, Mutani B, et al. Reproducibility and repeatability of central corneal thickness measurement in keratoconus using the rotating Scheimpflug camera and ultrasound pachymetry. Am J Ophthalmol. 2007;144:712-8.
51. Dingeldein SA, Klyce SD. The topography of normal corneas. Arch Ophthalmol. 1989;107:512-8.
52. Dubbelman M, Weeber HA, van der Heijde RG, et al. Radius and asphericity of the posterior corneal surface determined by corrected Scheimpflug photography. Acta Ophthalmol Scand. 2002;80(4):379-83.
53. Epstein RL, Chiu YL, Epstein GL. Pentacam HR criteria for curvature change in keratoconus and postoperative LASIK ectasia. J Refract Surg. 2012;28(12):890-4.
54. Feizi S, Jafarinasab MR, Karimian F, et al. Central and peripheral corneal thickness measurement in normal and keratoconic eyes using three corneal pachymeters. J Ophthalmic Vis Res. 2014;9(3):296-304.
55. Feng MT, Kim JT, Ambrósio R Jr, et al. International values of central pachymetry in normal subjects by rotating scheimpflug camera. Asia Pac J Ophthalmol (Phila). 2012;1(1):13-8.

56. Ferris J. Gross structure. Basic Sciences in Ophthalmology: A Self Assessment Text, 2nd edition. United Kingdom: BMJ Publishing Group; 1999. p. 18.
57. Fityo S, Buhren J, Shajari M, et al. Keratometry versus total corneal refractive power: Analysis of measurement repeatability with 5 different devices in normal eyes with low astigmatism. J Cataract Refract Surg. 2016;42:569-76.
58. Galletti JD, Ruiseñor Vázquez PR, Minguez N, et al. Corneal asymmetry analysis by pentacam scheimpflug tomography for keratoconus diagnosis. J Refract Surg. 2015;31(2):116-23.
59. Gatinel D, Haouat M, Hoang-Xuan T. A review of mathematical descriptors of corneal asphericity. J Fr Ophtalmol. 2002;25:81-90.
60. Gatinel D, Malet J, Azar ST. Corneal elevation topography: Best fit sphere, elevation distance, asphericity, toricity and clinical implications. Cornea. 2011;30(5):508-15.
61. Gatinel D, Malet J, Hoang-Xuan T, et al. Analysis of customized corneal ablations: Theoretical limitations of increasing negative asphericity. Invest Ophthalmol Vis Sci. 2002;43:941-8.
62. Gatinel D, Malet J, Hoang-Xuan T, et al. Corneal asphericity change after excimer laser hyperopic surgery: theoretical effects on corneal profiles and corresponding Zernike expansions. Invest Ophthalmol Vis Sci. 2004;45:1349-59.
63. Gatinel D, Racine L, Hoang-Xuan T. Contribution of the corneal epithelium to anterior corneal topography in patients having myopic photorefractive keratectomy. J Cataract Refract Surg. 2007;33(11):1860-5.
64. Gatinel D, Saad A. The Challenges of the detection of subclinical keratoconus at its earliest stage. Int J Keratoco Ectatic Corneal Dis. 2012;1(1):36.
65. Gharaee H, Shafiee, M, Hoseini R, et al. Angle Kappa Measurements: Normal Values in Healthy Iranian Population Obtained With the Orbscan II. Iranian Red Crescent Med J. 2015;17(1):e17873.
66. Gobbe M, Guillon M. Corneal wavefront aberration measurements to detect keratoconus patients. Cont Lens Anterior Eye. 2005;28:57-66.
67. Gomes JA, Tan D, Rapuano CJ, et al. Global consensus on keratoconus and ectatic disease. Cornea. 2015;34:359-69.
68. Gregoratos ND, Bartsocas CS, Papas K. Blue sclerae with keratoglobus and brittle cornea. Br J Ophthalmol. 1971;55(6):424-6.
69. Gridley MJ, Perlman EM. A form of variable astigmatism induced by pseudo pterygium. Ophthalmic Surg. 1986;17:794-5.
70. Gruenauer-Kloevekorn C, Fischer U, Kloevekorn-Norgall K, et al. Pellucid marginal corneal degeneration: Evaluation of the corneal surface and contact lens fitting. Br J Ophthalmol. 2006;90:318-23.
71. Guber I, McAlinden C, Majo F, et al. Identifying more reliable parameters for the detection of change during the follow-up of mild to moderate keratoconus patients. Eye Vis (Lond). 2017;4:24.
72. Gudmundsdottir E, Arnarsson A, Jonasson F. Five-year refractive changes in an adult population: Reykjavik Eye Study. Ophthalmology. 2005;112:672-7.
73. Guilbert E, Saad A, Grise-Dulac A, et al. Corneal thickness, curvature, and elevation readings in normal corneas: Combined Placido–Scheimpflug system versus combined Placido–scanning-slit system. J Cataract Refract Surg. 2012;38(7):1198-206.
74. Guillon M, Lydon DP, Wilson C. Corneal topography: A clinical model. Ophthalmic Physiol Opt. 1986;6:47-56.
75. Hall JN. Inter-rater reliability of ward rating scales. Br J Psychiatry. 1974;125:248-55.
76. Hansen A, Norn M. Astigmatism and surface phenomena in pterygium. Acta Ophthalmol. 1980;58:174-81.
77. Haouat M, Gatinel D, Duong MH, et al. Corneal asphericity in myopes. J Fr Ophtalmol. 2002;25:488-92.
78. Harvey EM, Dobson V, Miller JM. Prevalence of high astigmatism, eyeglass wear, and poor visual acuity among Native American grade school children. Optom Vis Sci. 2006;83:206-12.
79. Harvey W, Gilmartin B. Paediatric Optometry. Edinburg: Butterworth-Heinemann; 2004. p. 47.
80. Hashemi H, Beiranvand A, Yekta A, et al. Pentacam top indices for diagnosing subclinical and definite keratoconus. J Current Ophthalmology. 2016;28:21-6.
81. Hashemi H, Khabazkhoob M, Yazdani K, et al. Distribution of angle kappa measurements with Orbscan II in a population-based survey. J Refract Surg. 2010;26:966-71.
82. Hashemi H, Yekta A, Khabazkhoob M. Effect of keratoconus grades on repeatability of keratometry readings: Comparison of 5 devices. J Cataract Refract Surg. 2015;41:1065-72.
83. Hayashi K, Hayashi H, Nakao F, et al. Correlation between pupillary size and intraocular lens decentration and visual acuity of a zonal-progressive multifocal lens and a monofocal lens. Ophthalmology. 2001;108:2011-7.
84. Hick S, Laliberté JF, Meunier J, et al. Effects of misalignment during corneal topography. J Cataract Refract Surg. 2007;33(9):1522-9.
85. Holden BA, Sweeney DF, Vannas A, et al. Effect of long-term extended contact lens wear on the human cornea. Invest Ophthalmol Vis Sci. 1985;26:1489-501.

86. Holladay JT. Holladay Report Interpretation Guidelines 2016. Oculus;2016:pp.1-14.
87. Holladay JT, Hill WE, Steinmueller A. Corneal power measurements using scheimpflug imaging in eyes with prior corneal refractive surgery. J Refract Surg. 2009;25:863-8.
88. Holladay JT, Janes JA. Topographic changes in corneal asphericity and effective optical zone after laser in situ keratomileusis. J Cataract Refract Surg. 2002;28:942-7.
89. Holladay JT. Accuracy of Scheimpflug Holladay equivalent keratometry readings after corneal refractive surgery. J Cataract Refract Surg. 2010;36:182-3.
90. Holladay JT. Automated keratometry in routine cataract surgery: Comparison of Scheimpflug and conventional values. J Cataract Refract Surg. 2011;37:1738-9.
91. Holladay JT. Corneal topography using the Holladay Diagnostic Summary. J Cataract Refract Surg. 1997;23:209-21.
92. Holladay JT. Detecting Forme Fruste Keratoconus with the Pentacam. J Cataract Refract Surg. 2008;11:12.
93. Holladay JT. Effect of corneal asphericity and spherical aberration on intraocular lens power calculations. J Cataract Refract Surg. 2015;41(7):1553-4.
94. Holladay JT. Exact toric IOL calculations using currently available lens constants. Arch Ophthalmol. 2012;130(7):946-7.
95. Holladay JT. Quality of vision: Essential optics for the cataract and refractive surgeon. Thorofare: Slack; 2007. pp. 32-4.
96. Hoogewoud F, Gatzioufas Z, Hafezi F. Transitory topographical variations in keratoconus during pregnancy. J Refract Surg. 2013;29(2):144-6.
97. Huang J, Savini G, Hu L, et al. Precision of a new Scheimpflug and Placido-disk analyzer in measuring corneal thickness and agreement with ultrasound pachymetry. J Cataract Refract Surg. 2013;39(2):219-24.
98. Ishii R, Kamiya K, Igarashi A, et al. Correlation of corneal elevation with severity of keratoconus by means of anterior and posterior topographic analysis. Cornea. 2012;31(3):253-8.
99. Jacq PL, Sale Y, Cochener B, et al. Keratoconus, changes in corneal topography and allergy. Study of 3 groups of patients. J Fr Ophtalmol. 1997;20(2):97-102.
100. Jafri B, Li X, Yang H, et al. Higher order wavefront aberrations and topography in early and suspected keratoconus. J Refract Surg. 2007;23(8):774-81.
101. Jimenez JR, Anera RG, Diaz JA, et al. Corneal asphericity after refractive surgery when the Munnerlyn formula is applied. J Opt Soc Am A Opt Image Sci Vis. 2004;21:98-103.
102. Jinabhai A, Radhakrishnan H, O'Donnell C. Pellucid corneal marginal degeneration: a review. Cont Lens Ant Eye. 2011;34:56-63.
103. Jones-Jordan LA, Walline JJ, Sinnott LT, et al. Asymmetry in keratoconus and vision-related quality of life. Cornea. 2013;32(3):267-72.
104. Kanellopoulos AJ, Asimellis G. Revisiting keratoconus diagnosis and progression classification based on evaluation of corneal asymmetry indices, derived from Scheimpflug imaging in keratoconic and suspect cases. Clinical Ophthalmology. 2013;7:1539-48.
105. Kanellopoulos AJ, Moustou V, Asimellis G. Evaluation of visual acuity, pachymetry and anterior-surface irregularity in keratoconus and cross-linking intervention follow-up in 737 cases. J Kerat Ect Cor Dis. 2013;2(3):95-103.
106. Karabatsas CH, Cook SD. Topographic analysis in pellucid marginal corneal degeneration and keratoglobus. Eye. 1996;10(Pt 4):451-5.
107. Karhanova M, Jaresova K, Pluhacek F, et al. The importance of angle kappa for centration of multifocal IOLs. Cesk Slov Oftalmol. 2013;69(2):64-8.
108. Kennedy RH, Bourne WM, Dyer JA. A 48-year clinical and epidemiologic study of keratoconus. Am J Ophthalmol. 1986;101:267-73.
109. Kermani O, Schmeidt K, Oberheide U, et al. Hyperopic laser in situ keratomileusis with 5.5-, 6.5-, and 7.0-mm optical zones. J Refract Surg. 2005;21:52-8.
110. Khachikian SS, Belin MW, Ambrósio R Jr. Normative data for the oculus pentacam. Elevation Based Corneal Tomography, 2nd edition. Panama: Jaypee Highlights Medical Publisher, Inc; 2012. pp. 71-9.
111. Kiely PM, Carney LG, Smith G. Diurnal variations of corneal topography and thickness. Am J Optom Physiol Opt. 1982;59:976-82.
112. Kim H, Joo CK. Measure of keratoconus progression using Orbscan II. J Refract Surg. 2008;24(6):600-5.
113. Klyce SD, Karon MD, Smolek MK. Advantages and disadvantages of the Zernike expansion for representing wave aberration of the normal and aberrated eye. J Refract Surg. 2004;20:S537-41.
114. Klyce SD, Smolek MK, Maeda N. Keratoconus detection with the KISA% method-another view. J Cataract Refract Surg. 2000;26:472-4.

115. Klyce SD. Chasing the suspect: Keratoconus. Br J Ophthalmol. 2009;93:845-7.
116. Koch DD, Ali SF, Weikert MP, et al. Contribution of posterior corneal astigmatism to total corneal astigmatism. J Cataract Refract Surg. 2012;38(12):2080-7.
117. Kompella VB, Aasuri MK, Rao GN. Management of pellucid marginal corneal degeneration with rigid gas permeable contact lenses. CLAO J. 2002;28:140-5.
118. Krachmer JH, Feder RS, Belin MW. Keratoconus and related non-inflammatory corneal thinning disorders. Surv Ophthalmol. 1984;28:293-322.
119. Krachmer JH. Pellucid marginal corneal degeneration. Arch Ophthalmol. 1978;96:1217-21.
120. Krumeich JH, Daniel J, Knull A. Live-epikeratophakia for keratoconus. J Cataract Refract Surg. 1998;24:456-63.
121. Labiris G, Giarmoukakis A, Sideroudi H, et al. Variability in Scheimpflug image-derived posterior elevation measurements in keratoconus and collagen-crosslinked corneas. J Cataract Refract Surg. 2012;38:1616-25.
122. Lee BW, Jurkunas UV, Harissi-Dagner M, et al. Ectatic disorders associated with a claw-shaped pattern on corneal topography. Am J Ophthalmol. 2007;144(1):154-6.
123. Levy D, Hutchings H, Rouland JF, et al. Videokeratographic anomalies in familial keratoconus. Ophthalmology. 2004;111(5):867-74.
124. Li X, Rabinowitz YS, Rasheed K, et al. Longitudinal study of the normal eyes in unilateral keratoconus patients. Ophthalmology. 2004;111(3):440-6.
125. Li X, Yang H, Rabinowitz YS. Keratoconus: classification scheme based on Videokeratography and clinical signs. J Cataract Refract Surg. 2009;35(9):1597-603.
126. Li Y, Shekhar R, Huang D. Corneal pachymetry mapping with high-speed optical coherence tomography. Ophthalmology. 2006;113(5):792-9.
127. Li Y, Tang M, Zhang X, et al. Pachymetric mapping with Fourier domain optical coherence tomography. J Cataract Refract Surg. 2010;36(5):826-31.
128. Lim L, Wei RH, Chan WK, et al. Evaluations of keratoconus in Asians: Role of Orbscan II and Tomey TMS-2 corneal topography. Am J Ophthalmol. 2007;143:390-400.
129. Litoff D, Belin MW, Winn SS, et al. PAR technology corneal topography system. Inv Ophthalmol Vis Sci. 1991;32:922.
130. Liu Z, Pflugfelder SC. The effects of long-term contact lens wear on corneal thickness, curvature and surface regularity. Ophthalmology. 2000;107:105-11.
131. Lopes BT, Ramos IC, Faria-Correia F, et al. Correlation of topometric and tomographic indices with visual acuity in patients with keratoconus. J Kerat Ect Cor Dis. 2012;1(3):167-72.
132. Maeda N, Klyce SD, Smolek MK, et al. Automated keratoconus screening with corneal topography analysis. Invest Ophthalmol Vis Sci. 1994;35(6):2749-57.
133. Maguire LJ, Klyce SD, McDonald MB, et al. Corneal topography of pellucid marginal degeneration. Ophthalmology. 1987;94:519-24.
134. Mahmoud AM, Nuñez MX, Blanco C, et al. Expanding the cone location and magnitude index to include corneal thickness and posterior surface information for the detection of keratoconus. Am J Ophthalmol. 2013;156(6):1102-11.
135. Mahmoud AM, Roberts CJ, Herderick EE, et al. The cone location and magnitude index (CLMI). Invest Ophthalmol Vis Sci. 2005;82:1038-46.
136. Mahmoud AM, Roberts CJ, Lembach RG. CLMI: the cone location and magnitude index. Cornea. 2008;27(4):480-7.
137. Mahon L, Kent D. Can true monocular keratoconus occur? Clin Exp Optom. 2004;87:126.
138. Miller D, Gurland JE, Isby EK, et al. Human eye as an optical system. In: American Academy of Ophthalmology Basic and Clinical Sciences Course. San Francisco: American Academy of Ophthalmology; 1988-1990. pp. 108-9.
139. Miranda MA, Radhakrishnan H, O'donnell C. Repeatability of oculus pentacam metrics derived from corneal topography. Cornea. 2009;28:657-66.
140. Moshirfar M, Edmonds JN, Behunin NL, et al. Current options in the management of pellucid marginal degeneration. J Refract Surg. 2014;30(7):474-85.
141. Mosquera SA, Verma S, McAlinden C. Centration axis in refractive surgery. Eye Vis. 2015;2:4.
142. Muftuoglo O, Ayar O, Ozulken K, et al. Posterior corneal elevation and back difference corneal elevation in diagnosing forme fruste keratoconus in the fellow eyes of unilateral keratoconus patients. J Cataract Refract Surg. 2013;39:1348-57.
143. Muftuoglu O, Ayar O, Hurmeric V, et al. Comparison of multimetric D index with keratometric, pachymetric, and posterior elevation parameters in diagnosing subclinical keratoconus in fellow eyes of asymmetric keratoconus patients. J Cataract Refract Surg. 2015;41:557-65.

144. Mularoni A, Torreggiani A, di Biase A, et al. Conservative treatment of early and moderate pellucid marginal degeneration: a new refractive approach with intracorneal rings. Ophthalmology. 2005;112:660-6.
145. Murta J, Rosa AM. Measurement and topography guided treatment of irregular astigmatism. In: Goggin M (Ed). Astigmatism—Optics, Physiology and Management. Croatia: InTech; 2012. pp. 247-66.
146. Nilforoushan MR, Speaker M, Marmor M. Comparative evaluation of refractive surgery candidates with Placido topography, Orbscan II, Pentacam, and wavefront analysis. J Cataract Refract Surg. 2008;34:623-31.
147. O'Brart DP, Chan E, Samaras K, et al. A randomized, prospective study to investigate the efficacy of riboflavin/ultraviolet A (370 nm) corneal collagen cross-linking to halt progression of keratoconus. Br J Ophthalmol. 2011;95:1519-24.
148. O'Donnell C, Maldonado-Codina C. Agreement and repeatability of central thickness measurement in normal corneas using ultra-sound pachymetry and the OCULUS Pentacam. Cornea. 2005;24:920-4.
149. OCULUS. (2018). The topography maps of the Pentacam®. [online] Available from https://www.pentacam.com/int/technology/topography-maps.html [Accessed August 2018].
150. Oldenburg JB, Garbus J, McDonnell JM, et al. Conjunctival pterygia: Mechanism of corneal topographic changes. Cornea. 1990;9:200-4.
151. Oner FH, Kaderli B, Durak I, et al. Analysis of the pterygium size inducing marked refractive astigmatism. Eur J Ophthalmol. 2000;10:212-4.
152. Ozdemir M, Cinal A. Early and late effects of pterygium surgery on corneal topography. Ophthalmic Surg Las Imag. 2005;36:451-6.
153. Pande M, Hillman JS. Optical zone centration in keratorefractive surgery. Entrance pupil center, visual axis, coaxially sighted corneal reflex, or geometric corneal center? Ophthalmology. 1993;100:1230-7.
154. Park CY, Oh SY, Chuck RS. Measurement of angle kappa and centration in refractive surgery. Curr Opin Ophthalmol. 2012;23:269-75.
155. Perry HD, Buxton JN, Fine BS. Round and oval cones in keratoconus. Ophthalmology. 1998;87(9):905-9.
156. Pouliquen Y, Dhermy P, Espinasse MA, et al. Keratoglobus. J Fr Ophthalmol. 1985;8(1):43-5.
157. Prakash G, Prakash DR, Agarwal A, et al. Predictive factor and kappa angle analysis for visual satisfactions in patients with multifocal IOL implantation. Eye (Lond). 2011;25(9):1187-93.
158. Rabinowitz YS, Garbus J, McDonnell PJ. Computer-assisted corneal topography in family members of patients with keratoconus. Arch Ophthalmol. 1990;108(3):365-71.
159. Rabinowitz YS, Li X, Canedo ALC, et al. Optical coherence tomography (OCT) combined with videokeratography to differentiate mild keratoconus subtypes. J Refract Surg. 2014;30(2):80-7.
160. Rabinowitz YS, McDonnell PJ. Computer-assisted corneal topography in keratoconus. Refract Corneal Surg. 1989;5:400-8.
161. Rabinowitz YS, Nesburn AB, McDonnell PJ. Videokeratography of the fellow eye in unilateral keratoconus. Ophthalmology. 1993;100:181-6.
162. Rabinowitz YS, Rasheed K, Yang H, et al. Accuracy of ultrasonic pachymetry and videokeratography in detecting keratoconus. J Cataract Refract Surg. 1998;24(2):196-201.
163. Rabinowitz YS, Rasheed K. KISA% index: a quantitative videokeratography algorithm embodying minimal topographic criteria for diagnosing keratoconus. J Cataract Refract Surg. 1999;25:1327-35.
164. Rabinowitz YS, Yang H, Brickman Y, et al. Videokeratography database of normal human corneas. Br J Ophthalmol. 1996;80(7):610-6.
165. Rabinowitz YS. Keratoconus. Surv Ophthalmol. 1998;42(4):297-31.
166. Rabinowitz YS. Tangential vs sagittal videokeratographs in the "early" detection of keratoconus. Am J Ophthalmol. 1996;122(6):887-9.
167. Rabinowitz YS. Videokeratographic indices to aid in screening for keratoconus. J Refract Surg. 1995;11(5):371-9.
168. Ramos IC, Correa R, Guerra F, et al. Variability of subjective classifications of corneal maps from LASIK candidates. J Refract Surg. 2013;29(11):770-5.
169. Randleman JB, Trattler WB, Stulting RD. Validation of the Ectasia Risk Score System for preoperative laser in situ keratomileusis screening. Am J Ophthalmol. 2008;145(5):813-8.
170. Randleman JB. Etiology and clinical presentations of irregular astigmatism after keratorefractive surgery. In: Wang M (Ed). Irregular Astigmatism: Diagnosis and Treatment. Thorofare, NJ: Slack; 2008. pp. 73-84.
171. Rao SN, Raviv T, Majmudar PA, et al. Role of Orbscan II in screening keratoconus suspects before refractive corneal surgery. Ophthalmology. 2002;109:1642-6.
172. Rasheed K, Rabinowitz YS, Remba D, et al. Interobserver and intraobserver reliability of a classification scheme for corneal topographic patterns. Br J Ophthalmol. 1998;82:1401-6.

173. Rasheed K, Rabinowitz YS. Surgical treatment of advanced pellucid marginal degeneration. Ophthalmology. 2000;107:1836-40.
174. Read SA, Collins MJ, Carney LG. A review of astigmatism and its possible genesis. Clin Exp Optom. 2007;90(1):5-19.
175. Reinstein DZ, Gobbe M, Archer TJ. Anterior segment biometry: a study and review of resolution and repeatability data. J Refract Surg. 2012;28:509-20.
176. Robin JB, Schanzlin DJ, Verity SM, et al. Peripheral corneal disorders. Surv Ophthalmol. 1986;31:1-36.
177. Romero-Jimenez M, Santodomingo-Rubido J, Wolffsohn JS. Keratoconus: a review. Cont Lens Ant Eye. 2010;33:157-66.
178. Saad A, Gatinel D. Combining Placido and Corneal Wavefront Data for the Detection of Forme Fruste Keratoconus. J Refract Surg. 2016;32(8):510-6.
179. Saad A, Gatinel D. Evaluation of total and corneal wavefront high order aberrations for the detection of forme fruste keratoconus. Invest Ophthalmol Vis Sci. 2012;53(6):2978-92.
180. Saad A, Gatinel D. Topographic and tomographic properties of forme fruste keratoconus corneas. Invest Ophthalmol Vis Sci. 2010;51(11):5546-55.
181. Saad A, Gilbert E, Gatinel D. Corneal enantiomorphism in normal and keratoconic eyes. J Refract Surg. 2014;30(8):542-7.
182. Saad A, Lteif Y, Azan E, et al. Biomechanical properties of keratoconus suspect eyes. Invest Ophthalmol Vis Sci. 2010;51(6):2912-6.
183. Salabert D, Cochener B, Mage F, et al. Keratoconus and familial topographic corneal anomalies. J Fr Ophtalmol. 1994;17(11):646-56.
184. Saleh-Mabed I, Saad A, Gattine D. Topography of the corneal epithelium and Bowman Layer in low to moderately myopic eyes. J Cataract Refract Surg. 2016;42:1190-7.
185. Santhiago M, Giacomin NT, Smadja D, et al. Ectasia risk factors in refractive surgery. Clin Ophthalmol. 2016;10:713-20.
186. Santhiago MR, Smadja D, Wilson SE, et al. Role of percent tissue altered on ectasia after LASIK in eyes with suspicious topography. J Refract Surg. 2015;31(4):258-65.
187. Schlegel Z, Hoang-Xuan T, Gatinel D. Comparison of and correlation between anterior and posterior corneal elevation maps in normal eyes and keratoconus-suspect eyes. J Cataract Refract Surg. 2008;34(5):789-95.
188. Scholz K, Messner A, Eppig T, et al. Topography-based assessment of anterior corneal curvature and asphericity as a function of age, sex, and refractive status. J Cataract Refract Surg. 2009;35(6):1046-54.
189. Schwartz SH. Image formation: Point sources. Geometrical and Visual Optics: A Clinical Introduction, 2nd edition. USA: McGraw-Hill Education; 2013. p. 143.
190. Schweitzer C, Roberts CJ, Mahmoud AM, et al. Screening of forme fruste keratoconus with the ocular response analyzer. Invest Ophthalmol Vis Sci. 2010;51(5):2403-10.
191. Sefic kasumovic S, Racic-Sakovic A, Kasumovic A, et al. Assessment of the tomographic values in keratoconic eyes after collagen crosslinking procedure. Med Arch. 2015;69(2):91-4.
192. Seiler T, Quurke AW. Iatrogenic keratectasia after LASIK in a case of forme fruste keratoconus. J Cataract Refract Surg. 1998;24:1007-9.
193. Seitz B. Astigmatism after keratoplasty: prophylaxis and therapy. Ocular Surgery News US Edition;2000.
194. Shankar H, Taranath D, Santhirathelagan CT, et al. Anterior segment biometry with the Pentacam: comprehensive assessment of repeatability of automated measurements. J Cataract Refract Surg. 2008;34:103-13.
195. Shirayama-Suzuki M, Amano S, Honda N, et al. Longitudinal analysis of corneal topography in suspect keratoconus. Br J Ophthalmol. 2009;93:815-19.
196. Sideroudi H, Labiris G, Giarmoukakis A, et al. Contribution of reference bodies in diagnosis of keratoconus. Optom Vis Sci. 2014;91:676-81.
197. Sinjab MM, Cummings AB. Introduction to wavefront science. In: Sinjab MM, Cummings AB (Eds). Customized Laser Vision Correction. Heidelberg, Germany: Springer; 2018. pp. 65-93.
198. Sinjab MM, Youssef LN. Pellucid-like keratoconus. F1000Res. 2012;1:48.
199. Sinjab MM. A 12-point Algorithm to Master Corneal Tomography. CRSTEurope; 2017.
200. Sinjab MM. Classifications and patterns of keratoconus and keratectasia. Quick Guide to the Management of Keratoconus. Heidelberg, Germany: Springer; 2012. pp. 13-57.
201. Sinjab MM. Diagnosis of Keratoconus. Quick guide to the management of keratoconus. Heidelberg, Germany: Springer; 2012. pp. 1-11.
202. Sinjab MM. Introduction to astigmatism and corneal irregularitits. In: Sinjab MM, Cummings AB (Eds). Customized Laser Vision Correction. Heidelberg, Germany: Springer; 2018. pp. 1-64.
203. Sinjab MM. Patterns and classifications in ectatic corneal diseases. In: Sinjab MM, Cummings AB (Eds). Corneal Collagen Cross Linking. Heidelberg, Germany: Springer; 2017. pp. 23-62.

204. Skuta GL, Cantor LB, Weiss JS. Refractive surgery. In: American Academy of Ophthalmology Basic and Clinical Sciences Course. San Francisco: American Academy of Ophthalmology; 2011-2012. pp. 45-6.
205. Smadja D, Touboul D, Cohen A, et al. Decision of subclinical keratoconus using an automated decision tree classification. Am J Ophthalmol. 2013;156:237-46.
206. Smolek MK, Klyce SD, Hovis JK. The universal standard scale: proposed improvements to the American National Standard Institute (ANSI) scale for corneal topography. Ophthalmology. 2002;109:361-9.
207. Smolek MK, Klyce SD. Current keratoconus detection methods compared with a neural network approach. Invest Ophthalmol Vis Sci. 1997;38(11):2290-9.
208. Smolek MK, Klyce SD. Zernike polynomial fitting fails to represent all visually significant corneal aberrations. Invest Ophthalmol Vis Sci. 2003;44:4676-81.
209. Smolek, MK, Klyce SD. Goodness-of-prediction of Zernike polynomial fitting to corneal surfaces. J Cataract Refract Surg. 2005;31:2350-5.
210. Sorbara L, Dalton K. The use of videokeratoscopy in predicting contact lens parameters for keratoconic fitting. Cont Lens Anterior Eye. 2010;33(3):112-8.
211. Sparrow JM, Ayliffe W, Bron A, et al. Inter-observer and intra-observer variability of the Oxford clinical cataract classification and grading system. Int Ophthalmol. 1988;11:151-7.
212. Sridhar MS, Mahesh S, Bansal AK, et al. Pellucid marginal corneal degeneration. Ophthalmology. 2004;111:1102-7.
213. Srivannaboon S, Chotikavanich S. Corneal characteristics in myopic patients. J Med Assoc Thai. 2005;88:1222-7.
214. Stuphin JE. External diseases and cornea. In: American Academy of Ophthalmology Basic and Clinical Sciences Course. San Francisco: American Academy of Ophthalmology; 2006-2007.
215. Suzuki M, Amano S, Honda N, et al. Longitudinal changes in corneal irregular astigmatism and visual acuity in eyes with keratoconus. Jpn J Ophthalmol. 2007;51(4):265-9.
216. Swartz T, Duplessie M, Munir W, et al. Non ectatic corneal problems causing irregular astigmatism. In: Wang M (Ed). Irregular Astigmatism: Diagnosis and Treatment. Thorofare, NJ: Slack; 2008. pp. 145-73.
217. Sykakis E, Karim R, Evans JR, et al. Corneal collagen cross-linking for treating keratoconus. Cochrane Database Syst Rev. 2015;(3):CD010621.
218. Symes RJ, Ursell PC. Automated keratometry in routine cataract surgery: Comparison of Scheimpflug and conventional values. J Cataract Refract Surg. 2011;37:295-301.
219. Szczotka LB, Rabinowitz YS, Yang H. Influence of contact lens wear on the corneal topography of keratoconus. CLAO J. 1996;22:270-3.
220. Szczotka LB, Thomas J. Comparison of axial and instantaneous videokeratographic data in keratoconus and utility in contact lens curvature prediction. CLAO J. 1998;24:22-8.
221. Taglia DP, Sugar J. Superior pellucid marginal corneal degeneration with hydrops. Arch Ophthalmol. 1997;115:274-5.
222. Tomidokoro A, Oshika T, Amano S, et al. Changes in anterior and posterior corneal curvatures in keratoconus. Ophthalmology. 2000;107(7):1328-32.
223. Tomidokoro A, Oshika T, Amano S, et al. Quantitative analysis of regular and irregular astigmatism induced by pterygium. Cornea. 1999;18:412-5.
224. Tummanapalli SS, Maseedupally V, Mandathara P, et al. Evaluation of corneal elevation and thickness indices in pellucid marginal degeneration and keratoconus. J Cataract Refract Surg. 2013;39:56-65.
225. Twa MD, Parthasarathy S, Roberts C, et al. Automated decision tree classification of corneal shape. Optom Vis Sci. 2005;82:1038-46.
226. Tzelikis PF, Cohen EJ, Rapuano CJ, et al. Management of pellucid marginal corneal degeneration. Cornea. 2005;24:555-60.
227. Uçakhan ÖÖ, Cetinkor V, Özkan M, et al. Evaluation of Scheimpflug imaging parameters in subclinical keratoconus, keratoconus, and normal eyes. J Cataract Refract Surg. 2011;37:1116-24.
228. Uçakhan OO, Ozkan M, Kanpolat A. Corneal thickness measurements in normal and keratoconic eyes: Pentacam comprehensive eye scanner versus noncontact specular microscopy and ultrasound pachymetry. J Cataract Refract Surg. 2006;32:970-7.
229. Verrey K. Keratoglobe aigu. Ophthalmologica. 1947;114:284-8.
230. Vianna LM, Muñoz B, Hwang FS, et al. Variability in Oculus Pentacam tomographer measurements in patients with keratoconus. Cornea. 2015;34(3):285-9.
231. Walker RN, Khachikian SS, Belin MW. Scheimpflug imaging of pellucid marginal degeneration. Cornea. 2008;27(8):963-6.
232. Walland MJ, Stevens JD, Steele AD. The effect of recurrent pterygium on corneal topography. Cornea. 1994;13:463-4.

233. Wallang BS, Das S. Keratoglobus. Eye. 2013;27(9):1004-12.
234. Wang L, Koch DD. Custom optimization of intraocular lens asphericity. J Cataract Refract Surg. 2007;33:1713-20.
235. Wang X, McCulley JP, Bowman RW, et al. Time to resolution of contact lens-induced corneal warpage prior to refractive surgery. CLAO J. 2002;28(4):169-71.
236. Waring GO, Rabinowitz YS, Sugar J, et al. Nomenclature for keratoconus suspects. Refract Corneal Surg. 1993;9(3):219-22.
237. WaveLight GmbH. WaveLight® Allegro Oculyzer™ 1074 User Manual (English). Erlangen: WaveLight GmbH; 2001.
238. Williams R. Acquired posterior keratoconus. Br J Ophthalmol. 1987;71(1):16-7.
239. Wilson SE, Klyce SD, Husseini ZM. Standardized color-coded maps for corneal topography. Ophthalmology. 1993;100(11):1723-7.
240. Wittig-silva C, Chan E, Islam FM, et al. A randomized, controlled trial of corneal collagen cross-linking in progressive keratoconus: three-year results. Ophthalmology. 2014;121(4):812-21.
241. Wonneberger W, Sterner B, MacLean U, et al. Repeated same-day versus single tomography measurements of keratoconic eyes for analysis of disease progression. Cornea. 2018;37(4):474-9.
242. Zadnik K, Steger-May K, Fink BA, et al. Between-eye asymmetry in keratoconus. Cornea. 2002;21(7):671-9.
243. Ziemer Ophthalmic Systems AG. ZIEMER® GALILEI™ Software Version 5.2 Upgrade Information Package. Ziemer Ophthalmic Systems AG; 2010.

Index

Page numbers followed by *f* refer to figure and *t* refer to table.

A

Aberration 117*f*
   analysis of 131
   coma-like 120
   compensation, internal 120
   constant 122
   fourth order 129
   higher order 56, 107, 108, 118, 122, 124*f*, 125*f*, 129, 223
   lower-order 91, 123
   measurement of 118
   residual higher-order 137
   third order 129
   types of 118
   wavefront 117, 119
   with age, changes of 120
   Zernike description of 122, 123*t*
Aberrometers 118
   ingoing
      feedback 118
      reflective 118
   outgoing reflective 118
Aberrometry 223
   in cataract surgery 223
   wavefront 102
Achromatic axis 3
Alio-Shabayek
   classification 178*t*
   modification 177
Amsler-Krumeich
   classification 177, 177*t*
   grading system 177
   standards 178*t*
Angulated patterns 46
Anisometropia 101, 102*f*
Arcuate incision 224*f*
Asphericity
   patterns of 83
   posterior surface 120

Astigmatic aberration 129
Astigmatic cornea, normal high 210*f*
Astigmatic disparity, probabilities of 110*t*
Astigmatic dissociation 108, 146
   etiology 108
   types of 109
Astigmatic keratotomy 149, 225
Astigmatic lower-order aberration 130*f*
Astigmatism 33, 91
   against-the-rule 45, 45*f*, 52, 92
   axis of 13
   bioblique 226
   classifications of 91
   clinical manifest 108
   compound 91
   etiology of irregular 93
   evaluation of irregular 100
   mixed 92
      irregular 93, 94*f*
   posterior surface 149
   secondary 131, 135*f*
   simple 91
   tomographic 108, 110-113
   topographic 110
   unusual manifest 100
Asymmetric bowtie
   inferior steep 46*f*
   superior steep 46*f*
Asymmetric patterns 45

B

Belin ABCD keratoconus staging 161, 178, 179*t*, 184
Belin Ambrósio display 161, 168, 191, 194*f*, 197*f*, 199
   map 193
Belin/Ambrosio ectasia display 60, 61*f*-65*f*
Belin/Ambrosio enhanced ectasia 60, 60*f*
   applications of 66

Bell pattern 68*f*
Bent frown incision 224*f*
Best fit ellipsoid 56, 57*f*
Best fit sphere 53, 57*f*, 82
Best fit toric ellipsoid 56, 57*f*
Butterfly 48*f*

C

Camera, bad exposure to 23, 152
Cataract 109
   incision
      location of 224
      shape of 224
      size of 224
      type of 224
   surgery 41, 149
Central flat island 96*f*
Central steep island 96*f*
Chamber angle, anterior 35
Chamber depth
   anterior 35
   range, anterior 13
Chamber volume, anterior 35
Circular pattern 67*f*
Clown face 49*f*
Color map appearance 13
Color scale 17
   types of 17
Coma 129, 133*f*
   aberration, comet from 134*f*
Cone 10
Contact lens 23, 143
   soft 100*f*, 143, 144*f*
Conventional camera, imaging in 11*f*
Cornea 40, 50*f*, 214
   abnormal 167*t*, 176
   apparently normal 176
   back, posterior surface 34

Fourier analysis of normal 140f
front, anterior surface 33
Guttata and Fuchs' dystrophy 225
hyperprolate 84
infracentral 226
normal 86f, 176, 180f
   high-astigmatic 211
   low astigmatic 212, 213f
   thin 169f
oblate 84, 85
optical center of 209
peripheral 220
prolate 84
   shape of 131
thickness spatial profile 183
unclassified abnormal 176
volume 35
with abnormal elevation maps 64f
with high potential 167, 176
with normal elevation maps 63f
with suspicious posterior elevation map 65f
Corneal aberration 120
   compensation 120
Corneal aberrometry in cataract surgery 223
Corneal and pupillary level 119
Corneal apex 6
Corneal asphericity 6, 82, 83f
   affects 83
   in emmetropia 83
   in hypermetropia 84
   in myopia 84
   on curvature maps 84
   on elevation maps 84
   on refraction, effect of 83
   on vision, effect of 83
Corneal astigmatism 52, 52f, 58f, 91, 105, 137
   orientation of 45f
   regular 52f
   source of 6
Corneal asymmetry 85, 87f
   horizontal 86f
   on curvature maps 86
   on elevation maps 86
Corneal changes with age 120
Corneal coma 137
Corneal cross-linking 181
Corneal curvature 152
   map, patterns of 43
   patterns of 43

Corneal dimensions 4
Corneal dioptric power 137
   calculating objective 103
   objective 103
Corneal disease 99
   ectatic 87f
Corneal epithelium 6
   on corneal shape, effect of 6f
Corneal flattening, postoperative 226
Corneal geometry 4, 8
   measuring 8
   of right eye 4f
Corneal graft 149, 203
   after removal 98f
   before suture removal 97f
Corneal induced irregular astigmatism 94
Corneal irregular astigmatism, nonectatic 94
Corneal irregularities 96t
   reduces 6f
Corneal landmarks 34, 34f
Corneal maps and profiles 31
Corneal opacities 23, 149
Corneal optics and geometry 3
Corneal parameters 33, 34f
   consists of 33
Corneal pathologies 149
Corneal periphery 22f, 194
Corneal power 6
   maps 36
      measurements of 38, 38t
      measurement, factors affecting 36
Corneal refraction, understanding 89
Corneal refractive
   power map, total 41
   power, total 108
   principle, total 42f
Corneal scar 69f-73f, 224
   peripheral 99f
Corneal shape 5, 82
   left eye 5f
   oblate 37f
Corneal sphere 137
Corneal steepening
   incision-related 226f
   postoperative 226
   wound-related 226
Corneal surface
   anterior 6, 36, 120, 182
   posterior 4f, 34, 36
Corneal surgeries 149
   previous 149

Corneal thickness 5, 152, 168, 183
   central 183, 184
   map 25f, 67, 162, 209
      limitations 69
      overlay for 30f
      patterns 67
      principle 67
   profiles 67, 163, 183
   spatial profile 67, 73, 74f
      patterns 73
      principle 73
   thinnest 183, 214
Corneal tomography 102, 118, 165, 223
   role of 223
Corneal topography 102
Corneal topometry 82
   anterior 192, 193f, 195, 196f, 199f
Corneal toricity 82
   on curvature maps 82
   on elevation maps 82
Corneal trauma 98
Corneal warpage 143
Corneal wavefront 119
   aberrations 118
   Fourier analysis of 137, 138f
Corneal zones 5
Corrected distance visual acuity 101, 111, 170, 178, 225
Crab claw 48f
Crystalline lens 94
   changes with age 120
Curvature
   based devices (topographers) 8
   based topography, limitations of 10
   color scales for 20f
   minimum radius of 179
   posterior radius of 179, 184
   radius of 5, 13
Curvature map 59, 59f
   anterior 194, 196
      sagittal 21f, 38, 44f
      tangential 39
   changes in 145
   overlay 20
   sagittal and tangential 47
Cycloplegic refraction 107

D

Decentered ablated zone 95f
Decentration 137

Defocus 128*f*
    and pupil size 129*f*
Dioptric power, spherocylindric 103
Discrete pattern 202*f*
Droplet pattern 69, 69*f*
Dry eye 223
    caused by 100*f*
Duochrome test 113

E

Ectasia 66, 167, 194*f*, 195
    established 167
    progressive posterior 184
Ectatic corneal disease 61, 83, 86*f*, 98, 103, 143, 165, 167, 167*t*, 177, 181, 182*t*, 191, 223
    curvature asymmetry in 86*f*
    grading systems of 177
    per se 167
Ectatic corneal irregular astigmatism 94
Efficient optical zone 193*f*
Elevation maps 51, 59, 59*f*, 61*f*, 212
    anterior 192, 194, 196, 198*f*
    changes in 145
    color
        display in 55*f*
        scale of 51*f*
    irregular patterns on 58*f*
    overlay 23
    principle of 51, 51*f*
Elevation-based devices (tomographers) 10
Ellipse
    blue 54*f*
    red 54*f*
Emmetropic eyes 119
Enantiomorphism 153, 154*f*, 155*f*
    in anterior elevation maps 156*f*
    in curvature maps 156*f*
    in posterior elevation maps 157*f*
    in thickness maps 157*f*
Endothelium 13
Entities misdiagnosed ectasia 191
Epithelial basement membrane dystrophy 223
Examiner's error misalignment 144
Excess tears 152*f*
Eye
    for capture, preparing 23
    normal 61
    superior view of right 3*f*
    wavefront aberrations 118

F

Flat slope 73, 78*f*
Focal corneal opacities 199
Focal point 3*f*
Forme fruste keratoconus 66, 167, 207
Fourier analysis
    decentration component in 139*f*
    irregularity component in 139*f*
    spherical component in 139*f*
Fourier transform 137
Foveola 3*f*
Fuchs' endothelial dystrophy, diagnosis of 67

G

Geometric tomography 82
Geometrical landmarks 6*f*
Ghost images 131*f*
Glare 131*f*
Globus pattern 69, 69*f*

H

Halos 131*f*
Headscarves, tight 152
Height asymmetry, index of 182, 183
Height decentration, index of 183
Herpetic disease 99, 100
Holladay report 207, 208*f*, 210*f*
    general settings for 30*f*
    specific settings for 25
Hot spot pattern 202*f*
Hourglass 52
    shape 52*f*
Human eye 129
    aberrations 118
    optical system of 3
Hybrid devices 12
Hypermetropic correction 195
Hyperopic population 58*t*
Hyperopic shift 143
Hyperprolate cornea 85*f*
    shape 37*f*
Hyperprolate surface 83
Hypertrophy 99

I

Image quality control 160
    purpose 160
    steps 160
Incision, dimensions of 225*f*
Intereye asymmetry 25, 146, 163
Intereye corneal asymmetry score 153*t*
Intracorneal rings 67, 191
    implantation 199
Intraocular lens 38, 207, 223
    aspheric 224
    calculation 224
    phakic 94
    pseudophakic 94
    toric 224
    types 224
Intraocular pressure 35
Irregular astigmatism 92, 226
    intraocular-induced 94
    subjective evaluation of 100
    suspicion of 100
    types of 122
Irregular patterns 57

K

Keratoconic cornea 153, 180*f*
Keratoconic eye 61, 145*f*
Keratoconus 105, 167, 177*t*, 178*t*, 182, 214, 215*f*
    classification of 177
        stages of 178*t*
    index 179, 183
        center 183
    mild 223
    posterior 176
    progression 185*f*-190*f*
    suspect 143
    with normal thickness 168*f*
Keratoglobus 168, 172*f*
Keratometer 36, 41
Keratometric calibration index 38
Keratometric dioptric power 103
Keratometric index 108
Keratometric power
    deviation 35
    distribution of 22
Keratometry 8
Keratoplasty 96, 131
    penetrating 96

Keratorefractive
 procedures 94
 surgeries, after 41
Keratoscopy 8
K-reading
 map, equivalent 212, 214
 parameters, equivalent 211
 power map, equivalent 41, 211

L

Lamellar keratitis, diffuse 95
Lamellar keratoplasty 97
Laser in situ keratomileusis 41
Laser vision correction 4, 94-96, 108, 149, 161, 162, 167, 191, 224
 ectasia after 173f
Lens thickness 35
Limbal relaxing incisions 223, 225

M

Map overlay, thickness 23
Mercedes-Benz
 image 133f
 symbol 129
Meridional power of cornea 104f, 105f
Mesopic pupil, measurement of 108f
Misalignment 23, 148f, 149f
 clues of 146
 effect of 145, 147f, 148f
 patient's error 144
 types of 144
Modulation transfer function 119
Multifocal corneal opacities 203
Multifocal intraocular lens 4
Myopia 91
Myopic keratorefractive procedures 83
Myopic population 58t

N

Nasal temporal asymmetry in normal cornea 5f
Nonoptimum spectacle 101
Nonperiodic irregular astigmatism 93, 94f
Numeric scoring systems 153
Numeric values 66

O

Oblate cornea
 curvature pattern in 85f
 elevation pattern in 85f
Oblate surface 83
Oblique astigmatism 45, 45f, 92
 on elevation map 54f
Ocular surgeries, previous 119
Optical axis 3
Optical transfer function 120

P

Pachy apex 34
Pachymetric data 66
Pachymetric progression index 74f, 79
Pachymetry map 67, 196f, 212
Paraectasia 167, 168, 174f, 191
Parallel light rays 117
Patient noncooperation 152
Pellucid marginal degeneration 167, 170f, 218f, 219f
 hallmark of 68
Pellucid-like keratoconus 167, 171f, 216f, 217f
Periodic irregular astigmatism 93, 93f
Peripheral extrapolation, mild 22f
Peripheral scar 99f
Phakic intraocular lens 13
Phase transfer function 120
Photokeratoscopy 8
Piston 117, 126f
Placido disk 9f, 10
 projection 10f
Placido-based technology 12
Point spread function 119
Post-laser vision correction
 corneal irregularities 96
 ectasia 168
Post-astigmatic ablation pattern 198f, 199f
Post-corneal-graft 200f, 201f
Post-corneal-rings implantation, patterns of 199
Post-graft pattern 199
Post-hypermetropic
 ablation pattern 195f-197f
 astigmatic ablation 196
 laser vision correction 220, 220f, 221f
Postkeratorefractive procedures 41
Post-laser vision correction
 patterns 191
 study 66
Postmydriatic test 101, 107
Post-myopic
 ablation pattern 192f-194f
 laser vision correction 221, 222f
Power distribution map 107f
Practical subjective scoring system 160, 161
 detailed step 161
Prism 127f
Prolate cornea 85f
 curvature pattern in 84f
 shape 37f
Prolate surface 83
Pterygium 99, 100, 224
 bilateral 100f, 101f
Pupil
 and thinnest location coordinates 25
 center 34
  coordinates, unusual 146
  zones centered on 211
 diameter 35, 208
 entrance 3f
 size 119
Pupillary axis 3

Q

Quality of capture, checking 23
Quality specification 161f
Quick slope 75f
Q-value
 and spherical aberration 37f
 negative abnormal 195

R

Radial keratotomy 94, 149
Radius of curvature, anterior 179, 184
Reference surface 51
 parameters 52
 position 51
 principle 51
 types of 53, 56f
Refraction
 objective 120
 subjective 101
Refractive display, four maps 15f
Refractive effect 36
Refractive errors, spherocylindrical 123
Refractive index 38
Refractive map, four-composite 106f, 186f, 187f
Refractive power
 map 39
 principle and map, anterior 40f
Refractive surgery, previous 223

Regular astigmatism 91, 92f, 137
    component in fourier analysis 139f
Relative pachymetry 79, 163
    map 191, 192, 193f, 195, 197, 199f, 209, 212, 214
Relative thickness map 79f
    abnormal 81f
    suspicious 80f
Retinoscopy, irregular reflex on 100
Retrocorneal membrane 97
Rigid gas permeable contact lenses 143
Root mean square 96

S

Salzmann's nodular degeneration 223
Scanning-slit devices 10
Scheimpflug camera 11, 12
    lateral rotating 11f, 12f
Scheimpflug corneal imaging 178
Scheimpflug law states 11
Scheimpflug system 11
Scheimpflug-based devices 11
Scissoring reflex 100
Scleral incisions 224f
Screening guidelines 13
Sim-K measurement 8f
Skewed hourglass 153
Spherical aberration 83, 134f
    halos resulting from 135f
Spherical component 137
Spherical cornea 84
    curvature pattern in 84f
    elevation pattern in 85f
    shape 36f
Spherical power 182
Spherical surface 83
Starburst 131f
Sturm, interval of 92f
Surface variance, index of 179, 182
Symmetric bowtie inferior steep 153

T

Tangential map, anterior 191, 193f, 198f
Tear film
    deficiency 148
    disturbance 23, 148
    excess 149
Tears on tomography, effect of excess 152f
Testing system, normal noise of 181
Tetrafoil 131, 136f
Thickness map, changes in 145
Tilt 127f
Tissue altered, percent of 67
Tomographers, types of 10
Tomography 11, 12t
Topography 11, 12t
Topometric indices 182
Toxic keratopathy, central 95
Transitional zone 193f
Trefoil 129, 132f
    aberration 129, 133f
Trifolium plant 129

V

Vertical asymmetry, index of 183
Videokeratoscopy, computerized 10
Visual acuity 143, 183
    best corrected 96
    uncorrected distance 143
Visual axis 3
Vortex pattern 49f

W

Wavefront analysis 115
Wavefront and wavefront analysis, principles of 117
Wavefront principle 117f
Wavefront technology, clinical application of 120
With-the-rule astigmatism 44f, 45, 92
    on elevation map 53f
Wound-related flattening 226
Wounds, unsutured 226

Z

Zernike analysis 118, 122
Zernike coefficient 120
Zernike polynomials 117, 122
Zernike pyramid 118f, 122